Aging Gametes

Proceedings of the International Symposium on Aging Gametes
Seattle, Wash., June 13–16, 1973

Aging Gametes

Their Biology and Pathology

Editor: R. J. Blandau, Seattle, Washington

148 figures and 61 tables, 1975

S. Karger · Basel · München · Paris · London · New York · Sydney

S. Karger · Basel · München · Paris · London · New York · Sydney
Arnold-Böcklin-Strasse 25, CH-4011 Basel (Switzerland)

Emil Witschi 1890–1971

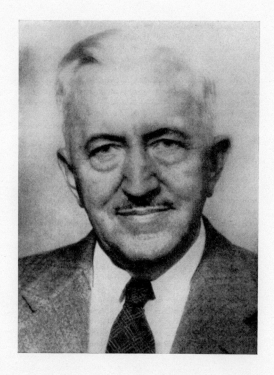

This volume is dedicated to the memory of
EMIL WITSCHI, *Mysterii Generationis Indagator Diligens*,
who throughout his lifetime encouraged these writers
and all other investigators of aging gametes.

Contents

Contents

Preface

Multicellular organisms are characterized by time-dependent, reproducible alterations in the structure and function of the cells composing them.
Aging is an accepted property of such organisms. Eggs and spermatozoa
share in this property but, in sharp contrast to multicellular organisms, do
not have the opportunity to throw off spontaneous or induced mutations.
Aging of gametes may lead to their partial deterioration or to loss of their
vitality; consequently their normal development may be interferred with
even at the earliest stages of segmentation. It is increasingly recognized that
only those eggs that are fertilized at the stage of optimal maturity and
vitality may develop normally and that conditions of overripeness of both
male and female gametes are a major cause of developmental failure. Gametes
become overripe either by retention in their storage chambers (ovaries in the
female and excurrent ducts in the male) or by delay in fertilization after
normal ovulation. Defective oocytes are more the cause of developmental
anomalies than is a hostile uterine environment. Thus, fertilization of a
devitalized egg may lead to abnormal development that may express itself
in death and spontaneous abortion or resorption of the embryo or, more
tragically, in the birth of a child with developmental abnormalities or with
subtle deficiencies, including the full range of mental retardation.

The exact time of ovulation in the human cannot as yet be determined.
Therefore the aging human gamete presents us with a key and timely problem. The use of the rhythm method in family planning may significantly
increase the number of aged oocytes that are fertilized. The ever-increasing
number of vasectomies have led to the formation of 'sperm banks' for
possible use in the production of progeny. There are insufficient data in the
human on the length of time sperms retain not only their fertilizing ability
but also, and more importantly, their ability to produce normal progeny

after prolonged periods of cryogenic preservation. For whatever value lies in the comparison of species, cryogenic sperm preservation has been carried out in cattle over many years. It is regrettable that the data from this gene pool have never been critically enough evaluated to be of much comparative use.

Although the phenomenon is well documented, we are utterly ignorant of the mechanisms that control the progressive degeneration of millions of oocytes in the ovaries of the human female between birth and menopause. In considering the mass destruction of intraovular oocytes, the possibility exists that some of the eggs released intermittently during the fertile years, may suffer damage from aging, thereby devitalizing ova, which, when fertilized, lead to reproductive wastage.

The inescapable characteristic common to all aging systems is progressive and irreversible change. Eggs and spermatozoa are ideal cells with which to explore these systems in detail. It was the primary objective of this symposium to stimulate thinking about the aging processes in gametes and, by extension, to all cells. Thirty-five scientists from a variety of disciplines met for three days of discussion, evaluation, and planning at the University of Washington in the hope of opening the way for new directions in the search for meaningful information on this and related areas. To the reader many of the facts presented here may seem repetitive, useless in prospect or in immediate retrospect. Without the wearisome steps up the mountain there is no view. Whatever success this book may achieve is owing solely to the efforts of its contributing authors.

Acknowledgments

This symposium was generously supported by the Population and Reproduction Grants Branch of the Center for Population Research, National Institute of Child Health and Human Development, by the Population Council, and by the Barren Foundation.

The editor is especially grateful to Mrs. IRENE WASNER, who, from its inception, carried the brunt of responsibility for the success of the conference. Special thanks are due Mrs. LUCILLE HOLT, Mr. GLEN GOODSON, Dr. RUTH RUMERY, Mrs. LYNN LANGLEY, Mrs. PATRICIA PIETERS, Miss FRANCINE HUHNDORF, Miss NANCY THOMAS, Miss SUSAN HAFFERTY, and Mr. ROY HAYASHI for their assistance in indexing, proofreading, and in evaluating and arranging the illustrations.

The skillful editing of Mrs. MARY ADAMS is especially appreciated.

Aging Gametes. Int. Symp., Seattle 1973, pp. 1–18 (Karger, Basel 1975)

Intrinsic Aging of Postmitotic Cells

ROBERT R. KOHN

Department of Pathology, School of Medicine, Case Western Reserve University, Cleveland, Ohio

Very little attention, in any systematic way, has been given to the question of what types of degenerative changes occur in cells that no longer divide. This subject does not appear to constitute a well-defined discipline, although it is easy enough to describe the borders of the area and list appropriate systems for study. A number of reported observations on these cells are scattered through the literature, and some findings have been reviewed in monographs on aging [COMFORT, 1956; STREHLER, 1962; KOHN, 1971]. This chapter will attempt to bring together some older and more recent observations and concepts and to define some major questions in relationship to practical biomedical problems.

Degenerative processes in postmitotic cells constitute aging processes. Such processes, as usually defined, must occur in all members of a population under study and are therefore normal processes. They are also progressive and physiologically irreversible. The criterion of irreversibility implies intrinsic changes – changes due to spontaneous processes within the cells themselves, not brought about by the environment or the influence of other tissues.

Cell aging could play a role in aging at higher levels of organization – i.e. in the aging syndrome in the intact animal or in degenerative diseases of aging. Neoplasia and growth abnormalities could result in part from failure of normal cell aging. Information on cellular aging processes could lead to a more effective use of postmitotic cells in various therapeutic and experimental procedures and might provide insight into the optimal time for certain cells to participate in highly specialized activities.

Probably over 90% of the total cell mass in a mammal consists of postmitotic cells. Many appear incapable of division, whereas some may undergo limited division under special circumstances. They are classified as postmitotic cells because they normally do not divide. Such cells are theoretically susceptible to a variety of aging processes. Components that are nonrenewable could undergo crystallization, cross linking, or denaturation. Insoluble or nondegradable substances might accumulate. Any minor imbalance between rates of synthesis and degradation of a molecule or organelle would result in conspicuous concentration changes over long periods of time. The fact that these cells survive for any time at all suggests that mechanisms have evolved that inhibit or reverse many potential aging processes of these types.

Almost all fixed postmitotic cells fall into two categories: long-lived fixed postmitotics are all present at around the time of birth and are not replenished by any population of stem cells; short-lived fixed postmitotics form populations that are more-or-less in steady states. Cells that die are continuously replaced by a progenitor population of dividing cells.

I. Observation of Cellular Aging Processes

To study changes in cell populations with time, use must be made either of cells maintained *in vitro* or of cell samples in animals. Generally, 4 types of measurements can be made as a function of time: the capacity to generate postmitotic cells, the ability of cells to carry out some special function, changes in the amount or rate of synthesis or degradation of some component, and rate of dying.

End points of cell death are of particular value in deciding whether a population of cells is aging and in inferring something about the time course of aging processes. If aging processes are occurring in a population of cells and eventually cause cell death, the survival curve will be rectangular. In other words, the longer cells have been in existence, the greater will be the probability of and rate of dying. In a homogeneous population, deaths will be over a narrow range of ages. If, on the other hand, deaths result from accidental or non age-related causes, the survival curve will be exponential, similar to that of a first order chemical reaction, and will originate at the time cells come into existence as a population of postmitotics. If a constant number of cells are killed at constant time intervals, the survival curve will be a straight line. These 3 types of curves are shown in figure 1. The primary cause of death could be either intrinsic or extracellular in the cases of aging or accidental deaths, but must be extrinsic to yield a straight line survival curve. In many real populations, survival curves are composites of these types, indicat-

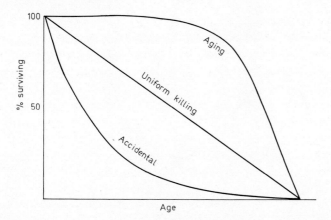

Fig. 1. Survival curves for populations dying out by different mechanisms.

ing that different mechanisms, possibly operating at different times over the life span, are responsible for cell death.

It is often very difficult to interpret observations made on aging cells. All cell populations maintained *in vitro* constitute highly artifactual systems as far as progressive and irreversible changes go. It is never certain that generalizing from *in vitro* cell populations to those *in situ* is justifiable. In some cases, the questions being asked are about processes occurring during storage, in which case experimental design is no problem.

Usually cell populations are studied at various times over the life span of an animal. Attempts are often made to correlate cellular changes with the period of senescence in the intact animal. When the questions deal with intrinsic cellular aging, such studies can give very misleading data. The life span of a mammal can be divided into two clearly defined periods. During growth and development there are many changes in cell populations and kinetics and in cell function. Other cellular phenomena are known or can be assumed to occur during senescence. Maturity, the point of significant slowing of growth, or its cessation, marks the borderline between development and aging in the intact animal. Overall physiologic efficiency is at a peak at maturity. Figure 2 shows physiologic capacity as a function of age in the mouse. Maturity by this measurement is around 7 months of age. This is also when bone growth subsides. It is clear that studying a given cell population in 3- and 18-month-old mice could result in the comparison of developing and middle-aged systems and, in the absence of other data, could be misleading in regard to animal aging which does not appear to start until after 7 months. On the other

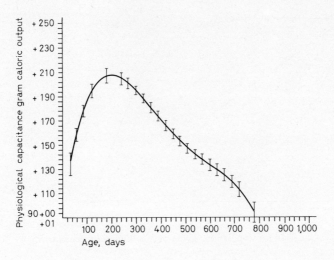

Fig. 2. Physiological capacitance as a function of age in mice. From Hensley *et al.* [1964].

hand, studies of long-lived fixed postmitotics from the time of birth would be of value if there were ways of distinguishing intrinsic processes from those dependent on the physiology of the animal.

A problem related to the above has to do with secondary effects and the question of reversibility of observed changes with age. After maturity, animals become progressively debilitated and diseased and undergo many changes in activity and feeding patterns. Understanding the causes of these changes is the goal of much aging research. Virtually all cell functions are controlled by a variety of mechanisms that depend on activity, stress, feeding schedules, etc. If a cell population is found to change in some way as animals age, there is usually no assurance that the change is intrinsic and irreversible. Determinations of the ultimate capacity of cells to do something are of more value than knowing the state they are in at any given time.

II. Aging of Short-Lived Fixed Postmitotics

Short-lived fixed postmitotic cell populations are in a more-or-less steady state over long periods, although their subpopulations may show diurnal rhythms or vary around some average value as environmental conditions vary. A population consists of a group of nonspecialized stem cells that di-

vide, giving rise to other stem cells, and more highly specialized cells that may
go through a small number of additional divisions before they attain their
highly specialized state and cease dividing. These nondividing cells are characterized by having some highly specialized function or by producing large
amounts of a special product. They have rather distinct life spans and die or
disappear on schedule, being replaced by cells from the progenitor pool.
There must be a very precise balance between rate of loss of the postmitotics
and the rate of their generation. Even a very slight imbalance over a long period causes a massive accumulation or disappearance of cells. Examples of
such postmitotic cells are all specialized cells of epithelial and endothelial surfaces, erythrocytes and granulocytes, holocrine gland cells, and spermatozoa.

There has been considerable interest in the ability of tissues to generate
postmitotic cells as a function of age of animals. It has been known for some
time that age made very little difference in the ability to regenerate liver after
partial hepatectomy [BUCHER and GLINOS, 1950] or to generate red blood
cells in response to bleeding or low oxygen tension [GRANT and LeGRANDE,
1964]. The generation time of intestinal epithelial cells in mice shows a moderate increase with advancing age. Since the number of cells remains constant, there is a slight prolongation of life span of the postmitotic cells [LESH-
ER, 1966]. Spermatogenesis in response to gonadotropin has been reported to
decrease with age in rabbits [EWING et al., 1972]. In tongue and palate epi-
thelia of rats, aging is associated with a decrease in the number of cells synthesizing DNA, but these cells divide more frequently with the result that the
number of fixed postmitotics generated remains rather constant with age.
CAMERON [1972 b] has reviewed a number of studies of these types and has
provided recent data on cell renewal. Although many progenitor cell populations show decreased proliferation in advanced age, there is no consistent
pattern; some populations, including some human cells, show increased mitotic activity with age. Total cellularity of tissues, where studied, was found
to remain constant with age, indicating the survival times of postmitotic cells
increased with age in those tissues with decreased cellular division rates. As
noted earlier and as mentioned by CAMERON [1972 b], old animals are debi-
liated and altered in many ways. There is no assurance that cellular changes
observed with age are intrinsic. As an example of the effect of environment, it
has been observed that transplanted mouse mammary gland from 3-week-old
and 12-month-old animals grew equally well in 3-week-old recipients but
grew poorly in older hosts [YOUNG et al., 1971].

The finding of HAYFLICK [1965] that diploid human fibroblasts died out
in culture after approximately 50 doublings in 1 year stimulated interest in

the possibility that animals aged and died because cell populations lost their capacity to divide. Recent data strongly suggest that these observations on tissue cultures have little or no relationship to cell kinetics with age *in vivo*. FRANKS [1970] cites studies in which serially transplanted mouse skin and prostate gland have survived for 7 and 6 years, respectively, in experiments still in progress. In other words, these populations of cells continue to proliferate 2–3 times longer than the mouse life span. Erythrocyte precursors serially transplanted in mice survive 13–21 months beyond the original donors' life spans [HARRISON, 1972]. Furthermore, *in vivo* labelling studies of mouse epithelial cell populations have shown the minimal number of doublings over a life span to be 146, with an average number of around 565 [CAMERON, 1972 a]. At present, there is no convincing evidence that stem cells in the types of tissues considered here lose their capacity to divide with increasing animal age.

The postmitotic cells constitute aging populations. Their probability of dying increases with the time they have been in existence, and the survival curve for a cohort of such cells resembles the rectangular curve in figure 1. Except for certain studies of gametes, discussed elsewhere in this volume, very few investigations have been carried out on the mechanisms and sequence of events in the deterioration and death of these cells *in vivo*. It has been assumed that deterioration is the price that must be paid for the great degree of specialization; so much of the energy-producing machinery and synthetic capacity of these cells is devoted to the special function that vegetative processes necessary for life cannot be maintained, or the accumulation of a special product interferes with these vital functions. Such a view appears reasonable when certain extreme examples are considered. Postmitotic cells of stratified squamous epithelium produce keratin until the entire cell finally consists of a keratin scale. Red blood cells lose their nuclei and become filled with hemoglobin. Reasons for the lack of survival of these cells are not difficult to imagine. If the role of specialization in cell death is a sound generality, the major question then is: What determines whether the daughter cells of a stem cell will be other stem cells or fixed postmitotics? This question is obviously central to problems of growth and neoplasia.

Most of what is known about the deterioration of short-lived fixed postmitotics has been learned from cells maintained *in vitro*. Conditions of culture or storage undoubtedly differ in important ways from physiological conditions, and these differences almost certainly play significant roles in the rates of deterioration and dying out of cell populations. However, conditions used *in vitro* are based on information on the natural environment and have

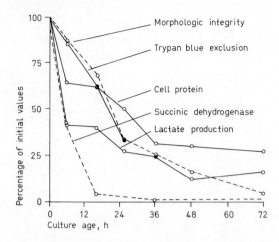

Fig. 3. Properties of rat leukocytes aging *in vitro*. From KOHN and FITZGERALD [1964].

been varied by trial and error to obtain maximal cell survival. It is likely, therefore, that the sequence of events *in vitro* bears some relationship to what happens in the animal.

Rat neutrophils, obtained from the peritoneal cavity, undergo rapid deterioration in culture. Since the cells are of different ages when obtained, a survival curve for a cohort is not available. When various cell properties are measured as a function of time *in vitro*, the curves obtained (fig. 3) resemble the curve for accidental, or non age-related, deaths and suggest that the cells are unstable when placed in culture and are equally susceptible to injury regardless of age. The earliest losses are in enzymatic activities. It is of interest that loss of morphologic integrity as determined by light microscopy and loss of the ability to exclude dye, which is a frequently used measure of cell viability, are late changes. Ultrastructural changes also occur early. During the first 8 h in culture a generalized structural deterioration occurs that is characterized by a blurring of membranes, granularity of nuclear material, and a disorganization and decrease in number of organelles [KOHN, 1964]. It is also of interest that during the first 27 h of culture, when many properties are rapidly deteriorating, the rate of incorporation of labelled amino acids into protein was found to remain constant [KOHN, 1964]. Such observations do not provide information on causes of deterioration but do serve to point out that all cell functions do not decrease according to the same time course and that no single kind of measurement yields reliable figures for overall viability.

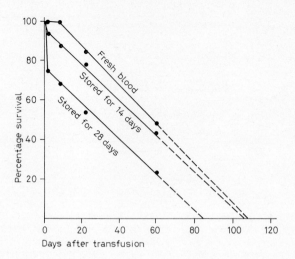

Fig. 4. Post transfusion survival of red cells of fresh blood compared with that of red cells stored for 14–28 days. From MOLLISON [1972].

Additional information on deterioration of cells has been obtained from work on red blood cells stored for transfusion purposes. Significant findings have been summarized by SCHMIDT [1969] and MOLLISON [1972]. Storage of cells is usually at 2–6°C in an acid-citrate-dextrose solution. Although glycolysis is markedly slowed at this temperature, there is sufficient production of lactate to lower pH, which causes decreased activity of hexokinase and phosphofructokinase. Consequently, glycolysis ceases, and there are decreases in levels of ATP and 2,3-diphosphoglyceric acid. A loss of one third of the ATP is associated with 50% loss in cell viability, with spherical cell shape, with increased cell rigidity, and with loss of membrane lipids. During storage, there is a loss of active transport of sodium and potassium; extra- and intracellular concentrations come to equilibrium.

A collection of circulating red cells contains cells of all different ages, with fractions of cells in every age category presumed to be the same. The survival curve for such a collection *in situ* is therefore linear, reaching zero survival at around 120 days, which is the maximum red cell life span. Stored red cells are also of all different ages. These can be transfused, and the effects of storage can be determined by following their survival.

The most abrupt loss of transfused cells is in the first 24 h, and the number disappearing is proportional to the time in storage. After the initial loss, survival curves become linear, but there is some inconsistency in data on the

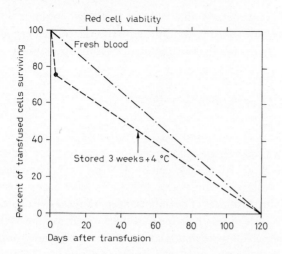

Fig. 5. Post transfusion survival of red cells of fresh blood compared with that of red cells stored for 3 weeks. From SCHMIDT [1969].

slopes of these curves. Curves for transfused cells have been reported to be below, but parallel to, the curve for nonstored cells, indicating either a selective injury of young cells or the aging of all cells as a result of storage (fig. 4). Other data show a convergence of survival curves for stored and nonstored cells, both reaching zero at around 120 days (fig. 5). This indicates that storage had no irreversible effects on most cells and that the cells that were injured by storage and disappeared during the first 24 h were of all ages. In either case, it appears that by the criterion of persistence after transfusion older cells are not selectively injured under storage conditions.

The mechanisms of cell disappearance and destruction are other questions about which very little is known. In the cases of epithelial surfaces, dead and dying cells are sloughed off. In other cell populations, it is likely that activated lysosomal hydrolytic enzymes degrade cell components. The components may become more susceptible to degradation in the course of deterioration. Also, degenerating cells or cell fragments may be taken up by the reticuloendothelial system and degraded.

It is clear from the foregoing that there is little detailed information available on the sequence of events leading to disappearance of any short-lived fixed postmitotics. There may be no theoretical or practical problems that are of sufficient concern to warrant any large scale investigation of this subject. The most important questions about these cell populations appear to deal with the kinds of events determining whether a cell will continue to divide or will differentiate into a fixed postmitotic and with the times and conditions for optimal viability of cells that are required for some special function.

III. Aging of Long-Lived Postmitotic Cells

The full complement of long-lived fixed postmitotics is present at around the time of birth. Whatever may subsequently happen to them, they are not replaced by cell division or from any cell pool. Some have a limited capacity to divide under certain circumstances and others have been reported to synthesize DNA in rare instances. The important point is that virtually all cells in these populations are normally in the postmitotic state as long as they are in existence. The major cell types in this category are neurons and cardiac and skeletal muscle cells. Smooth muscle cells could probably also be placed in this group; they do not normally divide but retain the capacity to do so rapidly when it is required, as in response to tissue injury. Ova represent a special case. These are composed of several different populations of postmitotic cells: primary oocytes that never undergo further development, secondary oocytes after ovulation, and polar bodies.

Progressive degenerative changes in fixed postmitotics would be expected to lead to cell loss over the life span of an animal. This question has been studied most often in cells of the nervous system. BRODY [1955] counted neurons at various sites in the human cerebral cortex in a small number of subjects of different ages. Figure 6 shows data for the two locations where he found the greatest age-changes. It is clear that if these curves truly represent numbers of cells remaining, such cell disappearance is not caused by cell aging but by some selective effect on younger cells; younger cells have a greater probability of dying than do older cells. Furthermore, some or most of the apparent fall in cell numbers during the period of growth could be an artifact caused by the growth of nonneuronal elements that diluted out the number of neurons counted. A thorough study by BRIZZEE et al. [1968] of neurons at various levels in the rat cerebral cortex indicated no significant change in the number of cells out to 972 days of age.

The total number of nerve cells in spinal cords of mice was determined as a function of age [WRIGHT and SPINK, 1959]. No change was found up to 50 weeks of age, but there was a decrease of 15–20% between 50 and 110 weeks. JOHNSON and ERNER [1972] counted total brain neurons in cell suspensions of mouse brain. Their data, shown in figure 7, suggest the dying out

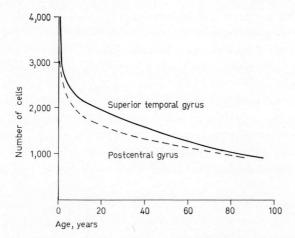

Fig. 6. Cell counts as a function of age in the 2 areas of human cerebral cortex that show the greatest change. Drawn from data of BRODY [1955].

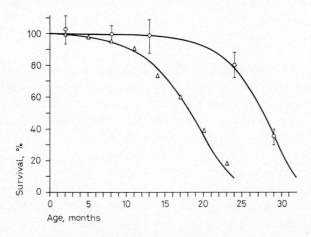

Fig. 7. Percent survival of mice (△) and their neurons (○) as a function of age. From JOHNSON and ERNER [1972].

of an aging population. However, the mouse survival curve, also in figure 7, indicates an unhealthy population of animals with a life span of around 2 years. The low figure for neurons at 29 months of age was obtained from about 1 % of survivors from the starting population. When 50 % of the mice had died, there was no decrease in cell number in the brains of the surviving mice.

No changes with age have been observed in fibers of ventral roots in rats, in sciatic nerve fibers of rats, or in the ventral root fibers of cats [cited by WRIGHT and SPINK, 1959]. The total number of nerve cells in the human olivary nucleus has been reported not to change from birth to middle age in human beings [MOATAMED, 1966].

Purkinje cells in the human cerebellum have been reported to decrease from around 600 at 20 years of age in males to around 400 in advanced old age and from around 520 to 310 in females [ELLIS, 1920]. Similarly, a linear loss of 15% of the Purkinje cells at 1,000 days of age has been observed in the rat [INUKAI, 1928]. These are old data and have been criticized by TOMASCH [1971].

To summarize, loss of neurons in some population probably occurs over an animal's life span. Loss of Purkinje cells may be the best example. This cannot be a general biological phenomena, however, because too many studies have indicated no change in cell number over very long periods. In those cases where losses have been observed, not enough information is available to determine whether cell death is caused by intrinsic mechanisms or is secondary to other degenerative processes.

Data on skeletal muscle cells and their significance are perhaps even more equivocal. ROWE [1969] compared 5 different muscles in a group of mice 126–137 days old with those in a group 750 days old and found only a suggestion of a loss of fibers, not enough to be statistically significant, and no difference in fiber diameter. On the other hand, TAUCHI et al. [1971] in comparing tibialis anterior muscle from 12-month-old rats with 24-month-old rats, found a very significant loss of red fibers with age but not of white fibers. Again, the loss of fibers does not appear to be a general phenomenon, and when it occurs it could be a secondary change.

In mammals, only a small fraction of oocytes present at birth are ovulated; the bulk of them undergo atresia. The rate at which they become atretic is probably greater earlier in life, indicating they are not dying because of aging processes but are being killed by some environmental factors. After ovulation, however, the cells are clearly aging; they become progressively less functional in fertilization and have a greater probability of dying the longer they have been in existence.

It is of interest that the depletion or diminution of oocytes is probably responsible for the evolutionary origins of aging of mammals. Survival of animals is required only until the last offspring are self-sufficient. There is no way natural selection could act on any life-prolonging process after this period. In other words, animals with defense reactions that were manifested only in the postreproductive period would not leave any more descendents than those without such processes. Selectivity would be at work to favor defenses against diseases that occur during the reproductive period, resulting in longer life span. Animals would then be left with degenerative processes against which no defenses would be likely to develop.

Although it appears that deaths of long-lived postmitotics are not, as a general biological phenomenon, caused by aging processes, progressive alterations over long periods of time in these cells are expected. It is known that muscle strength and endurance decline after maturity and that nervous system function similarly declines in terms of reaction time, psychomotor speed, perception, and velocity of conduction. It is, again, a problem to ascertain whether these are intrinsic cellular changes. The same problem is encountered in attempting to evaluate morphological and chemical changes with age.

Muscle atrophy, in which individual fibers become smaller, occurs with age. This atrophy may involve mainly white fibers [TAUCHI et al., 1971]. Muscle size is very labile and changes rapidly in response to variations in functional demands. Atrophy is almost certainly due, to a large extent, to the generalized physiological decline with age. Compensatory hypertrophy of muscle has been studied by exercising 45-day-old and 19-month-old rats [TO-MANEK and WOO, 1970]. Although these are not very satisfactory ages for comparison because the young animals are immature, hypertrophy in the 2 groups was equivalent. This suggests that when stimulated, the synthetic capacity of these cells is not diminished with age.

In a comparison of myocardial cells in 18- and 33-month-old rats [TRAVIS, 1972], increases with age were observed in numbers of residual bodies, lysosomes, and lipid droplets. Degradation of mitochondria and glycogen particles was seen in the old samples. Intranuclear inclusions have been described in the neurons of aged mice [FIELD and PEAT, 1971]. Increased numbers of microtubules and decreased numbers of neurofilaments and mitochondria have been described in 26-month-old mice as compared to 8-month-old animals [SAMORAJSKI et al., 1971]. The significance of these findings is not known.

Many studies of biochemical function in long-lived postmitotics that have been reviewed [KOHN, 1971] have revealed no pattern of change with age. More recent studies yield similar conclusions. For example, glutamic acid decarboxylase concentration shows no change with age in various regions of rat brain [EPSTEIN and BARROWS, 1969]; myofibrillar ATPase and creatine kinase are reported not to change with age in rat muscle [ERMINI,

1970 a, b]; and acid hydrolases were found to increase with age in rat heart and diaphragm muscle [COMALLI, 1971]. One of the more consistent changes with age appears to be an increase in such lysosomal enzymes. A very significant study was carried out on adult and old rats by MENZIES and GOLD [1971], who determined mitochondria turnover in a large number of tissues, including brain and heart. No differences with age were observed. Thus, the complex machinery responsible for mitochondria synthesis and degradation does not appear to be affected by aging processes.

Studies at the levels of transcription and protein synthesis are also inconclusive regarding intrinsic aging processes. Protein synthesis in isolated perfused mouse heart was found to decrease with age [GEARY and FLORINI, 1972]. As shown in figure 8, incorporation decreased with age to 27 months. However, the highest specific activity of intracellular precursors was in the youngest and oldest animals. Correcting for this, protein synthesis was found to be lowest in young and old mice and highest at maturity. In a study of dog

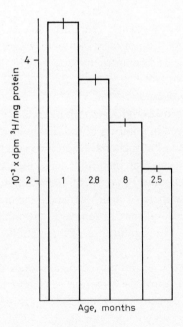

Fig. 8. The effect of age on ³H-leucine incorporation into proteins in mouse hearts. From GEARY and FLORINI [1972].

cardiac muscle [SHIREY and SOBEL, 1972], no age difference was found in protein/DNA or RNA/DNA ratios or in percentage of DNA transcribed.

RNA polymerase activity in muscle nuclei was found to decrease with age in mice (table I). A similar study of liver, in which solubilization of polymerase showed less difference with age, suggested that the major change with

Table I. Changes with age in RNA synthesis by nuclei isolated from mouse skeletal muscle. From BRITTON *et al.* [1972]

Experiment No.	Mouse age, months	^{3}H-UMP incorporated into RNA, pmol/10 min/mg DNA		
		polymerase I	polymerase II	total activity
1	2.8	3.84	10.3	21.6
	8.0	6.66	9.5	26.2
	25	0.99	2.3	5.3
2	9.0	5.00	9.80	22.0
	30	2.50	5.04	12.6

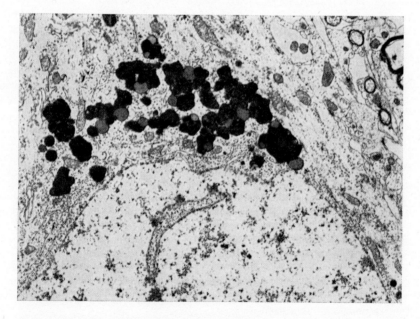

Fig. 9. A portion of a neuron from lamina V in a 605-day-old rat. Lipofuscin granules are clustered at one pole of the nucleus. × 7,500. From BRIZZEE *et al.* [1969].

age was in template activity of chromatin rather than in polymerase activity. On the other hand, RNA synthesis of brain nuclei showed no change between 5 and 22 months of age in the rat [GIBAS and HARMAN, 1970].

The most widespread and consistent age-change in long-lived fixed postmitotics is the accumulation of lipofuscin pigment. This material has long been known to accumulate in a variety of organs, but primarily in neurons, heart, and skeletal muscle. It consists largely of oxidatively polymerized unsaturated lipids plus components of lysosomes. With age, there is an increase in size and aggregation of granules. The granules do not appear to cause alterations in other cytoplasmic organelles (fig. 9).

Summary

In summary, there is no convincing evidence, as noted earlier, that long-lived fixed postmitotics die out because of aging processes. There is also no pattern of deterioration or decline in function that clearly represents intrinsic change or that characterizes these cell types. Lipofuscin accumulation appears to be a true aging change, but its significance is not known.

Additional studies are required of nonrenewable molecules and structures, perhaps including cell membrane components, likely to undergo changes over long periods of time. In the future search for age changes, the most useful information will come from studies in which animals of different ages have similar recent histories in terms of stress, activity, and diet.

Perhaps the best reason for studying aging of long-lived fixed postmitotics is to determine whether intrinsic aging of these cells has any causative relationship to aging of the whole animal. On the basis of evidence at hand, there is little reason for believing this is so.

References

BRITTON, V.L.; SHERMAN, F.G., and FLORINI, J.R.: Effect of age on RNA synthesis by nuclei and soluble RNA polymerase from liver and muscle of C57BL/6J mice. J. Geront. *27:* 188 (1972).

BRIZZEE, K.R.; CANCILLA, P.A.; SHERWOOD, N., and TIMIRAS, P.S.: The amount and distribution of pigments in neurons and glia of the cerebral cortex. J. Geront. *24:* 127 (1969).

BRIZZEE, K.R.; SHERWOOD, N., and TIMIRAS, P.S.: A comparison of cell populations at various depth levels in cerebral cortex of young adult and aged Long-Evans rats. J. Geront. *23:* 289 (1968).

BRODY, H.: Organization of the cerebral cortex. III. A study of aging in the human cerebral cortex. J. comp. Neurol. *102:* 511 (1955).

BUCHER, N.L.R. and GLINOS, A.D.: The effect of age on regeneration of rat liver. Cancer Res. *10:* 324 (1950).

CAMERON, I.L.: Minimum number of cell doublings in an epithelial cell population during the life span of the mouse. J. Geront. *27:* 157 (1972a).

CAMERON, I. L.: Cell proliferation and renewal in aging mice. J. Geront. *27:* 162 (1972b).

COMALLI, R.: Hydrolase activity and intracellular pH in liver, heart, and diaphragm of aging rats. Exp. Geront. *6:* 219 (1971).

COMFORT, A.: The biology of senescence (Rinehart, New York 1956).

ELLIS, R.S.: Norms for some structural changes in the human cerebellum from birth to old age. J. comp. Neurol. *32:* 1 (1920).

EPSTEIN, M.E. and BARROWS, C.H.: The effects of age on the activity of glutamic acid decarboxylase in various regions of the brains of rats. J. Geront. *24:* 136 (1969).

ERMINI, M.: Das Altern der Skelettmuskulatur. Gerontologia, Basel *16:* 72 (1970a).

ERMINI, M.: Kreatinkinase in der Muskulatur verschieden alter Ratten. Gerontologia, Basel *16:* 231 (1970b).

EWING, L.L.; JOHNSON, B.H.; DESJARDINS, C., and CLEGG, R.F.: Effect of age upon the spermatogenic and steroidogenic elements of rabbit testes. Proc. Soc. exp. Biol. Med. *140:* 907 (1972).

FIELD, E.J. and PEAT, A.: Intranuclear inclusions in neurones and glia. A study in the ageing mouse. Gerontologia, Basel *17:* 129 (1971).

FRANKS, L.M.: Cellular aspects of aging. Exp. Geront. *5:* 281 (1970).

GEARY, S. and FLORINI, J.R.: Effect of age on rate of protein synthesis in isolated perfused mouse hearts. J. Geront. *27:* 325 (1972).

GIBAS, M.A. and HARMAN, D.: Ribonucleic acid synthesis by nuclei isolated from rats of different ages. J. Geront. *25:* 105 (1970).

GRANT, W.C. and LEGRANDE, M.C.: The difference of age on erythropoiesis in the rat. J. Geront. *19:* 505 (1964).

HARRISON, D.E.: Normal function of transplanted erythrocyte precursors for 21 months beyond donor life span. Nature New Biol. *237:* 220 (1972).

HAYFLICK, L.: The limited *in vitro* lifetime of human diploid cell strains. Exp. Cell Res. *37:* 614 (1965).

HENSLEY, J.C.; McWILLIAMS, P.C., and OAKLEY, G.E.: Physiological capacitance. A study in physiological age determination. J. Geront. *19:* 317 (1964).

INUKAI, T.: On the loss of Purkinje cells, with advancing age, from the cerebellar cortex of the albino rat. J. comp. Neurol. *45:* 1 (1928).

JOHNSON, H.A. and ERNER, S.: Neuron survival in the aging mouse. Exp. Geront. *7:* 111 (1972).

KOHN, R.R.: Unpublished observations (1964).

KOHN, R.R.: Principles of mammalian aging (Prentice Hall, Englewood Cliffs, 1971).

KOHN, R.R. and FITZGERALD, R.G.: Rat leucocytes aging *in vitro*. A study of morphologic and metabolic degeneration. Exp. molec. Path. *3:* 51 (1964).

LESHER, S.: Chronic irradiation and ageing in mice and rats; in LINDOP and SACHER Radiation and ageing, pp. 183 (Taylor & Francis, London 1966).

MENZIES, R.A. and GOLD, P.H.: The turnover of mitochondria in a variety of tissues of young adult and aged rats. J. biol. Chem. *246:* 2425 (1971).

MOATAMED, F.: Cell frequencies in the human inferior olivary nuclear complex. J. comp. Neurol. *128:* 109 (1966).

MOLLISON, P.L.: Blood transfusion in clinical medicine; 5th ed. (Scientific Publications, Oxford 1972).

ROWE, R.W.D.: The effect of senility on skeletal muscle in the mouse. Exp. Geront. *4:* 119 (1969).

SAMORAJSKI, T.; FRIEDE, R.L., and ORDY, J.M.: Age differences in the ultrastructure of axons in the pyramidal tract of the mouse. J. Geront. *26:* 542 (1971).

SCHMIDT, P.J.: Safe and effective transfusions; in STEFANINI Progress in clinical pathology, vol. 2, pp. 168 (Grune & Stratton, New York 1969).

SHIREY, T.L. and SOBEL, H.: Compositional and transcriptional properties of chromatins isolated from cardiac muscle of young, mature and old dogs. Exp. Geront. *7:* 15 (1972).

STREHLER, B.L.: Time, cells, and aging (Academic Press, New York 1962).

TAUCHI, H.; YOSHIOKA, T., and KOBAYASHI, H.: Age change of skeletal muscles of rats. Gerontologia, Basel *17:* 219 (1971).

TOMANEK, R.J. and WOO, Y.K.: Compensatory hypertrophy of the plantaris muscle in relation to age. J. Geront. *25:* 23 (1970).

TOMASCH, J.: Comments on neuromythology. Nature, Lond. *233:* 60 (1971).

TRAVIS, D.F.: Ultrastructural changes in the left ventricular rat myocardial cells with age. J. Ultrastruct. Res. *39:* 124 (1972).

WRIGHT, E.A. and SPINK, J.M.: A study of the loss of nerve cells in the central nervous system in relation to age. Gerontologia, Basel *3:* 277 (1959).

YOUNG, L.; MEDINA, D., and DE OME, K.B.: The difference of host and tissue age on life span and growth rate of serially transplanted mouse mammary gland. Exp. Geront. *6:* 49 (1971).

Author's address: Dr. ROBERT R. KOHN, Department of Pathology, School of Medicine, Case Western Reserve University, *Cleveland, OH 44106* (USA)

Aging Gametes. Int. Symp., Seattle 1973, pp. 19–49 (Karger, Basel 1975)

The Mitotic Spindle[1]

HIDEMI SATO

Department of Biology, University of Pennsylvania, Philadelphia, Pa.

The subject of this chapter is the mechanism of mitotic spindle formation, and the ways in which the normal function of the spindle may be affected by various experimental conditions. The relationship between aging phenomena and abnormal spindle function will also be considered.

At each division of a eukaryotic cell a mitotic spindle is formed, and the chromosomes are oriented, aligned, and then separated regularly into 2 daughter cells. When the cell has divided, the mitotic spindle is disassembled.

Until recently, the mitotic spindle could be visualized only in fixed and stained material (fig. 1). In a living cell, the mitotic spindle is usually difficult to detect under the phase contrast microscope (fig. 2 A) because of the small difference between the refractive indices of the spindle region and the surrounding cytoplasm. However, owing to the weak birefringence of the living mitotic spindle, it can be visualized under the sensitive polarizing microscope (fig. 2 B). This birefringence reflects the amount of orderly aligned fibrous structure within the spindle. Thus, measuring spindle birefringence with the polarizing microscope allows us to establish the relationship between spindle fiber birefringence and the amount of fibrous structure present in cells affected by alteration of various physiological parameters.

Many conditions and agents have been found that systematically and reversibly alter spindle morphology and fiber birefringence. From various observations and experiments [cf. INOUÉ, 1964; INOUÉ and SATO, 1967] we postulated that spindle fibers are composed mainly of parallel arrays of microtubules formed by a reversible association of globular tubulin molecules. Thus, there

---

1   This research was supported by grants from NIH CA10171, NSF GB31739X, and NSF GF34908.

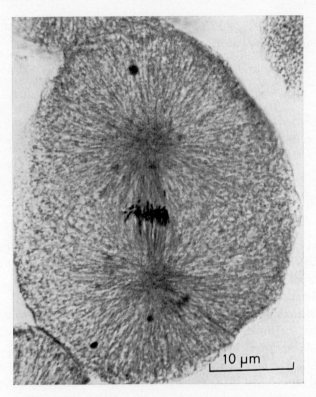

Fig. 1. Photomicrograph of mitosis in a dividing white fish blastomere that has been fixed, sectioned, and stained.

exists a dynamic equilibrium between the labile spindle fibers and a pool of unassociated molecules. The formation of microtubules by the association of tubulin molecules is more than likely controlled by the orienting centers [STE-PHENS, 1971], such as centrioles and kinetochores, and the available concentration of active pool material.

The directional association or dissociation of activated molecules was proposed as a mechanism for anaphase chromosome movement [INOUÉ and SATO, 1967]. The directionality could result from a minor shift of the state of equilibrium. However, the mechanism of chromosome movement will not be discussed in the present paper. (For that purpose, the reader is referred to articles by the following authors: BAJER and MOLÉ-BAJER [1971, 1972]; DIETZ [1972]; INOUÉ [1964]; INOUÉ and SATO [1967]; MAZIA [1961]; NICKLAS [1971]; SCHRADER [1953].) Rather, I shall discuss the following topics: (1)

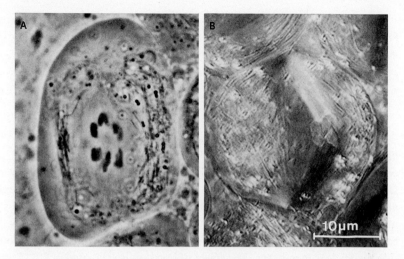

Fig. 2. The meiosis observed in the spermatocytes of the crane fly, *Nephrotoma suturalis*. *A* Phase contrast microscopy shows no detectable spindle structure. *B* Chromosomal spindle fibers can now clearly be seen under the sensitive polarization microscope owing to their birefringent nature.

visible changes of spindle birefringence in mitosis; (2) nature of form birefringence in the mitotic spindle; (3) effects of heavy water (D_2O), temperature, and mitotic poisons on spindle structure; (4) crystallization of spindle material *in vivo*, and (5) effects of maturity on spindle or crystal formation. Echinoderm gametes are used as the experimental material throughout the discussion.

I. Visible Changes of Spindle Birefringence in Mitosis

The mitotic spindle usually shows a positive birefringence if the direction from one aster to the opposite aster is considered to be the major structural axis. *In vivo*, the overall birefringence, or the measured retardation, of the metaphase spindle of various marine gametes is distributed within a range of but 1–5 nm. For this reason mitotic spindles can be clearly visualized with a sensitive polarizing microscope; even discriminating chromosomal spindle fibers, continuous spindle fibers, and astral rays can be seen. Thus, changes of fine structures during mitosis can be followed by interpreting measured changes in birefringence [cf. DIETZ, 1963, 1972; FORER, 1965; INOUÉ, 1964, 1969; INOUÉ and SATO, 1967].

With the exceptions of oocyte meiotic divisions and the first mitosis after fertilization, the major patterns of birefringence change in mitosis of marine gametes may be summarized as follows:

A. Prophase

Centrioles are activated and separate so as to form the spindle axis. Visually, asters are separated and grow during the migration of one aster, increasing in birefringence. The weakly birefringent central spindle generally forms between the separating asters. The prophase nucleus becomes larger and shows a more homogeneous structure but has no birefringence until the nuclear membrane breaks down. Nuclear membrane breakdown may be caused by the rapid invasion of birefringent bundles previously located outside the nuclear membrane. The speed of invasion is estimated at $10–12\,\mu m \cdot min^{-1}$ in the endosperm cell division of *Haemanthus katherinae* [SATO et al., 1970] and in spermatogenesis of grasshoppers. It has not been measured for marine gametes.

B. Prometaphase

More birefringent spindle material becomes oriented around the kinetochores and asters in the prometaphase. Although the major structure contributing to spindle birefringence at this stage is probably the oriented microtubules, the contribution of oriented sheath fibers around the chromosomes should not be ignored [DIETZ, 1963; WENT, 1966]. Birefringent chromosomal fibers are established parallel to the continuous spindle fibers in the direction of chromosome movement. The birefringence of these fibers fluctuates occasionally, reflecting decrease or increase of the oriented fine structure. Such changes may function in the alignment of chromosomes on the metaphase plate as the equilibrium position [INOUÉ, 1964; INOUÉ and SATO, 1967; ÖSTERGREN, 1951].

C. Metaphase

Whereas prometaphase may last 4–10 min, metaphase lasts 1.75–4 min in echinoderm gametes, depending on the specimen and the temperature of the environment. The pattern of birefringence established during prometaphase is sustained virtually without change during metaphase.

D. Anaphase and Telophase

Chromosomes are led by their strongly birefringent fibers to the poles of the spindle. The overall birefringence decreases gradually during anaphase, and the birefringence adjacent to kinetochores and in much of the chromosomal spindle fibers remains unchanged during the major part of anaphase movement. This suggests rapid dissociation of continuous spindle fibers in echinoderm gametes, whereas chromosomal fibers may or may not shorten during anaphase, depending on the mode of chromosome separation relative to spindle elongation. Although continuous spindle fibers are not so prominent in echinoderms, in many cases they become strongly birefringent in telophase and form the core of the stem, or Stem Körper, connecting the daughter cells. Many investigators show large numbers of microtubules in this region [cf. BAJER and MOLÉ-BAJER, 1972; BRINKLEY and CARTWRIGHT, 1971; MCINTOSH and LANDIS, 1971].

In summary, with the polarizing microscope we are able to follow the transition of birefringent material from one spindle component to another throughout mitosis. The directional centriole segregation and central spindle formation contribute to the orientation of subsequent fibers. The successive fibers formed appear to coorient and align the chromosomes on the metaphase plate, subsequently moving them apart to the poles (cf. fig. 2, 3) and establishing the correlation of cytokinesis with karyokinesis [COSTELLO, 1961; INOUÉ, 1964; INOUÉ and SATO, 1967; RAPPAPORT, 1971]. The events outlined for animal cell mitosis are illustrated schematically in figure 3. For comparison, figure 4 illustrates normal and abnormal spindles at various stages of mitosis as observed in demembranated and macerated echinoderm blastomeres in culture.

II. Nature of Form Birefringence of the Mitotic Spindle

The birefringence of the mitotic spindle may be produced by a system of highly oriented fine structures such as microtubules. However, a theoretical value for the form birefringence calculated by WIENER's equation [WIENER, 1912], on the basis of the number and the volume of the fraction of microtu-

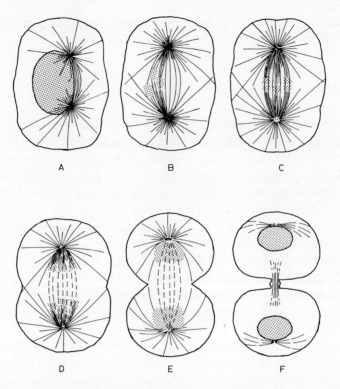

Fig. 3. Schematic diagrams of mitosis in animal cells. These figures were drawn specifically to illustrate change of birefringence distribution in various regions of spindle. They are composites of observations on a variety of living cells undergoing normal mitosis [INOUÉ and SATO, 1967].

bules, did not agree with what we observed. This discrepancy was thought to be due to the difficulties in preserving labile spindle microtubules.

To overcome these difficulties, several technical improvements were tried. Firstly, we chose metaphase arrested meiosis I spindles of *Pisaster ochraceus* oocytes as the experimental material because: (a) mass induction of such spindles can be achieved easily be applying either 10^{-5}M 1-methyl adenine or starfish motor nerve extract [CHAET, 1966; KANATANI *et al.*, 1969] to the isolated mature ovary, and (b) the spindle is large ($8 \times 8 \times 12$ μm), and has good physical stability and a rather strong birefringence (3.4 nm retardation). Secondly, we developed a technique to achieve a rather clean mass isolation of spindles without disturbing their initial size and birefringence (cf. fig. 5) [BRYAN and SATO, 1970].

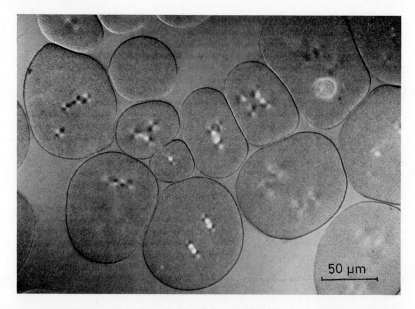

50 µm

Fig. 4. Normal and abnormal spindles at various stages of mitosis in demembranated and macerated blastomeres in culture. Note tripoler or tetrapoler spindles and a half spindle. The spindle abnormality is greatly enhanced in overmature zygotes by altering physiological parameters. Specimen: Fertilized eggs of *Dendraster exebticus*. Polarization microscopy.

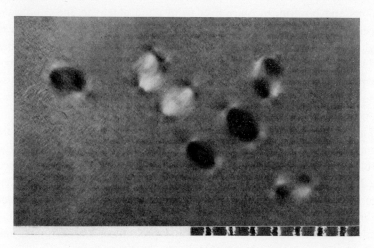

Fig. 5. Isolated metaphase spindles from mature oocytes of *Pisaster ochraceus* following the modified KANE [1965] technique. Polarization microscopy. Scale interval, 10 µm.

In order to effect the mass isolation of metaphase spindles, we pretreated mature oocytes with 0.53 M NaCl/KCl (19:1), pH 7.8, that contained Pronase and a sulfhydryl reducing agent to activate and remove the fertilization membranes. The dejellied and demembranated oocytes were then quickly exposed to the spindle-stabilizing medium, buffered in 12% hexylene glycol, pH 6.3, according to the technique described by KANE [1965]. Fixation with 3% gluturaldehyde for electron microscopic observation, post fixation with 1% OsO_4, and the initial dehydration steps were carried out in the presence of 12% hexylene glycol at pH 6.3.

The WIENER [1912] equation for the form birefringence derived for aligned multi-rods and described as

$$n_e{}^2 - n_0{}^2 = \frac{\delta_1 \delta_2 (n_1{}^2 - n_2{}^2)^2}{(\delta_1 + 1) n_2{}^2 + \delta_2 n_1{}^2}$$

was used to calculate the coefficient of birefringence ($n_e - n_0$). If we have the right values for the refractive indices of oriented rods (n_1 : microtubules), and medium (n_2 : saline solution), and the values of the fractional volumes as rods (δ_1) and medium (δ_2), the calculated ($n_e - n_0$) should match the coefficient of birefringence of the intact spindle, which is the retardation as measured directly by using the compensator divided by the specimen thickness.

We obtained a value of 1.51 for n_1 by using the matching index technique [SATO et al., 1971]. Clean isolated spindles that retain their original dimensions and birefringence are fixed with glutaraldehyde and sandwiched between thin gelatin layers. Reversible imbibition with a nonaqueous media of high refractive index (n), such as iodobenzene or nitrobenzene, was made possible by careful initial imbibition with dimethylsulfoxide. Spindle birefringence measured over a range of imbibing n from 1.332 to 1.622 plots as a paraboloid curve with maxima at the extremes ($n_e - n_0 = 5 \times 10^{-4}$ at n = 1.33 and 2×10^{-4} at 1.62) and the minimum at 4×10^{-5} for n = 1.51.

The fractional volume as microtubules, δ_1, was calculated from an electron microscopic survey. EM cross sections of these spindles (fig. 6) show microtubules (20 nm outer diameter and 12 nm inside diameter) almost exclusively distributed at an average density of $130/\mu m^2$. On the basis of 13 microtubule subunits or tubulin monomers per microtubule cross section, each tubulin monomer being a 4 nm sphere (based on hydrodynamic analysis), we can calculate the average volume of oriented protein per unit volume of spindle. The δ_1 value obtained was 0.021.

A theoretical curve for birefringence as a function of the refractive index of the medium calculated from WIENER's equation, with n_1 as 1.51 and δ_1 as

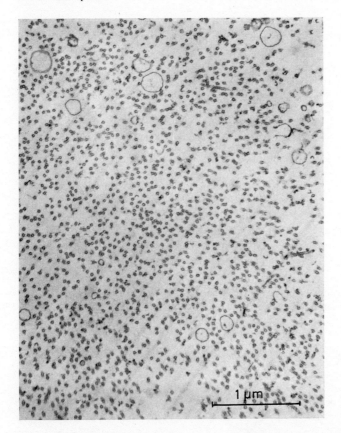

Fig. 6. Cross section of the isolated metaphase spindle of *Pisaster ochraceus* is mainly occupied by microtubules having an average density of $130/\mu m^2$. Vesicles in the photograph are the degenerated mitochondria caused by the stabilization and the isolation procedures.

0.021, gives an exact fit to the experimental curve over the measured range (fig. 7). Since the isolated spindles are not, or at most only minimally contaminated by other fine structures or protein aggregates (fig. 8), we concluded that the spindle birefringence in fact reflects the exact amount of oriented microtubules.

The intrinsic birefringence due to the molecular structure of the microtubules is not greater than 8% of the total birefringence at $n_2 = 1.33$. Fluctuation of birefringence during mitosis should, therefore, be interpreted as the result of the association, the dissociation, or the disorientation of microtubules.

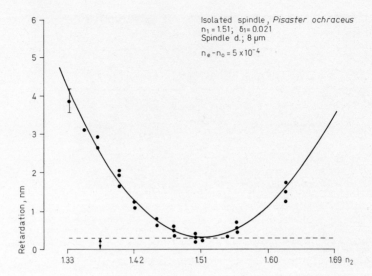

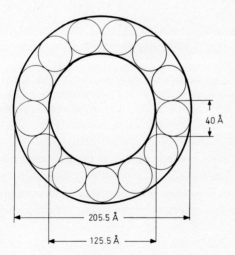

Fig. 7. Theoretical Wiener's curve for form birefringence matches with the actual spindle birefringence (black dots) measured at various refractive indices. Broken line corresponds with the estimated value of the intrinsic birefringence of subunits in the microtubules.

Fig. 8. Schematic diagram of the cross section of a microtubule. Subunit is considered to be a sphere holding 40 Å diameter. 13 subunits are arranged in one turn. Values calculated as 205.5 Å for outer diameter and 125.5 Å for inner diameter coincide with the actual dimension of spindle microtubules directly measured from electron micrograph.

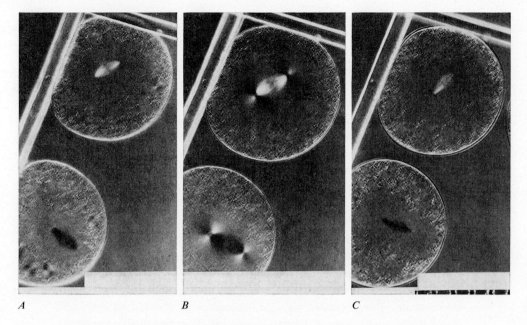

A   B   C

Fig. 9. Reversible enhancement of spindle volume and birefringence by heavy water
in arrested metaphase oocyte of *Pectinaria gouldi*. Cells supported by Butvar film and
slightly compressed. Polarization microscopy. Scale interval, 10 μm. *A* Before D$_2$O-sea
water perfusion. *B* Perfused for 2 min in 45% D$_2$O-sea water. *C* Approximately 3 min
after return to normal sea water perfusion [INOUÉ and SATO, 1967].

III. Effects of D$_2$O, Temperature, and Mitotic Poisons on Spindel Fine Structure

A. Effect of D$_2$O

Heavy water (D$_2$O) enhances spindle volume and birefringence. For
instance, using the metaphase arrested meiosis I spindle of the *Pectinaria
gouldi* oocyte as the experimental material, we observed an 8-fold increase in
spindle volume and practically a doubling in retardation (fig. 9) [INOUÉ *et al.*,
1965; INOUÉ and SATO, 1967]. The increase in volume and retardation depends on the concentration of D$_2$O and the stage of mitosis at the time of
application. The maximum increases are obtained by applying 45% D$_2$O
during metaphase. We have obtained this particular concentration of D$_2$O

over the past 10 years for various metaphase spindles of animals and plants. The changes are rapid, the new state of the dynamic equilibrium being reached within 2 min in *Pectinaria* oocytes and within 5 min in *Pisaster ochraceus*. The effect is completely reversible and repeatable on the same metaphase spindle.

Although pD = pH + 0.4 at 100% D_2O, we do not believe that the effect is due to a pH change. In fact, the pH of sea water can be varied from 7.2 to 8.6 with no detectable change in spindle size, shape, or retardation [INOUÉ and SATO, 1967]. Furthermore, H_2O_{18}, even at high concentrations, is totally inactive, whereas HDO and HDO_{18} have the same effect as 50% D_2O.

In many respects, the D_2O effect is quite similar to elevating temperature within an optimum range. However, the spindle will overstabilize, or freeze [MARSLAND and ZIMMERMAN, 1965], with the application of high concentrations of D_2O. To compare the effects of temperature and D_2O, we analyzed the association-dissociation reaction of the spindle in D_2O according to the thermodynamic approach [INOUÉ and MORALES, 1959], assuming that the birefringence reflects the concentration of oriented spindle fiber molecules or microtubules. For this study, we used the metaphase arrested meiosis I spindle of the mature oocyte of *Pisaster ochraceus*. Thermodynamic parameters were calculated from measurements of retardations of equilibrated metaphase spindles at various temperatures, both in living and rapidly isolated cells [SATO and BRYAN, 1968]. In sea water or in isotonic environment we obtained ΔH = 58.9 kcal/mol, ΔS = 209.5 eu, and ΔF = −1.1 kcal/mol. In 45% D_2O sea water the values were ΔH = 29.55 kcal/mol, ΔS = 106.3 eu, and ΔF = −0.9 kcal/mol. These values are similar to those obtained for *Chaetopterus* spindles [INOUÉ and MORALES, 1959] and *Pectinaria* spindles [CAROLAN *et al.*, 1965, 1966]. A summary of the data is given in figure 10.

Kinetic data were obtained from retardation measurements of rapidly isolated spindles after varying intervals following a temperature shift or addition of D_2O. Both association and dissociation processes appear to follow first-order kinetics. The activation energy for the temperature dependent association reaction in sea water is 41 kcal/mol; for 45% D_2O sea water, 39 kcal/mol; and for the dissociation reaction on removing D_2O, 15 kcal/mol. For each condition, these data are consistent with the hypothesis that the spindle birefringence measures the reversible association of protein molecules into linearly aggregated polymers in a first-order reaction. However, the difference of both ΔH and ΔS in sea water and in D_2O sea water and their similar high activation energy in the association reactions suggests that the spindle reaction, in fact, is a two step reaction, such as

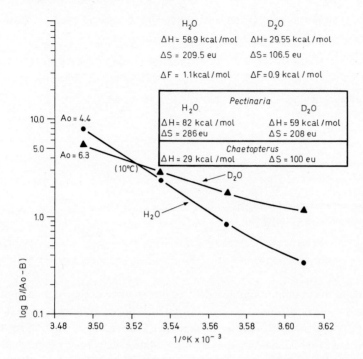

$$
\begin{array}{ll}
\mathrm{H_2O} & \mathrm{D_2O} \\
\Delta H = 58.9\ \mathrm{kcal/mol} & \Delta H = 29.55\ \mathrm{kcal/mol} \\
\Delta S = 209.5\ \mathrm{eu} & \Delta S = 106.5\ \mathrm{eu} \\
\Delta F = 1.1\ \mathrm{kcal/mol} & \Delta F = 0.9\ \mathrm{kcal/mol}
\end{array}
$$

	Pectinaria	
$\mathrm{H_2O}$		$\mathrm{D_2O}$
$\Delta H = 82$ kcal/mol		$\Delta H = 59$ kcal/mol
$\Delta S = 286$ eu		$\Delta S = 208$ eu
	Chaetopterus	
$\Delta H = 29$ kcal/mol		$\Delta S = 100$ eu

Fig. 10. A thermodynamic analysis of the effects of D_2O and temperature on the spindle association reaction. Material: Metaphase-arrested spindle in *Pisaster ochraceus* oocytes. Arrhenius plots [log B/(Ao-B) versus l/temperature where B is spindle retardation and Ao is the asymptote B could approach], show linear functions between 3 and 13°C [SATO and BRYAN, 1968]. Calculated values of ΔH and ΔS for the association reaction in metaphase-arrested spindle of *Pectinaria* oocytes [CAROLAN et al., 1965, 1966] and *Chaetopterus* oocytes [INOUÉ and MORALES, 1959] are framed in rectangle for comparison.

$$
\begin{array}{ccc}
& K_1 & K_2 \\
\text{spindle molecules} & \xrightarrow{\hspace{1cm}} \ \text{activated form} & \xrightarrow{\hspace{1cm}} \ \text{spindle fiber} \\
\text{(tubulin monomer)} & \xleftarrow{\hspace{1cm}} \ \text{(dimer?)} & \xleftarrow{\hspace{1cm}} \ \text{(polymer)}
\end{array}
$$

where K_1 and K_2 are primarily governed by temperature, but K_1 could be greatly regulated by D_2O and could provide a more available activated form of spindle molecules. The low activation energy for the back reaction of D_2O suggests the polymer may first break down into random oligomers.

The coefficient of birefringence (n_e-n_o) of both D_2O spindle and the control remains constant at 5×10^{-4}. This suggests that there is an increase in

Table I. Comparison of D_2O-spindle versus normal spindle. Material: *Pisaster ochraceus*

Condition of isolation	13°C, 12% HG	13°C, 45% D_2O to 12% HG
Pol. M.		
Retardation (Δx), nm	3.8	5.4
Spindle diameter (d), μm	8	12
$(n_e\text{-}n_o) = \Delta x/d$	$\simeq 5 \times 10^{-4}$	$\simeq 5 \times 10^{-4}$
E.M.		
Dimension of microtubules, Å		
OD	200	200
ID	120	120
Density of microtubules per μm²	130	130
Total number of microtubules		
per spindle	4,200	$\simeq 10,000$
$(n_e\text{-}n_o)$	5×10^{-4}	5×10^{-4}

microtubules in deuterated spindles with no disturbance of the original population density. Electron microscopy of isolated *Pisaster* spindles reveals that the total number of microtubules is increased from 4,500 in the control to 10,000 by D_2O spindle, holding the initial population density of $130/\mu m^2$. Microtubule length is also increased by D_2O. The reaction time is 5 min for the D_2O-dependent association reaction in *Pisaster* spindles and 3 min for the dissociation reaction. This is a quite rapid assembling reaction for a biological system. Based on the information described above, we calculated the estimated rate of tubulin association as 1×10^{-2} monomers · sec^{-1} microtubule. The comparison of D_2O spindle and normal spindle is summarized in table I.

Computer analysis of microtubule distribution in *Pisaster* mitotic spindle showed that the data fit a binominal distribution of microtubules, high density regions corresponding to chromosomal spindle fibers and low density regions to continuous fibers. We also determined that D_2O greatly increased the number of continuous fiber microtubules while the number of chromosomal fiber microtubule remained constant [SATO and DANIELS, 1971].

B. Temperature Shift

Spindle birefringence is abolished in a matter of seconds by treatment with low temperature in *Chaetopterus* oocytes [INOUÉ, 1952 a], in *Lilium* pollen mother cells [INOUÉ, 1964] and in sea urchin gametes [INOUÉ *et al.*, 1970].

Upon return to normal temperature, they recover in the course of a few minutes after which chromosome movement can continue [INOUÉ, 1964]. Low
temperature disintegration of the spindle can be repeated for as many as 10
times in the same cell. In *Chaetopterus* oocytes, *Lilium* pollen mother cells,
Halistaura developing eggs, and *Dissosteira* spermatocytes, the duration of
the chilling, even up to several hours, does not affect recovery [INOUÉ, 1952b
and unpublished data].

C. Antimitotic Poisons

Colchicine, Colcemid and many other antimitotic poisons eliminate the
spindle birefringence rapidly (fig. 11) [INOUÉ 1952a; INOUÉ *et al.*, 1965; IN-
OUÉ and SATO, 1967]. The effect is usually reversible and repeatable. For instance, when washed with normal sea water, *Pectinaria* oocytes treated with
10^{-5}M griseofulvin may recover their birefringent spindles in as little as $5 \frac{1}{2} \sim$
11 min. We could carry out this reversible dissolution repeatedly in a single
oocyte; recovery is complete even after treatment with 10^{-4}M griseofulvin
[MALAWISTA *et al.*, 1968].
    Electron microscopy at various intervals after treatment with Colcemid,
griseofulvin, or vinblastine clearly revealed that the diminished spindle size
noted in the living cells was the result of shortened microtubules. Diminished
spindle birefringence was the result of fewer microtubules. The randomly oriented microtubules in the region of the miniature spindle suggest that decreased birefringence represents a loss, rather than the disorientation of microtubules. At the completion of the action of antimitotic poisons, only a few
segmented microtubules were left near the chromosomes [INOUÉ and SATO,
1967; MALAWISTA *et al.*, 1968]. When the marine gametes were treated with
Colcemid or vinblastine and washed by sea water, their spindles recovered in
the course of 40–60 min, requiring a much longer time than when treated
with griseofulvin. Recovery is not accelerated or prolonged by D_2O. There
is no suggestion that protein synthesis is required for the recovery of spindle
fibers or microtubules. In fact, addition of the protein synthesis inhibitors,
actinomycin D, puromycin, cyclohexamid, or chloramphenicol, did not hin-
der spindle recovery. Actually, for some unknown reason both puromycin
and actinomycin D accelerated recovery.
    The Colcemid effect can be blocked locally in the spindle zone of the div-
iding *Lytechinus variegatus* egg by irradiating with 366 nm light. ARONSON
and INOUÉ [1970] believe that the near UV radiation causes a photochemical

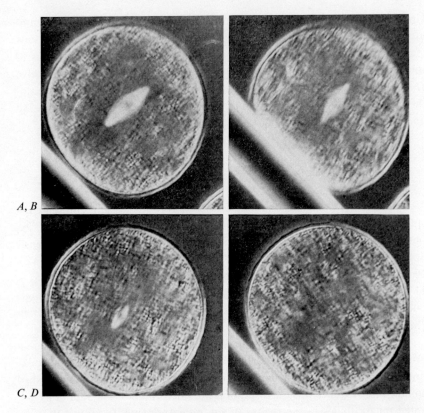

A, B

C, D

Fig. 11. Effect of 10^{-5} M Colcemid-sea water perfusion on the arrested metaphase spindle of *Pectinaria* oocyte. The eggs, without compression, were placed on a slide glass coated with a thin layer of Butvar film, to which the eggs adhere. They were surrounded by glass wool, which further prevents the eggs from flowing away during rapid perfusion. *A* 5 min before the perfusion. *B* 2 min 30 sec after the Colcemid perfusion was started. *C* 7 min 15 sec in Colcemid, the miniature spindle is still visible. *D* After 11 min 45 sec, the spindle has disappeared completely. P ↑ = Vibrating direction of polarized light; A → = direction of analyzer; applies to all figures in polarized light [INOUÉ and SATO, 1967].

rearrangement in the colchicine molecule that reduces or destroys its effect on the spindle. If colchicine or Colcemid act on the association-dissociation reaction of the microtubule protein, as seems reasonable from colchicine binding studies [BORISY and TAYLOR, 1967 a, b], then the photochemical in-activation of colchicine or Colcemid should be a means of varying the available pool size or the local concentration of polymerizable tubulin [ARONSON and INOUÉ, 1970].

The effectiveness of the antimitotic poisons can be summarized in the following order:

10^{-1}M mercaptoethanol > 10^{-5}M griseofulvin > 10^{-5}M vinblastine, 10^{-5}M Colcemid > 10^{-5}M colchicine, 10^{-5}M Vincrystine > 10^{-5}M Podophyllotoxin.

IV. Crystalization of Spindle Material in vivo

Spindle microtubule material can be crystallized in living mature oocytes. At least 2 different types of crystals can be classified: (1) SM crystals – spindle microtubule crystal [SATO and MAZIA, 1970], and (2) VB crystals – crystals induced by vinblastine [MALAWISTA and SATO, 1969; STRAHS and SATO, 1973].

A. SM Crystals

SM crystals (fig. 12) were successfully induced in the mature oocytes of *Pisaster ochraceus* or *Asterias forbesi* by using a combination of elevated temperature and mechanical compression. The timing for the preparation is rather critical, and oocytes collected at the germinal vesicle breakdown stage show the best yield. For this preparation, oocytes spread on a gelatin coated cover slip are gently compressed against fluorocarbon oils such as FC-47 (3-M) or Kel F-10 (3-M) and then incubated at a temperature 10°C higher than their initial environmental temperature.

Under these conditions, spindle formation is disrupted and, at first, highly birefringent aggregates are induced. Electron micrographs revealed that these aggregates consisted of well oriented annulate lamellae occasionally extending more than 30 µm (fig. 13). Crystal formation is limited to the central area of the aggregates, and the size of the birefringent aggregates decreases in association with the growth of the crystal. The whole process usually requires 3 h at 23°C in the case of *Pisaster* under the preparation conditions described above. During this time, the sign of birefringence changes dramatically. The aggregates, at first positive, become negative during the rapid development of annulate lamellae. The final rod-shape crystals have a positive form birefringence and easily reach dimensions of about 20 µm in length and 4 µm in width.

These crystals, which have a maximum absorbance at 280 nm, appear to be contained within a vesicle. Being fragile, heat-sensitive structures, they

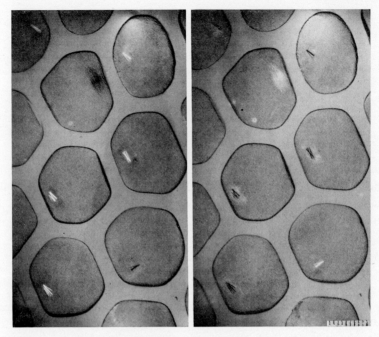

Fig. 12. SM crystals (spindle microtubule crystals) induced in mature oocytes of *Pisaster ochraceus* with 3 h incubation at 23°C. Note the different sign of birefringence of crystals and the surrounding aggregates. Polarization microscopy showing same field in reversed contrast by rotating compensator. Scale interval, 10 μm.

easily dissociate and reform within the vesicle. It is exceedingly difficult to stabilize these crystals, and it has not been possible to isolate them with various stabilizing media originally designed to isolate the mitotic apparatus. However, the direct conversion of a functional mitotic spindle to SM crystal and the reverse transformation have been observed [DANIELS, personal commun.]. SM crystals are readily induced by incubation in media lacking Na^+ but having increased K^+, Mg^{++}, and Ca^{++} concentrations. Subsequent transfer of the oocytes to sea water results in vesicle breakdown and crystal dissociation concomitant with spindle formation.

SM crystals may be liquid crystals, and the newly formed vesicles, or female pronuclei, may be acting as dialyzing biomembranes. Because pretreatment with mitotic poisons such as Colcemid, vinblastine, or griseofulvin, and incubation with $10^{-2}M$ mercaptoethanol prohibit crystal formation, these crystals are considered to be composed of highly oriented microtubule subunits. The molecular alignment of subunits could result from an acute con-

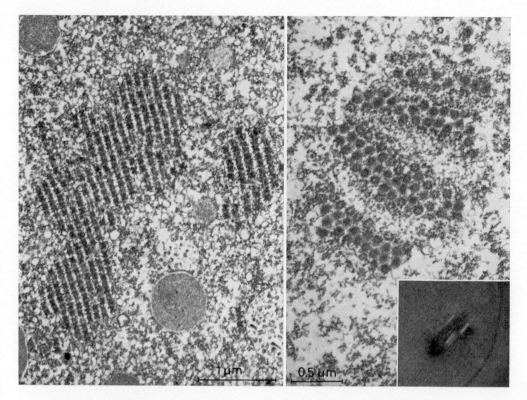

Fig. 13. Electron micrographs reveal that the negatively birefringent aggregates (right bottom) induced prior to the SM crystal formation in *Pisaster* oocytes are in fact the annulate lamellae. These lamellae structures, which are shown in both photographs as the longitudinal and cross sections, were quickly developed after the incubation started; however, they disappeared simultaneously after the completion of the SM crystal formation.

centration gradient within the vesicle. The coefficient of birefringence of the crystal has been calculated as 3×10^{-3}, which is much higher than that of the mitotic spindle. The birefringent nature of the SM crystal is demonstrated in figure 14 by rotating an oocyte within a crossed polarizer and analyzer axis.

B. VB Crystals

Vinblastine, a mitotic poison, has a short-term effect of dissociating all microtubules in the mitotic spindle. However, it was found that the pro-

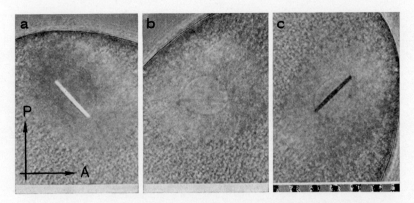

Fig. 14. Demonstrating the optical properties of the birefringent SM crystal induced in a *Pisaster* oocyte. P indicates the vibrating direction of polarized light; A, the direction of the analyzer. The slow axis of $\lambda/20$ mica-compensator is set at $+10°$ from the P axis. *a* The SM crystal positioned $+45°$ to P. *b* The stage has been rotated $45°$ so that the initial axis of SM crystal becomes perpendicular to P or parallel to A. Thus the birefringence of the crystal is extinguished. *c* The stage has been rotated an additional $135°$ in the same direction. The contrast of the SM crystal is now changed to black owing to the overcompensation by the mica compensator. Scale interval, 10 μm.

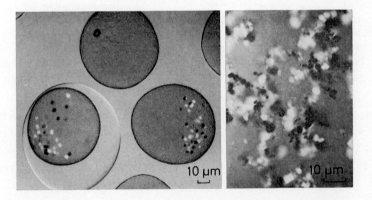

Fig. 15. Left photograph shows the VB crystals induced in the fertilized and unfertilized eggs of *Lythechinus pictus*. Right photograph demonstrates the clean mass isolation of VB crystals obtained from the unfertilized sea urchin eggs. The potentiation effect of Colcemid for VB crystal formation allows us to increase the yield of isolated crystals. Polarization microscopy.

longed incubation of living cells with vinblastine induced the formation of microtubular crystals within the cytoplasm [BENSCH and MALAWISTA, 1968, 1969; MALAWISTA and SATO, 1969]. The vinblastine induced microtubular crystals (VB crystals) were highly birefringent (fig. 15) and behaved as uniaxial crystals owing to the high degree of ultrastructural organization. As shown in figure 16, the honeycomb-like fine structure, having greater dimensions than the microtubule itself, was commonly found in a variety of cells, including echinoderm gametes and oocytes.

Within limits, crystal growth is a function of vinblastine concentration, temperature, and incubation time. For instance, the meiotic spindle of *Pisaster ochraceus* dissociates within about 7 min at 13°C in 10^{-4}M vinblastine sea water. Within a few hours, small birefringent spots appear all over the cytoplasm and gradually grow into square or rectangular crystals never seen in control cells. The maximum yield of VB crystals is reached at 18–24 h incubation. By comparison, in sea urchin gametes (*Lytechinus variegatus*) incubated with the same concentration of vinblastine at 22°C, 3.5 h are required to obtain the maximum yield. As an extreme case, the gametes of *Mespilia globulus* require only 30 min at 30°C incubation [SATO, unpublished].

Although other *Vinca* alkaloids such as vincrystine sulfate also induce microtubule crystals in living cells, no crystal induction is obtained by incubation with griseofulvin, colchicine, or Colcemid. However, colchicine and Colcemid do potentiate induction of VB crystals. In the case of the gametes of *Lytechinus variegatus*, 15% of the eggs successfully formed VB crystals during 3.5 h incubation in 10^{-4}M vinblastine at 22°C, whereas nearly 100% crystal induction is attained in 40 min when gametes are incubated with 10^{-4}M vinblastine and Colcemid. Actually, even 11 min pretreatment with 10^{-4}M Colcemid is ample to effect this potentiation of VB crystal formation. In fact, by pulse-incubating *Lytechinus* gametes with 10^{-4}M vinblastine and Colcemid for various time intervals, we found that a 30 min pulse was sufficient to activate maximum VB crystal induction. And though the percentage of crystals induced remained constant, each crystal increased in size and birefringence as incubation continued. Gametes pretreated with vinblastine and Colcemid maintain perfect fertilizability, but crystal formation proceeds without allowing spindle formation [FUJIWARA and SATO, 1972].

A general comparison of the physical properties of SM and VB crystals is made in tables II and III. The 2 kinds of microtubular crystals constitute distinctly different types of biocrystals. The VB crystal specifically requires vinblastine, has a much larger yield per gamete than the SM crystal, has a different morphology, has a definite readily fixed honeycomb-like cross section-

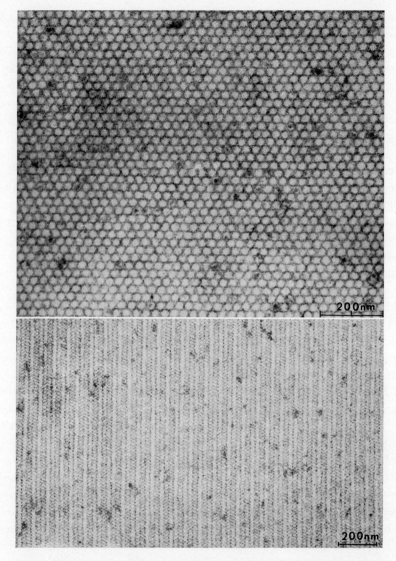

Fig. 16. Electron micrographs show a cross section (above) and a diagonal section (bottom) of the VB crystal. The average diameter of a tubular structure is 320 Å. The VB crystal was induced in unfertilized oocytes of *Strongylocentrotus purpuratus* by incubating with 10^{-4} M vinblastine sulfate and 10^{-4} M Colcemid in artificial sea water at 22 °C for 12 h. The eggs were treated with 1 M urea (pH 8.5 with Tris-HCl), and lysed in a medium containing 100 mM KCl, 1 mM MgCl$_2$, 0.1% Triton X-100 and 10^{-5} M vinblastine (pH 7.5 with Tris-HCl). The isolated VB crystals were fixed by 2% glutaraldehyde and tanic acid, and postfixed with 1% OsO$_4$. (Courtesy of Mr. Keigi Fujiwara, unpublished photograph.)

Table II. Physical properties of SM and VB crystals compared with MA (mitotic apparatus). Material: *Pisaster ochraceus*

	SM crystal	VB crystal	MA
Shape (side view)	bar	square	elliptical
Shape (cross section)	circular	rectangular	circular
Dimension at 13°C	20×3 μm (24°C)	$15 \times 15 \times 8$ μm	12×8 μm
Sign of BR	form BR	form and intrinsic BR	form and intrinsic BR
$(n_e\text{-}n_o)$	3×10^{-3}	3×10^{-3}	5×10^{-4}
Refractive index	1.52?	1.51	1.51
UV sensitivity	–	–	+

Table III. Comparison of SM and VB crystals with MA (mitotic apparatus). Material: *Pisaster ochraceus*

	SM crystal	VB crystal	MA
Induction			
Optimum temp., °C	24 ± 1	10 ± 5	13 ± 2
Time required	3 h	14 h	5 min
Flattening (comp.)	+	–	
Yield/mature oocyte, %	> 80	> 80	> 80
Yield/immature oocyte, %	< 2	< 20	< 20
Induction with			
10^{-1}M mercaptoethanol	–	±	–
10^{-5}M Colcemid	–	+++ (enhanced)	–
10^{-4}M VB or VC	–	+	–
Low temp., $\cong 4$°C	–	+	+
Stabilization			
Cold methanol	–	+	+
Cold HG, 12%	–	–	+
10^{-3}M DTDG	–	–	+
10^{-4}M VB or VC	–	+	–
10^{-4}M Colcemid	–	–	–
D_2O, 60%	+	–	–

al fine structure, and can be stabilized and isolated in quantity [Bryan, 1971].

The stoichiometry of VB crystals [Bryan, 1972] is such that 1 mol of vinblastine and 1 mol of colchicine are bound independently per mol of tubulin dimer, whereas 2 mol of guanosine nucleotide are bound per mol of dimer. Both the vinblastine and nucleotide are very tightly bound; they are not exchangeable under conditions in which the microtubule crystals are stable. From this data, Bryan [1972] postulates a heterodimer model of microtubule subunits, with each monomer containing a specific alkaloid binding site and one nucleotide site. And though this is a great step forward, still more information is certainly necessary for a complete understanding of VB crystals formation and the colchicine potentiation effect.

V. Effects of Maturity on Spindle or Crystal Formation

The yield of either SM crystals or VB crystals in marine gametes greatly depends on cellular maturity, and rather wide variations have been noted. SM crystals can be induced in more than 80% in mature oocytes of *Pisaster ochraceus* or *Asterias forbesi*, but in less than 2% in immature oocytes. For the most part, these crystals are not observed in either sea urchin or sea cucumber gametes. However, they can be induced in overmature summer sea urchin gametes by elevating the environmental temperature. For instance, the natural spawning of gametes in *Mespilia globulus* occurs twice per lunar month, and the maturation rhythm of the gonads is harmonized with the hemilunar periodicity [Kobayashi, 1967]. Recovery of gonads from spent to mature takes only a week. After disturbing the natural spawning rhythm of *Mespilia* with a temperature shift, we found that in overmature gametes (collected 5 days after the scheduled natural spawning) more than 30% possessed SM crystals. These natural SM crystals can be transformed either to functional mitotic spindles or to natural VB crystals even in the absence of vinblastine. However, like the VB crystals formed by vinblastine, these natural VB crystals cannot dissociate and transform to either SM crystals or spindles.

The different crystal characteristics presumably reflect a polymorphism of spindle microtubule subunits. Another example of this is that labile spindle microtubules can easily be split and dissociated by changing pH or osmolarity even during fixation. Figure 17 shows 'C tubules' induced by altering pH by ±0.5 units from the optimum. In this particular picture, 28% of the mi-

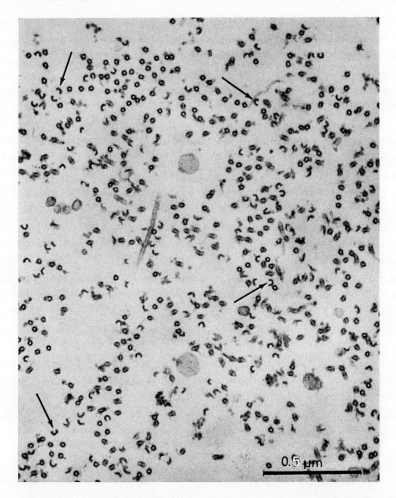

Fig. 17. Electron micrograph shows many 'C tubules' (indicated by arrows) in the cross section of an isolated meiosis I spindle of *Pisaster* oocyte. The lateral splits of microtubules are induced by quickly altering pH from 6.3 to 6.8 during the spindle isolation. 'C tubules' can be induced within the isolated spindles even during or after the glutaraldehyde fixation by changing pH or osmolarity.

crotubules present are split but otherwise retain their original dimensions. This suggests a possible lateral dissociation of the microtubules instead of the expected breakdown from the ends only. And it provides yet another polymeric manifestation of microtubule subunits.

As stated before, VB crystal formation also depends on cellular maturity. In fact, even the Colcemid potentiation of VB crystal induction is a function of cellular maturity. In the extreme case of overmature *Mespilia* gametes, incubation with vinblastine induces extremely high rates of VB crystal formation. Indeed, even the addition of Colcemid alone is sufficient to potentiate VB crystal induction at rates higher than normal.

Colcemid enhances VB crystal formation in at least 3 different ways. Firstly, it shortens the time of incubation in vinblastine required to induce crystals. Secondly, nearly 100% of the cells incubated in vinblastine with Colcemid give rise to the highly birefringent crystals. In vinblastine alone, the proportion of cells containing crystals rarely exceeds 60% in mature gametes, and in immature gametes the rate may be 5% or lower. Thirdly, Colcemid produces a 3-fold increase in crystal volume per cell.

Although the precise stoichiometric relationship between Colcemid and the microtubule subunits is not firmly established, one possible explanation for the potentiation effect of Colcemid might be its ability to favor the formation of subunit dimers from the cell's pool of monomers. The resulting dimers may bind vinblastine more readily, thus being incorporated into crystals more rapidly. However, this is speculation and needs to be tested experimentally [STRAHS and SATO, 1973].

The VB crystals formed in overmature gametes are often large and barrel-shaped, rather than the usual rectangular or square shape. As illustrated in figure 18, heavy contamination with ribosomes and polysomes is the characteristic feature and could be a typical sign of overmaturity in marine gametes.

VI. Concluding Remarks

The dynamic nature of the mitotic spindle under various physiological conditions is summarized in the present article. Based on *in vivo* observations of the behavior of the birefringent spindle fibers and on measurements of birefringence of spindle fibers under various experimental conditions, it is postulated that the dynamic living spindle is maintained as a steady-state equilibrium between a pool of spindle protein molecules (tubulins) and their linearly aggregated polymers, the microtubules. The analysis of the nature of the birefringence of the mitotic spindle shows that oriented microtubules are almost exclusively responsible for the observed birefringence. The close match between the theoretical Wiener's curve and experimental measure-

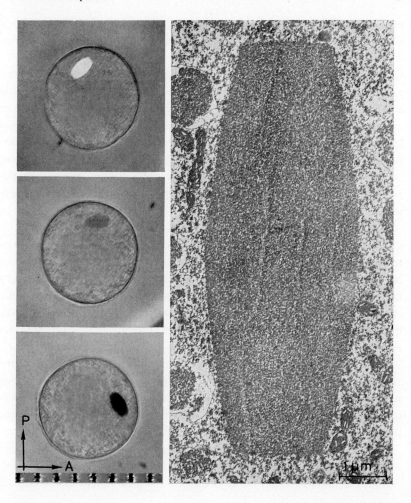

Fig. 18. The three polarization micrographs arranged on the left demonstrate the birefringent nature of the VB crystals induced in the overmature *Pectinaria* oocyte by rotating within a crossed polarizer and analyzer axis. However, as shown in the second photograph of left row, the VB crystal is barely extinguished optically because of the secondary disruption of the orderly arranged fine structure caused by the heavy contamination of ribosomes. Electron micrograph on the right shows the longitudinal section of the VB crystal induced in the overmature *Pectinaria* oocyte. Heavy accumulation of ribosomes is shown. Scale interval, 10 μm.

ment of spindle birefringence at various refractive indices indicates that the contribution of intrinsic birefringence of the protein itself is low and at most 8% at n = 1.33.

The association of molecules into polymers is rather weak in living cells, and the equilibrium is readily shifted. Dissociation is favored by low temperatures, high pressures, or reduction of D_2O concentration, whereas polymerization is enhanced by elevating temperature or the addition of D_2O. In the case of D_2O equilibriated spindles of *Pisaster* oocytes, the number of microtubules more than doubles without changing the initial population density per unit volume. The association-dissociation reaction in mitotic spindle is reversible and repeatable and is thought to be a first-order reaction on the basis of kinetic analysis.

Antimitotic poisons also dissociate spindle microtubules. However, this dissociation reaction does not follow simple first order kinetics, and further research is needed here. In the extreme case, microtubule subunits can be crystallized *in vivo* by altering physical or chemical parameters. The VB crystal, produced by prolonged incubation with vinblastine, is physically different from the SM crystal. The stable VB crystal has a distinct honeycomb-like fine structure whereas the labile SM crystal is thought to be a liquid crystal. However, both crystals are birefringent and composed of microtubule subunits.

The yield of VB crystals is greatly enhanced by colchicine and its derivatives, probably owing to the existence of a large pool of available tubulin monomers in marine gametes. The VB crystal never dissociates within the living cell and the microtubule subunits appear to be irreversibly bound. Knowing this extreme stability and the complication of ribosome contamination in overmature gametes, we conclude that we should be extremely cautious in applying mixtures of antimitotic poisons to overmature gametes or tissues as this may terminate forever many of the physiological functions of living substance at various levels.

Acknowledgments

The H_2O_{18} was a gift from Dr. D. SAMUEL, the Weizmann Institute of Science, and the vinblastine sulfate a gift from Eli Lilly and Company.

Parts of this work were done at the Friday Harbor Laboratories (USA), courtesy of Dr. R. FERNALD, and the Seto Marine Biological Laboratory (Japan), courtesy of Dr. T. TOKIOKA. Thanks are due to Mr. G. DANIELS for discussion and advice, Mr. K. FUJIWARA for the use of his unpublished photograph, and Mrs. D. BUSH, Mrs. Y. SATO and Mrs. B. WOODWARD for technical assistance.

References

ARONSON, J. and INOUÉ, S.: Reversal by light of the action of *N*-methyl-*N*-desacetyl colchicine on mitosis. J. Cell Biol. *45:* 470 (1970).

BAJER, A.S. and MOLÉ-BAJER, J.: Architecture and function of the mitotic spindle; in DuPRAW Advances in cell and molecular biology, vol. 1, pp. 213–266 (Academic Press, New York 1971).

BAJER, A.S. and MOLÉ-BAJER, J.: Spindle dynamics and chromosome movements. Int. Rev. Cytol., suppl. 3 (Academic Press, New York 1972).

BENSCH, K.G. and MALAWISTA, S.E.: Microtubule crystals. A new biophysical phenomenon induced by *Vinca* alkaloids. Nature, Lond. *218:* 1176 (1968).

BENSCH, K.G. and MALAWISTA, S.E.: Microtubular crystals in mammalian cells. J. Cell Biol. *40:* 95 (1969).

BORISY, G.G. and TAYLOR, E.W.: The mechanism of action of colchicine binding of colchicine-³H to cellular protein. J. Cell Biol. *34:* 525 (1967a).

BORISY, G.G. and TAYLOR, E.W.: The mechanism of action of colchicine-colchicine binding to sea urchin eggs and the mitotic apparatus. J. Cell Biol. *34:* 535 (1967b).

BRINKLEY, B.R. and CARTWRIGHT, J., jr.: Ultrastructural analysis of mitotic spindle elongation in mammalian cells *in vitro*. Direct microtubule counts. J. Cell Biol. *50:* 416 (1971).

BRYAN, J.: Vinblastine and microtubules. I. Induction and isolation of crystal from sea urchin oocytes. Exp. Cell Res. *66:* 129 (1971).

BRYAN, J.: Definition of three classes of binding sites in isolated microtubule crystals. Biochemistry *11:* 2611 (1972).

BRYAN, J. and SATO, H.: The isolation of the meiosis I spindle from the mature oocyte of *Pisaster ochraceus*. Exp. Cell Res. *59:* 371 (1970).

CAROLAN, R.M.; SATO, H., and INOUÉ, S.: A thermodynamic analysis of the effect of D_2O and H_2O on the mitotic spindle. Biol. Bull. *129:* 402 (1965).

CAROLAN, R.M.; SATO, H., and INOUÉ, S.: Further observations on the thermodynamics of the living mitotic spindle. Biol. Bull. *131:* 385 (1966).

CHAET, A.B.: Neurochemical control of gamete release in starfish. Biol. Bull. *130:* 43 (1966).

COSTELLO, D.P.: On the orientation of centrioles in dividing cells and its significance. A new contribution to spindle mechanics. Biol. Bull. *120:* 285 (1961).

DIETZ, R.: Polarisationsmikroskopische Befunde zur chromosomeninduzierten Spindelbildung bei der *Tipulide pales crocata* (Nematocera). Zool. Anz. *26:* suppl., p. 131 (1963).

DIETZ, R.: Anaphase behavior of inversions in living crane-fly spermatocytes. Chromosomes Today. Proc. Oxford Chromosome Conf., Oxford 1972.

FORER, A.: Local reduction of spindle fiber birefringence in living *Nephrotoma suturalis* (loew) spermatocytes induced by ultraviolet microbeam irradiation. J. Cell Biol. *25:* 95 (1965).

FUJIWARA, K. and SATO, H.: VB-crystal formation in sea urchin eggs by short term VB-col incubation. J. Cell Biol. *55:* part 2, abstract 79a (1972).

INOUÉ, S.: The effect of colchicine on the microscopic and submicroscopic structure of the mitotic spindle. Exp. Cell Res., suppl. *2*, p. 305 (1952a).

INOUÉ, S.: Effect of temperature on the birefringence of the mitotic spindle. Biol. Bull. *103:* 316 (1952b).

INOUÉ, S.: Organization and function of the mitotic spindle; in ALLEN and KAMIYA Primitive motile systems in cell biology, p. 549 (Academic Press, New York 1964).

INOUÉ, S.: The physics of structural organization in living cells; in DEVONS Biology and the physical sciences, p. 139 (Columbia Univ. Press, New York 1969).

INOUÉ, S.; ELLIS, G.W.; SALMON, E.D., and FUSELER, J.W.: Rapid measurement of spindle birefringence during controlled temperature shifts. J. Cell Biol. *47:* 95a (1970).

INOUÉ, S. and MORALES, M. F.: in INOUÉ Motility of cilia and the mechanism of mitosis. Rev. Mod. Phys. *31:* 402 (1959).

INOUÉ, S. and SATO, H.: Cell motility by labile association of molecules. The nature of mitotic spindle fibers and their role in chromosomal movement. J. gen. Physiol. *50:* 259 (1967).

INOUÉ, S.; SATO, H., and ASCHER, M.: Counteraction of colcemid and heavy water on the organization of the mitotic spindle. Biol. Bull. *129:* 409 (1965).

KANATANI, H.; SHIRAI, H.; NAKANISHI, K., and KUROKAWA, T.: Isolation and identification of meiosis inducing substance in starfish *Asterias amurensis.* Nature, Lond. *221:* 459 (1969).

KANE, R.E.: The mitotic apparatus. Physical-chemical factors controlling stability. J. Cell Biol. *25:* 137 (1965).

KOBAYASHI, N.: Spawning periodicity of sea urchins at Seto. I. *Mespilia globulus.* Publ. Seto Marine Biological Laboratory *14:* 403 (1967).

MALAWISTA, S.E. and SATO, H.: Vinblastine produces uniaxial, birefringent crystals in starfish oocytes. J. Cell Biol. *42:* 596 (1969).

MALAWISTA, S.E.; SATO, H., and BENSCH, K.: Vinblastine and griseofulvin reversibly disrupt the living mitotic spindle. Science *160:* 770 (1968).

MARSLAND, D. and ZIMMERMAN, A.M.: Structural stabilization of the mitotic apparatus by heavy water in the cleaving eggs of *Arbacia punctulata.* Exp. Cell Res. *38:* 306 (1965).

MAZIA, D.: Mitosis and the physiology of cell division; in BRACHET and MIRSKY The cell, vol. 3: Meiosis and mitosis, p. 77. (Academic Press, New York 1961).

MCINTOSH, J.R. and LANDIS, S.C.: The distribution of spindle microtubules during mitosis in cultured human cells. J. Cell Biol. *49:* 468 (1971).

NICKLAS, R.B.: Mitosis; in PRESCOTT, GOLDSTEIN and MCCONKEY Advances in cell biology, p. 225 (Appleton-Century-Crofts, New York 1971).

ÖSTERGREN, G.: The mechanism of co-orientation in bivalents and multivalents. Hereditas *37:* 85 (1951).

RAPPAPORT, R.: Cytokinesis in animal cells. Int. Rev. Cytol. *31:* 169 (1971).

SATO, H.; BAJER, A.S., and BAJER, J.M.: Birefringence in endosperm cell division; film (1970).

SATO, H. and BRYAN, J.: Kinetic analysis of association-dissociation reaction in the mitotic spindle. J. Cell Biol. *39:* 118a (1968).

SATO, H. and DANIELS, G.: Analysis of microtubule distribution in the mitotic spindle. Abstract. Amer. Zool. *11:* 684 (1971).

SATO, H.; INOUÉ, S., and ELLIS, G.W.: The microtubular origin of spindle birefringence.

Experimental verification of Wiener's equation. Abstr. Proc. 11th Annu. Meet. Amer. Soc. Cell Biology, 1971, p. 216.

SATO, H. and MAZIA, D.: Crystallization of spindle material in living mature oocytes. J. Cell Biol. *47:* 179a (1970).

SCHRADER, F.: in DUNN Mitosis, the movements of chromosomes in cell division; 2nd ed. (Columbia Univ. Press, New York 1953).

STEPHENS, R.E.: Microtubules; in TIMASHEFF and FASMAN Biological macromolecules, vol. 5: Subunits in biological systems, Part A, pp. 355–391 (Marcel Dekker, New York 1973).

STRAHS, K.R. and SATO, H.: Potentiation of vinblastine crystal formation *in vivo* by puromycin and colcemid. Exp. Cell Res. *80:* 10 (1973).

WENT, M.A.: The behavior of centrioles and the structure and formation of the achromatic figure. Protoplasmatologia *6:* G 1 (1966).

WIENER, O.: Die Theorie des Mischkörpers für das Feld der stationären Strömung. Die Mittelwertsätze für Kraft, Polarisation und Energie. Abhandl. math.-phys. Kl. Königl. Sächs. Ges. Wiss. *32:* 505 (1912).

Author's address: Dr. HIDEMI SATO, Department of Biology, University of Pennsylvania, *Philadelphia, PA 19104* (USA)

Aging Gametes. Int. Symp., Seattle 1973, pp. 50–71 (Karger, Basel 1975)

Normal and Abnormal Chromosomal Behavior in the Meiotic Divisions of Mammalian Oocytes

ROGER P. DONAHUE

Departments of Obstetrics and Gynecology and of Medicine, School of Medicine, University of Washington, Seattle, Wash.

In man, nearly 7% of all recognized conceptions have an abnormal chromosomal constitution (see contribution by BOUÉ). JACOBS [1972] has estimated that a minimum of 0.07%, and probably 1 or 2% of these are due to a chromosomal abnormality carried by the fertilizing spermatozoon. Suspicion falls on the egg as the origin of chromosomal aberrations mainly because of the association of some aberrations, e.g., trisomies 13, 18, and 21, with advanced maternal age. Other factors, radiation exposure [ALBERMAN et al., 1972] and thyroid autoimmunity [FIALKOW et al., 1971], also suggest a maternal origin. There has been difficulty, however, in determining whether maternally associated chromosomal abnormalities arise before, during, or after the meiotic divisions and few human oocytes have been examined. Most studies have used oocytes of the laboratory mouse with the profound hope their chromosomal behavior adequately represents that of human oocytes. This review will be limited to direct cytological observations of meiotic chromosomal behavior in mammalian oocytes, primarily those of the mouse.

I. Normal Chromosomal Behavior

A. The First Meiotic Division

In most mammals, oogonia in the fetal ovary enter the first meiotic division [PETERS, 1970] at which time pairing of homologous chromosomes occurs and exchange of genetic material (crossing over) takes place. By the time of birth, these primary oocytes have progressed only as far as late prophase of the first meiotic division and further progression then stops. Since the chromosomal configuration at this stage of arrest is not the same in all mam-

mals, being at diplotene in some species and at dictyate in others [BAKER and
FRANCHI, 1967], the term germinal vesicle, first used in 1875 by VAN BENE-
DEN in describing rabbit oocytes, remains a useful one to denote the nucleus
of oocytes during the extended period of meiotic arrest. Normally, the first
meiotic division is resumed under the influence of gonadotrophins in sexually
mature females; once germinal vesicle breakdown commences, the nucleus
completes the first division and arrests at second meiotic metaphase, a process called oocyte maturation. The entire sequence of oocyte maturation
from germinal vesicle to metaphase II takes between 10–24 h, depending on
the species. Maturation usually is synchronized so that metaphase II formation coincides with ovulation [DONAHUE, 1972 a].

Oocytes will also mature 'spontaneously' when removed from the follicle and placed into a suitable culture medium [DONAHUE, 1972 a], although
the reason they do so remains unexplained. Mouse and human oocytes matured *in vitro* are morphologically normal [CALARCO *et al.*, 1972; ZAMBONI *et
al.*, 1972] and normal fertile animals have been obtained from mouse oocytes
matured *in vitro* [MUKHERJEE, 1972].

Germinal vesicle breakdown begins with a shortening of the chromatin
fibers, and, within 2 h in mouse oocytes maturing *in vitro*, distinct chromosomes are visible (fig. 1–2). Condensation continues for approximately another hour, until the bivalents (tetrads) reach their maximum state of contraction, at which time they are arranged peripherally around the nuclear
membrane (fig. 3). This is the circularly arranged bivalent stage and probably
corresponds to the classical chromosomal stage of diakinesis. Interference-
contrast in living specimens [SORENSEN, 1973] and electron microscopy have
shown [CALARCO *et al.*, 1972] that the nuclear membrane by this time has become very convoluted.

Before complete dissolution of the nuclear membrane, two centromeres
per half bivalent appear, presumably occurring as one per chromatid (fig. 4)
[CALARCO, 1972]. Spindle microtubules are found in the cytoplasm and penetrate through the perforations in the nuclear membrane, making contact
with the forming centromeres [CALARCO *et al.*, 1972].

Subsequent to spindle formation, bivalents align on the spindle at prometaphase I and attain equilibrium at metaphase I when the centromeres of a
half bivalent lie above the equator (or 'metaphase plate') and centromeres of
the other lie below the equator (fig. 5). This bipolar orientation (also called
coorientation) is probably crucial for proper separation (disjunction) of bivalents at anaphase I, ensuring that homologous half bivalents will proceed to
opposite poles. Nondisjunction, or passage of the entire bivalent to one pole,

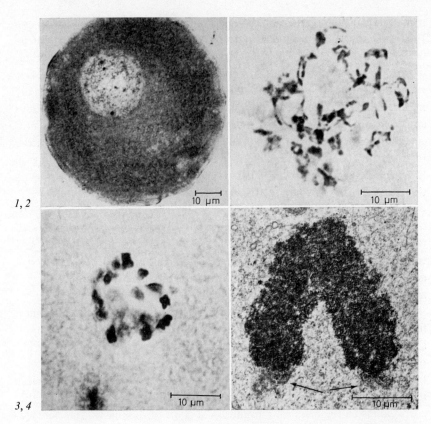

Fig. 1–4. Early stages of germinal vesicle breakdown in the mouse oocyte. Intact germinal vesicle (fig. 1), condensing chromosomes (fig. 2), and the circularly arranged bivalent stage (fig. 3). Each bivalent by this time (fig. 4) has two terminal centromeres (arrows) associated with each homolog (half bivalent). Figures 1–3 from DONAHUE [1968a], figure 4 from CALARCO [1972].

leads to one product of the first meiotic division being deficient one univalent, the other product containing an extra univalent. The mechanisms responsible for bipolar orientation are poorly understood. After bivalents in grasshopper spermatocytes are physically detached from the metaphase I spindle, they reassume this bipolar configuration on the spindle [NICKLAS and KOCH, 1969]. These and other studies involving micromanipulation on living spermatocytes have led to several models of chromosome movement and spindle behavior [NICKLAS and KOCH, 1972; see also contribution by

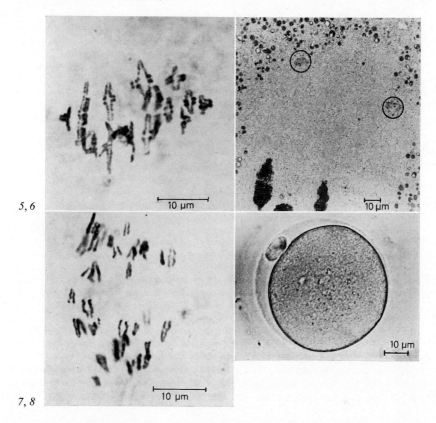

5, 6

7, 8

Fig. 5–8. At metaphase I, bivalents show a bipolar orientation (fig. 5) on the first meiotic spindle that, instead of centrioles, has microtubule foci (circled, fig. 6). Figure 7: Anaphase I. The first meiotic division is completed with formation of the first polar body (fig. 8) seen in this human oocyte photographed prior to fixation. The oocyte and first polar body are enclosed by the zona pellucida. Figures 5 and 7 from DONAHUE [1968a], figure 6 from SZOLLOSI *et al.* [1972], figure 8 from KENNEDY and DONAHUE [1969].

SATO]. Structural alterations in chromosomes can lead to multivalent formation, and their meiotic behavior is discussed elsewhere [FORD and CLEGG, 1969].

Although mammalian oogonia and oocytes early in meiosis (through pachynema) have centrioles, these organelles are absent in subsequent meiotic stages and are even lacking in the early cleavage divisions [SZOLLOSI *et al.*, 1972]. In their place are many (the actual number is unknown) electron-dense areas, termed microtubule foci or microtubule organizing centers, lo-

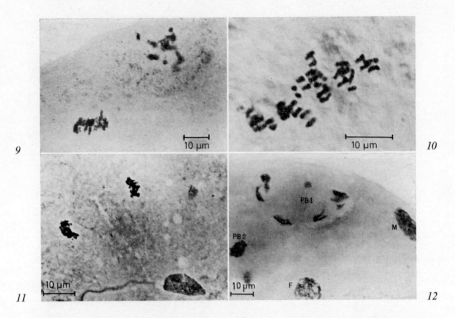

Fig. 9–12. Figure 9: Metaphase II and clumped first polar body chromosomes (above) in a human oocyte. Figure 10: Metaphase II in a mouse oocyte. Figure 11: Anaphase II in a mouse oocyte with a transforming sperm head. Figure 12: Completion of meiosis in a mouse zygote. PB1, First polar body; PB2, second polar body. F, Female chromatin; M, transforming sperm head. Figure 9 from Kennedy and Donahue [1969], figure 10 from Donahue [1968a], figures 11–12 from Donahue [1972b].

cated in the polar regions from which microtubules emanate (fig. 6). An unanswered question is the distribution of spindle fibers between the microtubule foci and the centromere: Are the two centromeres of the half bivalent linked to more than one such focus?

Bivalent separation occurs at anaphase I (fig. 7), and the first meiotic division is completed with formation of two cells of very unequal size – the first polar body (PB1) and the secondary oocyte (fig. 8). There is no intervening prophase II in the oocyte, and chromosomes immediately assume a metaphase configuration on the newly formed second meiotic spindle (fig. 9, 10).

The newly formed PB1 does not appear to be deficient in cytoplasmic organelles [Zamboni, 1971], but, unfortunately for cytogeneticists, its chromosomes rapidly become fuzzy, and frequently the entire chromosomal complement consists only of clumped chromatin masses (fig. 9) [Long and Mark, 1911; Donahue, 1968 a, 1972 d]. The entire PB1 itself is usually lost, presumably by cytolysis, within several hours. Of 100 'young' and 100 'old' secondary mouse oocytes, 14% of the young and 67% of the old had no PB1 [LONG and MARK, 1911]. Formation of a spindle in a normal-size PB1 is rare, and true division, if it occurs at all, must be rarer still. Fragmentation does occur, however, with unequal chromatin distribution.

B. The Second Meiotic and First Cleavage Divisions

The haploid number of chromosomes, now called univalents or dyads, are arranged on the second meiotic spindle such that all centromeres lie on the equator of the spindle, so-called auto-orientation. Chromosome alignment is, therefore, mechanically like that in mitotic divisions. Subsequent to sperm penetration, chromatid separation takes place (fig. 11) and the second meiotic division is completed with formation again of two cells of unequal size – the second polar body (PB2) and the egg (fig. 12). Thus, for several hours the egg is at the same time a secondary oocyte (still in meiosis) and a zygote (having been fertilized).

The PB2 differs from the PB1 in at least four respects: it is haploid, a nuclear membrane encloses a well-formed nucleus [ZAMBONI, 1971], DNA synthesis occurs [SZOLLOSI, 1966; LUTHARDT and DONAHUE, 1973], and it is retained within the zona pellucida for several days. The PB2 has so far been unavailable for chromosomal analysis for it has not been reported to form chromosomes and divide in any mammalian embryo.

The chromatin of the egg and of the sperm head form separate nuclei (pronuclei) (fig. 13). The two pronuclei in mouse zygotes differ in size, the larger being derived from the fertilizing sperm and having less condensed chromatin than the smaller, female pronucleus [DONAHUE, 1972 b, c]. Within 8 h after fertilization in the mouse, pronuclear DNA synthesis commences. In each zygote, the period of DNA synthesis is about 4 h with synthesis beginning and terminating slightly earlier in the male pronucleus [LUTHARDT and DONAHUE, 1973].

With the onset of first cleavage prophase, chromatin fibers simultaneously begin to contract in the two pronuclei. The differential chromosome contraction between the male and female nuclei is retained through much of first cleavage prophase (fig. 14–15) but is lost by the time the two chromosome groups unite to form first cleavage metaphase (fig. 16). Completion of the first cleavage division in mouse oocytes takes place about 16 h after fertilization.

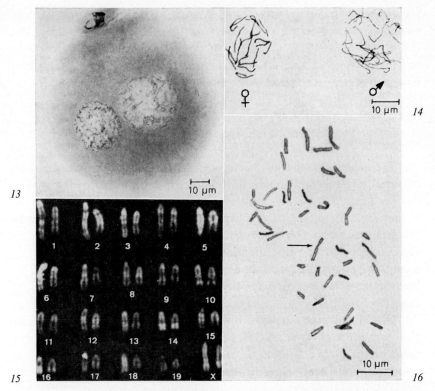

Fig. 13–16. Figure 13: Mouse zygote with the larger, male pronucleus on the right and second polar body at top. Figure 14: Prophase of the first cleavage division in a mouse oocyte exposed to a hypotonic solution to spread the chromosomes. A difference of chromosome contraction can be seen with those in the male nucleus (right) being less condensed. Figure 15: Karyotype of a mouse zygote at first cleavage prophase. In each pair the less condensed paternal chromosome has been placed on the left. Stained with quinacrine mustard to reveal chromosome bands. Figure 16: First cleavage metaphase chromosomes in a mouse zygote. Arrow indicates the submetacentric T163H chromosome introduced through the spermatozoon. Figure 13 from DONAHUE [1972b], figures 14 and 16 from DONAHUE [1972c], figure 15 from NESBITT and DONAHUE [1972].

II. Abnormalities of the First Meiotic Division

A. Evidence for Chromosomal Errors

Errors of disjunction or anaphase movement at the first meiotic division can be ascertained by direct examination of metaphase II chromosomes. Unfortunately, there are still far too few reports to establish a frequency (spontaneous or otherwise) of chromosomal errors occurring in mammalian oocytes. Mouse oocytes have received the most attention; in this species, JAGIELLO and her co-workers [JAGIELLO et al., 1972; JAGIELLO and DUCAYEN, 1973; JAGIELLO and LIN, 1973] failed to find other than the normal 20 metaphase II chromosomes in more than 1,400 oocytes matured in vivo and in vitro (age of the females did not exceed 200 days). Only a few human oocytes at metaphase II (all normal) have been reported to date [JAGIELLO et al., 1968; YUNCKEN, 1968; EDWARDS and FOWLER, 1970; UEBELE-KALLHARDT and KNORR, 1971] although many more reports may be expected in the future.

Instead of direct examination of meiotic chromosomes, an alternative approach is available in the pre- and postnatal individual to determine whether an error occurred at the first meiotic division. Since homologous chromosomes, i.e., half bivalents, normally separate at anaphase I, the presence in a trisomic individual of both these homologs indicates nondisjunction at the first meiotic division. However, since homologs usually look alike with usual cytological procedures, the problem has been to distinguish one from the other. With the new techniques for producing bands on chromosomes (fig. 15), it has been found that some homologs have a somewhat different banding pattern and that these differences are inherited. By use of these techniques, five cases (as of this writing) of trisomy-21 were shown to have both maternal No. 21 chromosomes, indicating nondisjunction at the first meiotic division in the oocyte [LICZNERSKI and LINDSTEN, 1972; ROBINSON, 1973]. This is the first strong evidence that trisomy-21 is indeed meiotic in origin. Other cases so far have been uninformative since the banding of homologs was identical. Even this type of evidence must be interpreted with caution, however, for the occurrence of crossing over could lead to erroneous identification of a first meiotic error when, in fact, a second meiotic division error was responsible.

Use of the Xg^a red cell antigen, whose locus is on the X chromosome, indicates that a meiotic origin during oogenesis at least cannot be excluded in some cases of Klinefelter's (XXY) and Turner's (XO) syndromes. Klinefelter's (but not Turner's) is associated with increased maternal age. In 60% of Klinefelter's, the two X chromosomes are maternal in origin, i.e. X^mX^mY; in 25% of Turner's, the paternal X is the one present (X^pO) indicating loss (meiotic?) of the maternal X [RACE, 1970]. In these cases, however, a mitotic loss during embryogenesis is also possible.

Theoretically, a number of different meiotic division errors involving entire chromosome sets are possible [discussed in BEATTY, 1957; RUSSELL,

Table I. Anomalies of mouse oocyte maturation and fertilization involving whole chromosome sets

Anomaly	'Spontaneous' frequency, %[1]	Percent frequency in old tubal eggs[2]	Chromosomal complement in the embryo
First meiotic division			
Large PB1	0.04–0.4	–	diploid mosaicism?
Suppression of PB1	0.08–0.3	–	triploid
All chromatin in PB1[3]	0.08	–	haploid
Fertilization and second meiotic division			
Large PB2	rare	7–10	haploid/diploid mosaicism
Suppression of PB2	0.3–0.6	0.9–1.7	triploid
All ♀ chromatin in PB2[3]	0.1	5–8	haploid
Other mononucleate	0.5–1.6	4	haploid
Dispermy	0.3–0.8	1.2	triploid

1 From BRADEN [1957] and DONAHUE [1970, 1972b].
2 From MARSTON and CHANG [1964] and DONAHUE and KARP [1973].
3 In these cases, there are two polar bodies with equal chromatin content.

1962] and a low frequency has been found in mouse oocytes (table I). When an exceptionally large PB1 forms, its chromosomes assume a normal-appearing metaphase II configuration (fig. 17). Fertilization might occur in both cells leading to genetic mosaicism in the embryo [DONAHUE, 1970]. Even more rare are suppression of PB1 formation and extrusion of all female chromatin into two first polar bodies (fig. 18). Similar errors occur at the second meiotic division (q.v.).

B. Asynchrony of Nucleolar-Associated Chromosomes

Trisomies for the D and G chromosomes are among the most common human trisomies. Since these chromosomes have secondary constrictions, features often associated with formation of the nucleolus, the hypothesis was advanced that the association of D and G chromosomes with the nucleolus was responsible in some way for the origin of D and G trisomies [FERGUSON-SMITH and HANDMAKER, 1961; OHNO et al., 1961]. Subsequent evidence, the reported nucleolar association of these chromosomes in human spermatoge-

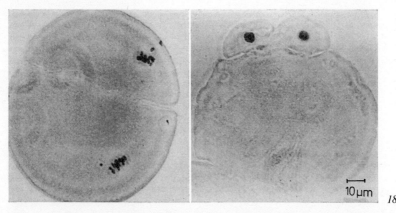

Fig. 17–18. Figure 17: Exceptionally large first polar body and mouse oocyte, each with organized metaphase II chromosomes. Figure 18: Mouse oocyte after maturation in which all chromatin has been expelled from the egg and is contained in two first polar bodies. From DONAHUE [1970].

nesis [FERGUSON-SMITH, 1964] and the presence of ribosomal RNA synthesizing sites at their satellited ends [HENDERSON *et al.*, 1972], has strengthened this association of D and G chromosomes with the nucleolus. Because of the association of some trisomies, especially trisomy-21, with advanced maternal age, suspicion naturally fell on the nucleolus of the oocyte. EVANS [1967] suggested that with the increasing duration of meiotic arrest in the oocyte, there was an increased probability that the nucleolus would not completely break down during oocyte maturation but instead persist, causing aberrant disjunction of the nucleolar associated chromosomes at the first meiotic division. In a number of mammalian cell lines, nucleoli do indeed persist through mitosis [HSU *et al.*, 1965]. One probable case of delayed nucleolar dissolution in a mammalian oocyte has been found and is described below.

When mouse ovarian oocytes at the germinal vesicle stage are placed in a culture medium [DONAHUE, 1968 a] containing the protein synthesis inhibitor puromycin (1 µg/ml), oocyte maturation will proceed only as far as the circularly arranged bivalent stage and stop without spindle formation and further meiotic progression. This arrest is reversible. If, however, oocytes are placed in a puromycin-containing medium after the first meiotic spindle has formed, e.g., at metaphase I, the division continues with PB1 formation, but maturation is again halted, this time just prior to formation of the second meiotic spindle [DONAHUE, 1968 b]. These observations suggest that protein synthesis is necessary for the assembly of both meiotic spindles. Puromycin

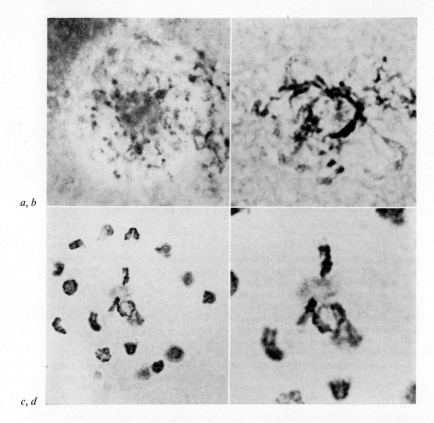

a, b

c, d

Fig. 19. Nucleolar-associated chromosomes in whole-mount preparations of mouse oocytes (orcein stain). *a* Intact germinal vesicle with two or three larger heterochromatic knobs adjacent to the single nucleolus. *b* Early germinal vesicle breakdown with forming bivalents around the nucleolus (center). *c, d* Oocyte cultured for 17 h in a puromycin-containing medium. In the center are three bivalents attached to what is assumed to be nucleolar material; the other bivalents are in the usual peripheral location.

does indeed inhibit protein synthesis during mouse oocyte maturation [Stern *et al.*, 1972].

Fig. 19 c and d show a mouse oocyte from a 2-month-old female that was placed into a puromycin-containing medium at the germinal vesicle stage and incubated for 17 h. Arrest at the circularly arranged bivalent stage has occurred as expected, but unexpectedly, in the center are three bivalents attached (at their noncentromeric ends?) to what appears to be nucleolar material. Normally, the nucleolus has completely broken down by this time. The finding of three bivalents associated with the nucleolus agrees with the evidence of BENNETT [1966] suggesting that three pairs of chromosomes are associated with the nucleolus in mouse somatic cells. Since no other oocytes with this anomaly were found after culture in puromycin or cycloheximide, the inhibition of protein synthesis *per se* apparently does not cause delayed nucleolar dissolution, and the reason for aberrant nucleolar dissolution in this oocyte is not known.

If nuclear progression had continued in this oocyte, the three nucleolar-associated bivalents probably would have been out of synchrony with the other bivalents in attaching to the spindle, a situation possibly leading to faulty spindle alignment and nondisjunction at the first meiotic division. Nondisjunction of one, two, or all three would presumably lead to a single, double, or triple monosomy or trisomy in the embryo. A few cases of single trisomy have been reported in the mouse, most arising after exposure of the male to triethyleneamine or radiation [GRIFFEN and BUNKER, 1967]. A multiple trisomic condition would probably lead to early embryonic death. Whether delayed nucleolar dissolution or an asynchrony of its associated chromosomes in the oocyte are indeed a cause of chromosomal anomalies must await further evidence.

C. Increase of Univalents in Older Females

The only observed anomalous chromosomal behavior at the first meiotic division associated with advanced maternal age is a decrease in the number of chiasmata accompanied by an increase in the number of univalents in mouse oocytes maturing both *in vivo* and *in vitro* (fig. 20–21). HENDERSON and EDWARDS [1968] and more recently LUTHARDT *et al.*, [1973] have shown that chiasmata, resulting from exchange of material between homologous chromosomes earlier in meiosis and thought to be responsible for holding half bivalents together, are fewer in number at metaphase I in older females. Some bivalents have apparently lost all chiasmata and have separated to varying degrees, resulting in physically separate half bivalents (univalents) (fig. 22). The cause and significance of these observations remain obscure.

Chiasmata are known to change in position by moving toward the ends of bivalents, a poorly understood process called terminalization. Since movement of chiasmata occurs during diplotene in some plants [DARLINGTON, 1965] movement might also take place in mammalian oocytes during the prolonged germinal vesicle stage, with loss of chiasmata by the time metaphase I is finally reached. Rather than accounting for the lower chiasma frequency

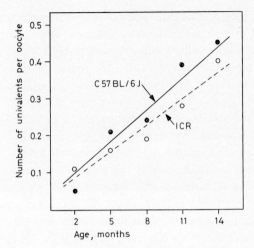

Fig. 20. Regression of the percentage of oocytes with univalents on age in 2 strains of mice. From LUTHARDT *et al.* [1973].

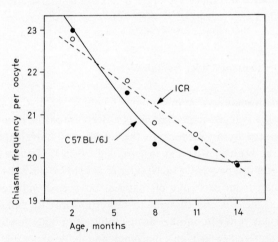

Fig. 21. Regression of chiasma frequency per oocyte on age for two strains of mice. From LUTHARDT *et al.* [1973].

by terminalization loss at the prolonged germinal vesicle stage, HENDERSON and EDWARDS advanced the hypothesis that those oogonia that are slower to enter meiosis in the fetal ovary actually form fewer chiasmata and are the last to ovulate in older females. Critical support for this 'production line' theory

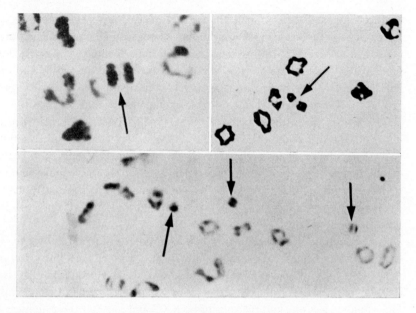

Fig. 22. Univalents (arrows) in mouse oocytes at metaphase I. From LUTHARDT *et al.* [1973].

comes from an observed decrease in genetical recombination in older female mice [FOWLER and EDWARDS, 1973].

HENDERSON and EDWARDS [1968] suggested that with the presumed misorientation of univalents on the metaphase I spindle, nondisjunction would result, accounting for the increase of trisomy (especially trisomy-21) with advanced maternal age in women. The difficulties in obtaining human oocytes have so far precluded determination of whether an increased univalent frequency also occurs in older women. A demonstration of extra or missing chromosomes at metaphase II in older female mice would be a crucial test of whether nondisjunction does indeed occur, but such examinations have yet to be made.

D. Nonrandom Chromosomal Segregation

Unexpected meiotic behavior leading to preferential inclusion (or exclusion) of certain chromosomes into functional gametes has been found in certain plants and animals, especially *Drosophila*. The term meiotic drive was introduced for such cases and is the subject of a review [ZIMMERING et al., 1970]. A possible case of such nonrandom segregation in a mammalian oocyte has been reported. In mice lacking an X chromosome (XO) one would predict that one half the oocytes at metaphase II would bear an X and one half lack an X. Breeding records, however, indicate a deficiency of XO progeny from XO females and one possible explanation would be formation of an excess of X-bearing oocytes. KAUFMAN [1972] found about twice as many oocytes at metaphase II with 20 as those with 19 chromosomes, and it was assumed those with 19 lacked the X chromosome. The first polar bodies would, therefore, be expected to bear a deficiency of X chromosomes, but the PB1 is not generally available for cytogenetic analysis, as previously stated. The mechanism responsible for this apparent nonrandom X chromosome segregation is not known.

Although no proven cases of nonrandom segregation are known to occur in human oocytes, an example might exist in women with three X chromosomes (XXX). Four such women are known to have produced offspring. All 17 children were normal XX females or XY males whereas, theoretically, one would expect one half the sons to be XXY and one half the daughters to be XXX [HAMERTON, 1971, vol. 2, p. 106]. However, whether the germ cells of these women are indeed XXX has not been verified.

III. Abnormalities of the Second Meiotic Division

A. Evidence for Chromosomal Errors

Direct evidence for single chromosomal errors arising at the second meiotic division is more difficult to obtain than for the first meiotic division. The next succeeding metaphase – that of the first cleavage division – includes the paternally introduced chromosomes, and one cannot distinguish between the maternally and paternally derived chromosomal complement, except possibly by banding or structural differences between a few chromosomes. At prophase, however, when the two chromosome groups are still separate, one can distinguish between the two when a coiling difference is still present, as it is in about half of mouse zygotes at prophase when collected for chromosome examination [DONAHUE, 1972 c]. Whether this coiling difference exists in human zygotes has not been established. In addition, there is an intervening DNA synthesis between completion of the second meiotic division and first cleavage metaphase, and conceivably chromosomal errors could arise during this period. To distinguish between second meiotic and later mitotic division nondisjunction in pre- or postnatal individuals, one would have to show nonidentical maternal chromosomes (e.g. in trisomy-21) to disprove a mitotic origin and, having demonstrated this, to distinguish a second from a first meiotic error!

In the only two studies to date of the first cleavage division, no evidence of single chromosomal errors was found in 776 mouse zygotes, except for some hypodiploids, which probably represent artifactual loss during preparation for chromosome examination [DONAHUE, 1972 c; DONAHUE and KARP, 1973].

Errors involving whole chromosome sets at the second meiotic division occur with a low frequency in mouse zygotes (table I). The frequency of 'spontaneous' triploidy in the mouse is about 1 %, the same frequency as that reported for human abortuses [CARR, 1971]. Results from whole-mount preparations, the different pronuclear sizes being used as indicators, have shown that dispermy and suppression of PB2 contribute about equally to produce triploidy in the mouse [BRADEN, 1957; DONAHUE, 1972 b], and similar estimates have been made for the origin of human triploids, sex chromosome constitution being used [SCHINDLER and MIKAMO, 1970]. UCHIDA and LIN [1972] used fluorescent banding patterns to prove a double paternal contribution (either by dispermy or a diploid sperm) in a live-born 69, XXY triploid. Other ploidy anomalies are increased in aging postovulatory oocytes and are discussed below.

B. Abnormalities Associated with Postovulatory Oocyte Aging

The fertilizable life of the mouse oocyte at metaphase II after it has entered the fallopian tube is estimated to be at least 15 h [MARSTON and CHANG, 1964; see also contribution by CHANG], and that for the human egg is probably close to this figure. Before fertilizability is lost, however, cytological changes take place including rotation of the metaphase II spindle [SZOLLOSI, 1971], precocious separation of sister chromatids [RODMAN, 1971], and detachment of chromosomes from the spindle (fig. 23) [AUSTIN, 1967]. Fertilization of old tubal eggs has been studied in various mammals and leads to multiple sperm penetration, suppression of PB2 formation, abnormal embryonic development, and decreased litter size [AUSTIN, 1970]. In these studies, old oocytes were obtained by postovulatory delaying of either artificial insemination or exposure to a male (delayed mating).

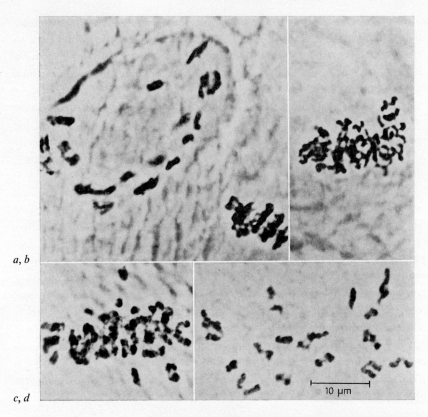

a, b

c, d

Fig. 23. Stages of chromosome degeneration in mouse oocytes at metaphase II. *a* Normal metaphase II with scattered first polar body chromosomes; *b* chromosome swelling; *c* further degeneration; *d* scattered chromosomes. From DONAHUE [1972a].

In the oldest fertilizable mouse oocytes there is a striking increase in three anomalies and another two may be increased (table I). All these aberrations involve whole chromosome sets. An aberrant orientation of the metaphase II spindle appears to be the cause of two anomalies. One, with a frequency of 5–8%, is the expulsion from the egg during the second meiotic division of both chromatin groups on the spindle, each group being included in a separate PB2. All the female chromatin is, therefore, expelled, leaving only the spermatozoon-introduced chromatin. This interpretation has been verified by chromosome examination at first cleavage metaphase, spermatozoa bearing a chromosomal marker being used [DONAHUE and KARP, 1973]. The second anomaly, with a frequency of 7–10%, associated with aberrant spindle position is the formation of an exceptionally large PB2 so that the zygote consists of two approximately equal-sized cells. Again, this was verified at first cleavage metaphase: one cell has a haploid complement of maternal origin (the PB2), and the other cell is fertilized and diploid [DONAHUE and KARP, 1973]. Both these anomalies also occur at the first meiotic division (fig. 17, 18).

The third anomaly associated with old tubal eggs is the presence of only one nucleus (table I). At first cleavage metaphase, the frequency of haploid groups of sperm origin (androgenesis) was increased, although not significantly so. Significantly increased were haploid cells of maternal origin indicating either parthenogenesis or gynogenesis [DONAHUE and KARP, 1973]. The increased frequency of two other aberrations, suppression of PB2 formation and dispermy, did not reach a statistically significant level when zygotes were examined just after fertilization or at first cleavage metaphase [MARSTON and CHANG, 1964; DONAHUE and KARP, 1973].

Although ploidy errors are one consequence of fertilization of aging tubal oocytes, it is not known whether single chromosome errors are produced. GERMAN [1968] has proposed that trisomy-21 in man arises from fertilization of such old oocytes by nondisjunction at the second meiotic division. However, in the only examination to date of first cleavage metaphases in mammalian zygotes developing from the oldest fertilizable oocytes, no evidence of nondisjunction at the second meiotic division was found in 152 mouse zygotes [DONAHUE and KARP, 1973]. Obviously many more zygotes must be examined before any definitive statement can be made regarding the effect of oocyte age on second meiotic nondisjunction.

Summary

This chapter is a review of chromosomal behavior, normal and abnormal, during the first and second meiotic divisions of mammalian (primarily mouse) oocytes.

Counts of metaphase II and first cleavage chromosomes have so far failed to reveal any evidence of single chromosomal errors, spontaneous or otherwise, arising during the first or second meiotic division. The number of cells examined, however, is still far too few to draw any conclusions.

'Spontaneous' ploidy errors have been found in both meiotic divisions: (1) formation of exceptionally large first and second polar bodies with presumably functional nuclei; (2) passage of all egg chromosomes into the first or second polar bodies, and (3) incomplete divisions so that the first or second polar bodies are not formed and their chromosomes are retained within the egg cytoplasm.

One new anomaly is described. In a mouse oocyte maturing in a medium containing puromycin, meiosis stopped prior to first spindle formation (a known effect of puromycin) but atypically, three bivalents remained attached to what is assumed to be a persistent nucleolus. One consequence of such behavior might be nondisjunction of the nucleolar-associated bivalents.

The only effects so far reported of maternal age are a decrease in the number of chiasmata and an increase in the number of univalents at metaphase I in older mice. The behavior of univalents at anaphase I has not been determined.

Postovulatory aging of mouse oocytes leads to an increased frequency of large second polar bodies, to expulsion of all egg chromosomes into the second polar body, and to zygotes with only one nucleus–found to be haploid and maternal in origin when examined at first cleavage metaphase. Whether suppression of second polar body formation is significantly increased is not clear.

Acknowledgments

I thank Mrs. W. DIANNE SMITH for technical assistance and Drs. LAURENCE KARP and FREDERICK LUTHARDT for valuable criticism. The author's research is supported by a grant from the National Institutes of Health (GM 15253) and the Ford Foundation. The author is an Investigator of the Howard Hughes Medical Institute.

References

ALBERMAN, E.; POLANI, P.E.; FRASER ROBERTS, J.A.; SPICER, C.C.; ELLIOTT, M., and ARMSTRONG, E.: Parental exposure to X-irradiation and Down's syndrome. Ann. hum. Genet. 36: 195 (1972).

AUSTIN, C.R.: Chromosome deterioration in ageing eggs of the rabbit. Nature, Lond. 213: 1018 (1967).

AUSTIN, C.R.: Ageing and reproduction. Post-ovulatory deterioration of the egg. J. Reprod. Fertil. Suppl. 12: 39 (1970).

BAKER, T.G. and FRANCHI, L.L.: The structure of the chromosomes in human primordial oocytes. Chromosoma, Berl. 22: 358 (1967).

BEATTY, R.A.: Parthenogenesis and polyploidy in mammalian development (Cambridge University Press, Cambridge 1957).

BENNETT, D.: Non-random association of chromosomes during mitotic metaphase in tissue cells of the mouse. Cytologia, Tokyo 31: 411 (1966).

BRADEN, A.W.H.: Variation between strains in the incidence of various abnormalities of egg maturation and fertilization in the mouse. J. Genet. 55: 476 (1957).

CALARCO, P.G.: The kinetochore in oocyte maturation; in BIGGERS and SCHUETZ Oogenesis, p. 65 (University Park Press, Baltimore 1972).

CALARCO, P.G.; DONAHUE, R.P., and SZOLLOSI, D.: Germinal vesicle breakdown in the mouse oocyte. J. Cell Sci. 10: 369 (1972).

CARR, D.H.: Chromosome studies in selected spontaneous abortions: polyploidy in man. J. med. Genet. *8:* 164 (1971).

DARLINGTON, C.D.: Cytology (Little, Brown, Boston 1965).

DONAHUE, R.P.: Maturation of the mouse oocyte *in vitro*. I. Sequence and timing of nuclear progression. J. exp. Zool. *169:* 237 (1968a).

DONAHUE, R.P.: Maturation of the mouse oocyte *in vitro*. Stage specific protein synthesis. Genetics *60:* Abstr., p. 173 (1968b).

DONAHUE, R.P.: Maturation of the mouse oocyte *in vitro*. II. Anomalies of first polar body formation. Cytogenetics *9:* 106 (1970).

DONAHUE, R.P.: The relation of oocyte maturation to ovulation in mammals; in BIGGERS and SCHUETZ Oogenesis, p. 413 (University Park Press, Baltimore 1972a).

DONAHUE, R.P.: Fertilization of the mouse oocyte. Sequence and timing of nuclear progression to the 2-cell stage. J. exp. Zool. *180:* 305 (1972b).

DONAHUE, R.P.: Cytogenetic analysis of the first cleavage division in mouse embryos. Proc. nat. Acad. Sci., Wash. *69:* 74 (1972c).

DONAHUE, R.P.: Control of meiosis and germ cell selection; in WRIGHT, CRANDALL and BOYER Perspectives in cytogenetics, p. 5 (Thomas, Springfield 1972d).

DONAHUE, R.P. and KARP, L.E.: Chromosomal anomalies after fertilization of aged, post-ovulatory mouse oocytes. Amer. J. hum. Genet. *25:* 24a (1973).

EDWARDS, R.G. and FOWLER, R.E.: The genetics of human preimplantation development; in EMERY Modern trends in human genetics, vol. 1, p. 181 (Appleton Century Crofts, New York 1970).

EVANS, H.J.: The nucleolus, virus infection, and trisomy in man. Nature, Lond. *214:* 361 (1967).

FERGUSON-SMITH, M.A.: The sites of nucleolus formation in human pachytene chromosomes. Cytogenetics *3:* 124 (1964).

FERGUSON-SMITH, M.A. and HANDMAKER, S.D.: Observations on the satellited human chromosomes. Lancet *i:* 638 (1961).

FIALKOW, P.J.; THULINE, H.C.; HECHT, F., and BRYANT, J.: Familial predisposition to thyroid disease in Down's syndrome. Controlled immuno-clinical studies. Amer. J. hum. Genet. *23:* 67 (1971).

FORD, C.E. and CLEGG, H.M.: Reciprocal translocations. Brit. med. Bull. *25:* 110 (1969).

FOWLER, R.E. and EDWARDS, R.G.: The genetics of early human development; in STEINBERG and BEARN Progr. med. genet., vol. 9, p. 49 (Grune & Stratton, New York 1973).

GERMAN, J.: Mongolism, delayed fertilization and human sexual behavior. Nature, Lond. *217:* 516 (1968).

GRIFFEN, A.B. and BUNKER, M.C.: Four further cases of autosomal primary trisomy in the mouse. Proc. nat. Acad. Sci., Wash. *58:* 1446 (1967).

HAMERTON, J.L.: Human cytogenetics, vol. 1 and 2 (Academic Press, New York 1971).

HENDERSON, A.S.; WARBURTON, D., and ATWOOD, K.C.: Location of ribosomal DNA in the human chromosome complement. Proc. nat. Acad. Sci., Wash. *69:* 3394 (1972).

HENDERSON, S.A. and EDWARDS, R.G.: Chiasma frequency and maternal age in mammals. Nature, Lond. *218:* 22 (1968).

HSU, T.C.; ARRIGHI, F.E.; KLEVECZ, R.R., and BRINKLEY, B.R.: The nucleoli in mitotic divisions of mammalian cells *in vitro*. J. Cell Biol. *26:* 539 (1965).

JACOBS, P.A.: Chromosome abnormalities and fertility in man; in BEATTY and GLUECK-SOHN-WAELSCH The genetics of the spermatozoon. Proc. Int. Symp., Edinburgh 1972, p. 346.

JAGIELLO, G. and DUCAYEN, M.: Meiosis of ova from polyovular (C58/J) and polycystic (C57 L/J) strains of mice. Fertil. Steril. *24:* 10 (1973).

JAGIELLO, G.; DUCAYEN, M., and LIN, J.S.: Meiosis suppression by caffeine in female mice. Molec. gen. Genet. *118:* 209 (1972).

JAGIELLO, G.; KARNICKI, J., and RYAN, R.J.: Superovulation with pituitary gonadotrophins – method for obtaining meiotic metaphase figures in human ova. Lancet *i:* 178 (1968).

JAGIELLO, G. and LIN, J.S.: An assessment of the effects of mercury on the meiosis of mouse ova. Mutation Res. *17:* 93 (1973).

KAUFMAN, M.H.: Non-random segregation during mammalian oogenesis. Nature, Lond. *238:* 465 (1972).

KENNEDY, J.F. and DONAHUE, R.P.: Human oocytes. Maturation in chemically defined media. Science *164:* 1292 (1969).

LICZNERSKI, G. and LINDSTEN, J.: Trisomy 21 in man due to maternal nondisjunction during the first meiotic division. Hereditas *70:* 153 (1972).

LONG, J.A. and MARK, E.L.: The maturation of the egg of the mouse (Carnegie Institution, Washington, D.C. 1911).

LUTHARDT, F.W. and DONAHUE, R.P.: Pronuclear DNA synthesis in mouse eggs. An autoradiographic study. Exp. Cell Res. *82:* 143 (1973).

LUTHARDT, F.W.; PALMER, C.G., and YU, P.-L.: Chiasma and univalent frequencies in aging female mice. Cytogenet. Cell Genet. *12:* 68 (1973).

MARSTON, J.H. and CHANG, M.C.: The fertilizable life of ova and their morphology following delayed insemination in mature and immature mice. J. exp. Zool. *155:* 237 (1964).

MUKHERJEE, A.B.: Normal progeny from fertilization *in vitro* of mouse oocytes matured in culture and spermatozoa capacitated *in vitro*. Nature, Lond. *237:* 397 (1972).

NESBITT, M.N. and DONAHUE, R.P.: Chromosome banding patterns in preimplantation mouse embryos. Science *177:* 805 (1972).

NICKLAS, R.B. and KOCH, C.A.: Chromosome micromanipulation. III. Spindle fiber tension and the reorientation of mal-oriented chromosomes. J. Cell Biol. *43:* 40 (1969).

NICKLAS, R.B. and KOCH, C.A.: Chromosome micromanipulation. IV. Polarized motions within the spindle and models for mitosis. Chromosoma, Berl. *31:* 1 (1972).

OHNO, S.; TRUJILLO, J.M.; KAPLAN, W.D., and KINOSITA, R.: Nucleolus-organisers in the causation of chromosomal anomalies in man. Lancet *ii:* 123 (1961).

PETERS, H.: Migration of gonocytes into the mammalian gonad and their differentiation. Philos. Trans. roy. Soc. B *259:* 91 (1970).

RACE, R.R.: The Xg blood groups and sex-chromosome aneuploidy. Philos. Trans. roy. Soc. B *259:* 37 (1970).

ROBINSON, J.A.: Origin of extra chromosome in trisomy 21. Lancet *i:* 131 (1973).

RODMAN, T.C.: Chromatid disjunction in unfertilized ageing oocytes. Nature, Lond. *233:* 191 (1971).

RUSSELL, L.B.: Chromosome aberrations in experimental mammals; in STEINBERG and BEARN Progr. med. Genet., vol. 3, p. 230 (Grune & Stratton, New York 1962).

SCHINDLER, A. and MIKAMO, K.: Triploidy in man – report of a case and a discussion on etiology. Cytogenetics 9: 116 (1970).

SORENSEN, R.A.: Cinemicrography of mouse oocyte maturation utilizing nomarski differential-interference microscopy. Amer. J. Anat. 136: 265 (1973).

STERN, S.; RAYYIS, A., and KENNEDY, J.F.: Incorporation of amino acids during maturation in vitro by the mouse oocyte. Effect of puromycin on protein synthesis. Biol. Reprod. 7: 341 (1972).

SZOLLOSI, D.: Time and duration of DNA synthesis in rabbit eggs after sperm penetration. Anat. Rec. 154: 209 (1966).

SZOLLOSI, D.: Morphological changes in mouse eggs due to aging in the fallopian tube. Amer. J. Anat. 130: 209 (1971).

SZOLLOSI, D.; CALARCO, P., and DONAHUE, R.P.: Absence of centrioles in the first and second meiotic spindles of mouse oocytes. J. Cell Sci. 11: 521 (1972).

UCHIDA, I.A. and LIN, C.C.: Identification of triploid genome by fluorescence microscopy. Science 176: 304 (1972).

UEBELE-KALLHARDT, B. und KNORR, K.: Meiotische Chromosomen der Frau. Humangenetik 12: 182 (1971).

YUNCKEN, C.: Meiosis in the human female. Cytogenetics 7: 234 (1968).

ZAMBONI, L.: Fine morphology of mammalian fertilization (Harper & Row, New York 1971).

ZAMBONI, L.; THOMPSON, R.S., and SMITH, D.: Fine morphology of human oocyte maturation in vitro. Biol. Reprod. 7: 425 (1972).

ZIMMERING, S.; SANDLER, L., and NICOLETTI, B.: Mechanisms of meiotic drive; in ROMAN, SANDLER and CAMPBELL Annual review of genetics, vol. 4, p. 409 (Annual Reviews, Palo Alto 1970).

Author's address: Dr. ROGER P. DONAHUE, Departments of Obstetrics and Gynecology and of Medicine, School of Medicine, University of Washington, Seattle, WA 98195 (USA)

Aging Gametes. Int. Symp., Seattle 1973, pp. 72–97 (Karger, Basel 1975)

Chromosomal Disorder Caused by Preovulatory Overripeness of Oocytes

Kazuya Mikamo and Hideo Hamaguchi

Biomedical Division, The Population Council, New York, N.Y. and Department of Biological Science, Asahikawa Medical College, Asahikawa

The arrest of normal sequence of oogenesis exerts a deleterious effect on the ovum when the delay exceeds a certain limit of time. The degenerative change of the ovum following such detrimental arrest of the meiotic process may be called aging, or overripeness of oocytes. Overripeness of oocytes caused by delayed fertilization has long been known in many species and has been well established as a teratogenetic factor [Austin, 1970; Lanman, 1968; Witschi, 1952]. Recent studies on amphibia and mammals suggest that overripeness leads to chromosomal anomalies effected at the time of the second meiotic and the cleavage divisions [Austin, 1967; Rodman, 1971; Shaver and Carr, 1967, 1969; Vickers, 1969; Witschi and Laguens, 1963; Yamamoto and Ingalls, 1972].

Overripeness exerts a deleterious effect on the ovum not only after, but also before, ovulation. Preovulatory overripeness of oocytes has been recognized as a cause of developmental and possibly of chromosomal anomalies in *Xenopus laevis* [Mikamo, 1961, 1968 a, b; Witschi and Laguens, 1963] and in the rat [Butcher and Fugo, 1967; Fugo and Butcher, 1966]. This type of deterioration develops at the very end of the germinal vesicle stage [Freeman *et al.*, 1970; Mikamo, 1968 b], unlike postovulatory overripeness. Aging may influence the first and second meiotic divisions and fertilization as well as later stages.

This chapter briefly reviews the developmental and chromosomal studies on the effects of preovulatory overripeness of the oocytes in *Xenopus* and reports new observations on the chromosomal constitution of 1.5- and 4.5-day rat preimplantation embryos developing from the eggs aged in follicles.

I. Studies in Xenopus

A. Delay in Ovulation and Developmental Anomalies

Developmental anomalies are common in *Xenopus* under laboratory conditions and are closely related to the arrest of the maturation process of oocytes associated with the lack of sufficient stimulus to induce ovulation of fully developed follicles. *Xenopus* does not maintain its seasonal periodicity of oogenesis under laboratory conditions. The ovaries always contain oocytes in all stages of oogenesis. Hormonal induction of ovulation is possible any time of the year. The same female may produce thousands of eggs, 2, 3, 4, or more times a year. On the other hand, if ovulation is not induced, fully grown follicles accumulate in the ovary and eventually regress and degenerate. Evidently, there must be a time when follicular eggs switch their status from 'ripe' to 'overripe'.

After the arrest of ovulation over an extended period of time, female *Xenopus*, when stimulated with injected gonadotropic hormones, spawns a large number of dead eggs along with fertile ones. A great number of fertilized eggs show obvious irregularities in early embryogenesis, such as abnormal cleavage, gastrulation, and neurulation, and upon continued growth frequently develop acephaly, microcephaly, cyclopia, spina bifida, twinning,

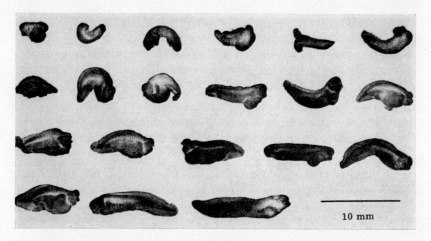

Fig. 1. Various types of developmental anomalies in *Xenopus* embryos deriving from eggs that had undergone preovulatory overripeness. The mother frog had not ovulated for at least one year. From MIKAMO [1968b].

edema, and lateral and dorso-ventral flexion (fig. 1). Most affected embryos die before attaining metamorphosis, but some with acromicrocephaly, scoliosis, polymelia, or oligomelia survive.

B. Arrested Meiotic Stage and Abnormal Meiotic Chromosomal Behavior

Observations on the meiotic process in the ovaries of both HCG treated and untreated females reveal the stage at which the preovulatory overripeness develops. In the untreated *Xenopus* all full sized eggs are at the germinal vesicle stage. There is no sign of germinal vesicle breakdown or of formation of the first meiotic spindle. The ovaries of hormone treated females contain eggs with a dispersing and vanishing germinal vesicle, which indicates clearly the resumption of the maturation process. These observations suggest that deterioration of the egg due to aging is established at the very end of the germinal vesicle stage and that a clear distinction exists between the effect of preovulatory and postovulatory overripeness on the meiotic stage at which time overripeness develops.

Unusual behavior of meiotic chromosomes and degeneration of spindles are seen in the eggs collected from the body cavity and the oviducts of females stimulated with HCG after a long-term arrest of ovulation. The abnormal chromosomal behavior includes precocious movement of 1 or 2 undivided chromosomes to the outer or inner spindle poles and loss of polarization of the displaced chromosomes (fig. 2A-H). The unusual poleward displacement of chromosomes and their lack of polarization indicate an imbalance between the power of the spindle fibers on the 2 sides of the displaced chromosomes. Degeneration of some of these fibers is thought to be the cause of the disturbed balance. Such chromosomal behavior can be observed in both the first and the second meiotic spindles (fig. 2A-H). The precocious moving of chromosomes to the outer and to the inner spindle pole occur at about the same frequency (table I).

The unusual behavior of the meiotic chromosomes may be an expression of the process leading to chromosomal nondisjunction that results in an uneven distribution of chromosome numbers in the polar body and the egg nucleus. Other affected spindles show hypertrophy and scattering of degenerating chromosomes outside the equatorial plane (fig. 2I). In eggs with visible degenerative changes, disintegration of the spindle fibers is clearly shown. The fibers are no longer bundles at the poles, and the hypertrophy of the

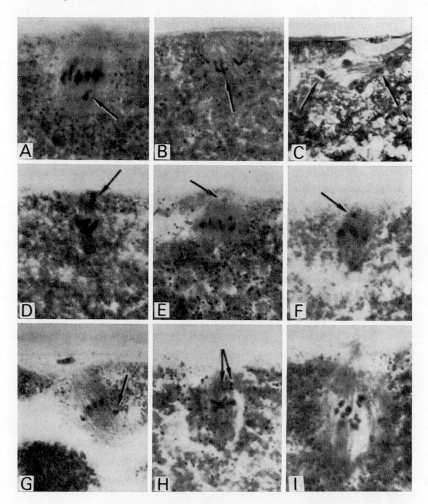

Fig. 2. A, B First meiotic spindle at metaphase in eggs of *Xenopus*. *A* Note the abnormal position of an undivided tetrad (arrow) and its lost polarization. *B* Note the lost
polarization of 3 tetrads. The arrow points to a tetrad (slightly out of focus) with normal
polarization. *C–I* Second meiotic metaphase in eggs of *Xenopus. C* Note 2 dyads (arrows)
in opposite spindle poles and the first polar body near the spindle. *D* Two dyads (arrow),
which are partly overlapped, are located near the outer spindle pole. *E* One dyad (arrow)
is nearly in the outer pole. *F* One dyad (arrow) is about half way to the outer pole. *G* One
dyad (arrow) is about half way to the inner pole. Note the clear structure of the dyad
and its lost polarization. *H* Two dyads (arrows) are about half way to the outer pole.
I Many chromosomes are located abnormally. Note their deformation and fuzzy appearance and hypertrophy of the spindle body. × 900. From MIKAMO [1968b].

Table I. Frequencies of precocious movement of undivided meiotic chromosomes to the outer or the inner poles of spindles

Meiotic stage	Outer pole	Inner pole
First metaphase	1	1
Second metaphase	11	10
Total	12	11

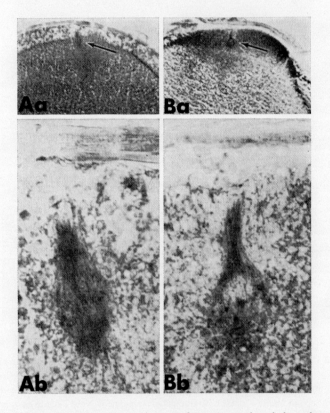

Fig. 3. Aa Degenerating uterine egg of *Xenopus* sectioned along the axis of the second meiotic spindle. Note the cytoplasmic modification near the egg surface of the animal hemisphere. × 65. *Ab* The same spindle shows disorganization of the spindle fibers and discontinuity of the fibers with the poles. Degeneration of chromosomes and hypertrophy of the spindle are also seen. × 650. *Ba* Degenerating uterine egg sectioned along the second meiotic spindle. × 65. *Bb* The same spindle shows degeneration of spindle fibers and of chromosomes, the spindle body is also hypertrophic. × 650. From MIKAMO [1968b].

spindle body is especially conspicuous (fig. 3A, B). The cytoplasmic degeneration is localized near the surface of the animal pole in many eggs. It is noteworthy that even in this advanced stage of deterioration the meiotic activity is still maintained and is able to progress as far as the second meiotic metaphase. These observations suggest that the degeneration due to aging begins in the surface area of the animal hemisphere within the cytoplasm. The process may advance to the nuclear elements secondarily when a meiotic spindle is formed near the area.

C. Chromosomal Anomalies in Developing Embryos

The hypothesis that preovulatory overripeness of the oocytes causes chromosomal abnormalities in *Xenopus* was confirmed by WITSCHI and LAGUENS [1963]. Acting on the finding that these females spawn a large number of preovulatory overripe eggs, they obtained many malformed larvae from females that had been prevented from spawning for several months. Their karyotype analysis revealed 22 chromosomal abnormalities in 23 malformed larvae, and none in 20 normal larvae. These anomalies included 1 case of trisomy, 6 of monosomy, and 15 of mosaicism with two cell lines of 35 and 37 chromosomes, respectively, instead of the normal 36. The result clearly showed that these anomalies derived from nondisjunction of either a meiotic chromosome or a somatic chromosome of the first cleavage. The high incidence of mosaicism suggests that overripeness indeed influences the mechanism of the cleavage spindle. Judging from the high incidence of monosomy, anaphase lag of a meiotic chromosome should also be considered as the result of damaged function of the meiotic spindle.

II. Studies in the Rat

A. Effects of Delay in Ovulation on Development

FUGO and BUTCHER [1966] investigated the occurrence of preovulatory overripeness of the ovum in mammals following delayed ovulation. In order to postpone ovulation in normally cycling rats, they used pentobarbital, a method first used by EVERETT and SAWYER [1950] to suppress the midcycle surge of luteinizing hormone. A series of extensive studies by FUGO, BUTCHER and co-workers have shown that arrest of ovulation at 48 h in the normal

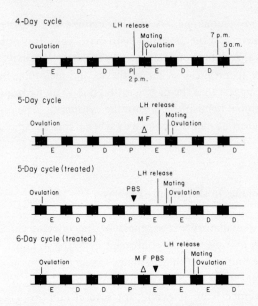

Fig. 4. Control and pentobarbital-treated estrous cycles in the rat. PBS = Pento-barbital sodium injection; MF = mating failure; E = estrus; D = diestrus; P = pro-estrus; LH = luteinizing hormone.

4-day estrous cycling rat resulted in a decrease in fertilization rate and a 3-fold increase of polyspermy [FUGO and BUTCHER, 1966]. The treatment was recognized as the cause of developmental and chromosomal anomalies and of implantation loss [BUTCHER and FUGO, 1967; BUTCHER *et al.*, 1969; FUGO and BUTCHER, 1966]. Observation of the preovulatory follicles in the rats with prolonged cycles revealed that the ovum remained at the germinal vesicle stage during the term of the prolongation [FREEMAN *et al.*, 1970], just as it did in *Xenopus* [MIKAMO, 1968 b]. TOYODA and CHANG [1969], in a simi-lar experiment of delayed ovulation with pentobarbital, found a reduction of the number of implantation sites and viable fetuses. However, they were un-able to detect a significant effect on fertilization or on the development of 1- and 2-cell embryos. Their failure in confirming a demonstrable effect of over-ripeness is evidently due to the small case number and to the unsuitable stage (too early) for detecting morphological anomalies in preimplantation em-bryos. Developmental anomalies occurred frequently in the offspring of the aged rats with spontaneously prolonged estrous cycles as well [FUGO and BUTCHER, 1971]. This observation was supplemented by our study of young rats mated during a 6-day cycle, which occurs occasionally in laboratory

Table II. Effect of pentobarbital-induced delay of ovulation on fertilization and embryonic development in the rat

	Number of litters	Number of corpora lutea	Number of eggs collected (%)	Number of normal blastocyst (%)	Number of abnormal blastocyst (%)	Number of morula (%)	Number of 2~7-cell (%)	Number of unfertilized eggs (%)
4-day cycle	44	524	504 (96.2)	454 (90.1)	29 (5.8)	15 (3.0)	3 (0.6)	3 (0.6)
5-day cycle	41	469	453 (96.6)	394 (87.0)	37 (8.2)	14 (3.1)	2 (0.4)	6 (1.3)
Treated 5-day cycle	40	497	476 (95.8)	410 (86.1)	34 (7.1)	23 (4.8)	4 (0.8)	5 (1.1)
Treated 6-day cycle	53	678	544* (80.2)	314** (57.7)	80** (14.7)	84*** (15.4)	28*** (5.1)	38*** (7.0)

* Significant difference from each of other groups (p <0.05).
** Highly significant difference from each of other groups (p <0.01).
*** Highly significant difference from each of other groups (p <0.001).

raised rats [Mikamo, unpublished]. Mating during such prolonged cycles often resulted in a reduction of implantation rates and in an increase of degenerated or amorphic embryos. It may also produce embryos with delayed organogenesis and those with a small body size for the age. Thus, it seems that the teratogenic effect of spontaneous delay of ovulation in the rat for 2 days is not necessarily associated with advanced maternal age.

The effects of preovulatory overripeness on the fertilization and the development of the rat were further confirmed in our present study. As shown in figure 4, 4- and 5-day estrous cycle rats were used as the control groups. A 6-day cycle was induced by an injection of sodium pentobarbital in the afternoon of the 4th day of the 5-day cycle. Pentobarbital-treated 5-day cycling rats were studied also in order to find out whether the injected chemical had any effect on the embryonic development.

As shown in table II, delay in ovulation had a decided effect on the embryonic development. The incidence of unfertilized, degenerating ova and of various developmental anomalies was much higher only in the induced 6-day cycle group (fig. 5). These developmental anomalies included zygotes with delayed or arrested development (remaining between 2-cell and morula

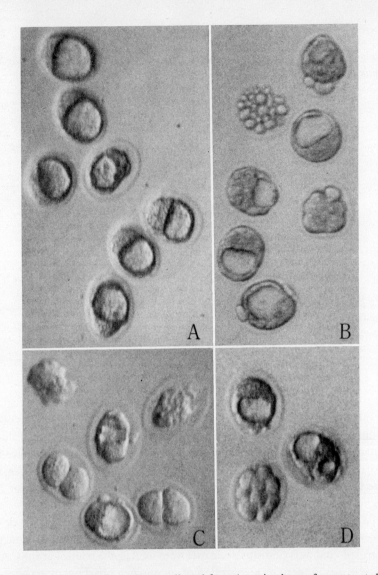

Fig. 5. A 4.5-day rat embryos collected from 1 uterine horn of an untreated 5-day cycle mother, showing all normal features of the rat blastocyst. *B–D* 4.5-day rat embryos from pentobarbital-treated 6-day cycle, including various anomalous embryos. *B* The fragmenting egg (the second uppermost) is unfertilized and obviously degenerating. One egg (middle) is a retarded embryo showing only several blastomeres and an unusually large polar body. The possible large polar bodies are also seen in the uppermost and the lowermost blastocyst. *C* Two eggs are arrested at the 2-cell stage. The other 2 exhibit a considerable number of live blastomeres but no blastocele. *D* An abnormal blastocyst (right) clearly shows 2 separate blastoceles. The other abnormal egg is arrested at the morula stage, having only 9 cells. × 200.

stage), blastocysts with 2 or more blastoceles, those with unusually large cells
that may possibly be abnormally large polar bodies, and those lacking blastoceles (fig. 5B-D). There was no significant difference between the pentobarbital treated 5-day cycle group and the untreated 4- and 5-day cycle groups.

B. Polyploidy Due to Errors in Fertilization

As mentioned earlier, FUGO and BUTCHER [1966] observed a significant
increase of polyspermy following the delay of ovulation. They, therefore, expected an increase of polyploidy. However, their chromosomal study with
11-day embryos revealed no increase of the anomaly following delayed ovulation [BUTCHER and FUGO, 1967]. We attempted to test whether the increase
in polyspermy is related to the production of polyploidy. Counts of the first
cleavage chromosomes and the spermatozoa in eggs were made in the same
slides prepared from the 1-celled embryos. The 4-day and the pentobarbital
treated 6-day estrous cycle groups were compared (fig. 4). Theoretically, it
should be possible to detect all polyploid embryos reaching the first cleavage
metaphase, and the polygynic or polyspermic origin of each polyploidy can
be judged by confirming the number of fertilized and incorporated spermatozoa.

In about 60% of the collected and prepared eggs, the remnant of the
head and tail of fertilizing spermatozoa and either a metaphase plate or a

Table III. Incidences of polyploidy in the rat at 1-cell zygotic stage

	Number of litters	Number of eggs collected (number/ lit.)	Number of eggs studied (%)	Diploid (%)	Triploid (%)	Tetra- ploid (%)	Penta- ploid (%)
Control	41	451 (11.0)	280 (62.1)	278 (99.3)	2 (0.7)	0	0
Experimental	50	482 (9.6)	276 (57.3)	256 (92.8)	16* (5.8)	3 (1.1)	1 (0.4)

* Highly significant difference from control (p <0.01).
Control: Eggs fertilized in the 4-day estrous cycle.
Experimental: Eggs fertilized in the 6-day estrous cycle that was induced by an injection
of pentobarbital.

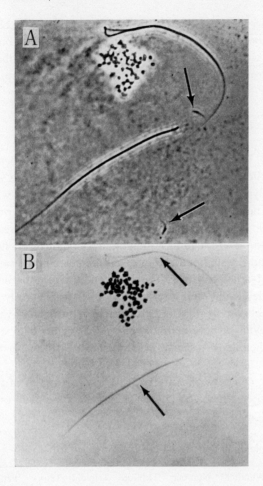

Fig. 6. Metaphase of the first cleavage division in a triploid rat egg caused by dispermic fertilization. *A* The tails and the head remnants (arrows) of 2 fertilized spermatozoa are clearly shown in the phase contrast microphotograph taken from an unstained and un-covered slide. *B* Photograph taken from the same slide after staining shows a triploid chromosome set in which approximately 63 chromosomes are countable. The 2 sperm tails (arrows) are also demonstrable in this picture, whereas the head remnants are invisible with the oil-immersion lens. × 500. From MIKAMO and IFFY, Obstetrics and Gynecology Annual 1974, Appleton-Century-Crofts, New York.

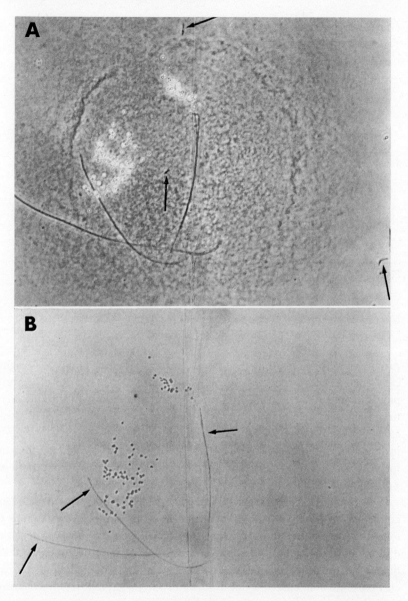

Fig. 7. Metaphase of the first cleavage division of a tetraploid rat egg caused by trispermic fertilization. *A* The tails and the head remnants (arrows) of 3 fertilizing spermatozoa are clearly shown under a phase contrast microscope. *B* The same slide shows a tetraploid chromosome set after staining. Three sperm tails are also demonstrable, but the head remnants are not visible with the oil-immersion lens. × 500.

Table IV. Nuclear condition of the rat eggs shown in table III

Ploidy	Nuclear condition	Control number of eggs (%)	Experimental number of eggs (%)
Diploid	2 N	264	246
	1 N + 1 pronucleus	4	3
	2 pronuclei	10	7
Total		278 (99.3)	256 (92.8)
Triploid	3 N	2	11
	2 N + 1 pronucleus	–	1
	1 N + 2 pronuclei	–	2
	3 pronuclei	–	2
Total		2 (0.7)	16 (5.8)
Tetraploid	4 N	–	3 (1.1)
Pentaploid	5 pronuclei	–	1 (0.4)
Grand total		280	276

N = An exact or an approximate haploid chromosome set.

pronuclei were successfully preserved. Incidence of polyploidy was significantly increased in the experimental group (table III). A total of 22 polyploids included 18 triploids, 3 tetraploids, and 1 pentaploid. Without exception, they were all polyspermic and the increased number of ploidy always equalled the number of fertilizing spermatozoa (fig. 6, 7). There was no instance of diploid embryos caused by polyspermy. It is quite certain that the polyploids were all caused by polyspermic fertilization and that there was no polyploid of digynic origin.

In some instances, pronuclear development was arrested. In such eggs, condensation of chromosomes of one or more pronuclei lagged behind the expected stage of development (table IV). They appeared infrequently in the diploid embryos of both the control and the experimental groups, but frequently in the triploids of the experimental group. All tetraploids showed chromosome condensation but 5 nuclei of the pentaploid remained pronuclear. It is assumed that such unsynchronized or arrested development may lead to early death of embryos. This also suggests that the same factor that induces polyspermy, and therefore polyploidy, may reduce the viability of the fertilized eggs.

In the experimental group it was clearly shown that the perivitelline

Table V. Incidences of supplementary sperm (perivitelline sperm), studied with 1-cell eggs

	I Number of eggs collected	II Number of eggs fertilized (%)	III Number of eggs with supplemen- tary sperm (%)	IV Total number of supplemen- tary sperm	V Average number of supplemen- tary sperm IV/III
Control	451	385 (85.4)	66 (17.1)	100	1.5
Experimental	482	383 (79.5)	142* (37.1)	314	2.2

* Highly significant difference from control (p <0.001).

space was filled with more supernumerary spermatozoa, as shown in table V. Delay of ovulation may disturb the normal function of the barrier system of zona pellucida against supernumerary penetration of spermatozoa and further reduce the similar function of vitelline surface, thereby encouraging polyspermic fertilization.

The study with 4.5-day embryos revealed an increase of polyspermy also. Preparations of the chromosomes of the cells of the blastocysts exhibited clearly degenerating tails of spermatozoa (fig. 8). An increase of polyspermy occurred again only in the 6-day estrous cycle group among 4 groups analyzed (fig. 4, table VI). The negative result with the pentobarbital treated 5-day cycle rats suggests that the medication may have no, or little, influence on the fertilization process.

Among a total of 40 polyspermic embryos some exhibited a reduced viability. They were delayed in development, remaining much younger than the blastocyst stage (table VII). Especially in the group of the 6-day cycle about half of the embryos were in the 2- or 3-cell stage and had no mitotic activity. Frequently they showed degeneration of nuclei suggesting death of the total embryo. About half of the polyspermic embryos were chromosomally confirmed to be triploid (fig. 9). Incidences of chromosomally confirmed triploidy did not differ among the 4 groups (table VIII). A large number of polyspermic embryos of the 6-day cycle group had no mitotic cells; accordingly, it was not possible to confirm a triploid number of chromosomes.

A small number of triploids were not ascertained to be dispermic because no tail of an extra spermatozoon could be detected (table VIII). Considering the overscattering of the blastomeres of these embryos in the slides,

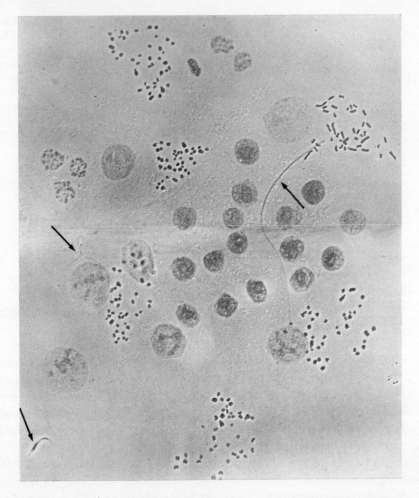

Fig. 8. A chromosome preparation of a blastocyst with 6 well-spread metaphase plates. Arrows indicate a fertilizing sperm tail with a fine, filamentous structure, and separated head and tail of a supplementary spermatozoon. Note that the supplementary spermatozoon is maintained in the perivitelline space without undergoing degeneration for a considerably long time. × 550.

it is likely that the degenerating sperm tail was lost during the process of preparing the slides. Therefore, there is no reason to assign a digynic origin to these triploid embryos. Evidently the study with 1-cell embryos, in which all polyploids were polyspermic, strongly favors the dispermic origin of triploidy in the rat.

Table VI. Incidences of polyspermy in 4.5-day embryo

	Number of zygotes analyzed	Number of zygotes with polyspermy (%)
4-day cycle	482	7 (1.5)
5-day cycle	444	5 (1.1)
Treated 5-day cycle	463	7 (1.5)
Treated 6-day cycle	497	21* (4.2)

* Significant difference from each of the other groups ($p < 0.05$).

Table VII. Developmental stages of polyspermic embryos at 4.5 days of age

	Blastocyst	Morula	4~7-cell	3-cell	2-cell	Total
4-day cycle	3	4	0	0	0	7
5-day cycle	3	2	0	0	0	5
Treated 5-day cycle	2	3	1	0	1	7
Treated 6-day cycle	2	5	2	3	9	21

C. Aneuploidy Due to Chromosomal Errors of Meiosis

The damaging effects of preovulatory overripeness on the chromosome constitution of developing embryos was indicated by the presence at 11 days of age of 18 anomalies in 390 treated embryos as opposed to 6 in 410 in the control group [BUTCHER and FUGO, 1967]. In the treated group there were 5 aneuploids (3 cases of monosomy and 2 of trisomy), whereas there was none in the control group. This suggests that the aging of the ovum in matured follicles may cause aneuploidy by influencing meiotic chromosomal behavior, i.e., by inducing nondisjunction or anaphase lag.

We attempted to detect such aneuploids in the preimplantation embryos in which anomalies were ordinarily eliminated at implantation or in early postimplantation stages and thus escaped from detection on the 11th day of

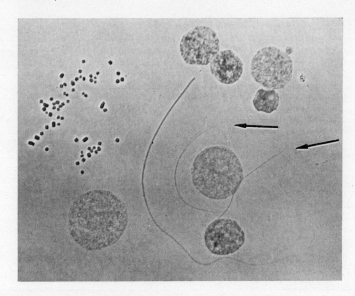

Fig. 9. A chromosome preparation of a triploid embryo at 4.5 days: Arrows indicate tails of 2 fertilizing spermatozoa. Tail of a supplementary spermatozoon (not indicated by arrow) is clearly shown, indicating a good maintenance of the original form. ×600.

Table VIII. Incidences of polyploidy in 4.5-day embryo

	Number of zygotes with metaphase	Triploid (%)	Dispermy confirmed
4-day cycle	480	8 (1.7)	7
5-day cycle	437	5 (1.1)	4
Treated 5-day cycle	455	6 (1.3)	5
Treated 6-day cycle	453	7 (1.5)	6
Total		26	22

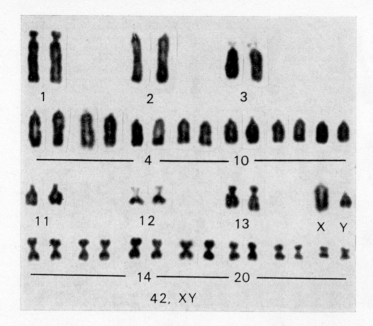

Fig. 10. Normal karyotype of the male rat prepared from a normal blastocyst at 4.5 days. × 2,500.

Table IX. Chromosome abnormalities in 4.5-day embryos

	Total number of embryos analyzed[1]	Diploid	Aneuploid 41 43 44 45				Mosaic[2]	Mixoploid 42/84	Total number of anomalies
Control (4- or 5-day cycle)	231	230	–	–	–	–	1	–	1
Treated 5-day cycle	233	225	1	1	–	–	6	–	8
Treated 6-day cycle	252	237	3	1	1	1	7	2	15

1 Number of embryos in which at least 2 metaphase plates were analyzed.
2 4- or 5-day cycle: 1 41/42. Treated 5-day-cycle: 2 41/42; 1 42/43; 3 41/42/43. Treated 6-day cycle: 3 41/42; 2 42/43; 1 41/43; 1 41/42/43.

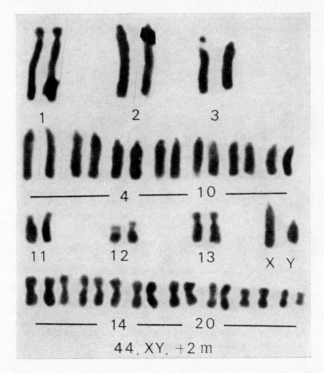

Fig. 11. An aneuploid karyotype with 44 chromosomes including 2 extra metacentric chromosomes obtained from an externally normal rat blastocyst at 4.5 days. ×3,000.

gestation. The purpose was to obtain a more accurate figure for the effect of preovulatory overripeness on the meiotic chromosomal behavior. The embryos studied were the same as those shown in table II. About 70 % of the slides that have thus far been studied showed that at least 2 mitotic figures were analyzable (fig. 10). Table IX includes only these cases.

The chromosome anomalies caused by disorders of the meiotic division or divisions were found more frequently in the blastocysts of the delayed group (table IX). They included both hyperdiploidy (fig. 11) and hypodiploidy (fig. 12). The incidence of our study was about twice as high as that of the 11-day embryos studied by BUTCHER and FUGO [1967]. There was no aneuploid in the control group and only 2 in the pentobarbital treated 5-day cycle group. In most of the aneuploids of our study, only 4–8 cells were analyzable owing to the small number of blastomeres (10–30; normally 30–40). Therefore, we cannot exclude the possibility that mosaicism existed in this material. However, chromosome anomalies that might have had a reduced mitotic

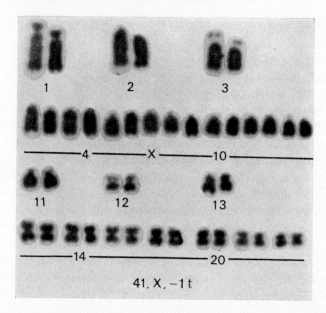

1

2

3

———— 4 ———— X ———— 10 ————

11   12   13

———— 14 ———————— 20 ————

41, X, −1 t

Fig. 12. An aneuploid karyotype with 41 chromosomes obtained from a 4.5-day rat embryo of which development was arrested at the morula stage. The missing chromosome is one of telocentric chromosomes. × 2,500.

activity also may not show; it is assumed that the above incidence is minimum. In fact, we excluded some cases of possible aneuploids from the figure for the 6-day cycle group because of the uncertainty of diagnosis due to the small number of analyzable metaphase plates. Considering such a technical limitation, we think that the true incidence of aneuploids in the experimental 6-day cycle group might be higher than the figure shown in table IX. It is certainly preferable to analyze the metaphase of the first somatic division for the purpose of detecting the aneuploids.

In this study of blastocysts, the treated 5-day cycle group had a much lower incidence of aneuploids than did the 6-day group, and the untreated 4- and 5-day cycle groups had no aneuploid embryo. It seems that medication with pentobarbital may have no, or little, influence on the meiotic division. The increased incidence in the 6-day cycle group is very likely due mainly to the delay of ovulation causing overripeness of the ovum, but it is not conclusive with this limited material.

D. Mosaicism Due to Errors in Somatic Chromosomal Behavior

BUTCHER and FUGO [1967] found 10 mosaic embryos in 390 cases of 11-day embryos (2.6%) in the pentobarbital treated 6-day cycle group and 3 in 410 cases (0.7%) in the nontreated 4-day cycle group. Since mosaicism is induced by nondisjunction or by anaphase lag of early somatic divisions, the results of this study strongly suggest that the pentobarbital treatment causes these abnormal chromosomal behaviors. As shown in table IX, mosaicism occurred frequently in the pentobarbital treated 5-day and 6-day cycle groups; in the 5-day group 6 in 233 embryos (2.6%) and in the 6-day group 9 in 252 (3.6%), including 2 mixoploids. Only 1 case in 231 occurred in the control embryos (0.4%). Pentobarbital treatment, therefore, may produce mosaic embryos but not solely because of delay of ovulation, that is, over-ripeness of the eggs.

The fact that all mosaics except one in our study showed normal features of blastocyst indicates that mosaics are generally more viable than aneu-ploids. This interpretation is supported by the similar incidence of mosaicism in our study with 4.5-day embryos and in BUTCHER and FUGO's study with 11-day embryos. Elimination of mosaics due to death may have occurred infrequently during the time lapse between the 2 developmental stages. The pentobarbital treatment in our study seemed to have no effect on the meiotic divisions and the fertilization, but possibly some effect on somatic division. Although our case number was too limited to draw conclusions, a change of tubal condition brought about by the medication should be considered in relation to nondisjunction or anaphase lag of the early somatic division.

III. Discussion

The experimental observations in *Xenopus* and the rat strongly suggest that preovulatory overripeness of the oocytes caused by delayed ovulation results in a significant reduction of fertility of the ovum, in its diminished capacity for development, and in a telling increase in developmental anomalies, thereby enhancing the frequency of early embryonic death.

In the rat, at least in the case of delayed ovulation, the mechanism producing triploidy and other polyploids was proven to be almost exclusively polyspermy. The mechanism varies, however, in different species and under different experimental conditions. In the mouse, rabbit, hamster, pig, and even in the rat, both digyny and diandry have been observed in the eggs examined shortly after fertilization, although the incidences are variable under different experimental conditions [AUSTIN, 1960, 1970]. In chromosome studies after delayed fertilization, SHAVER and CARR [1967, 1969] in the rabbit, VICKERS [1969] in the mouse, and YAMAMOTO and INGALLS [1972] in the hamster failed to detect triploidy with an XYY sex chromosome constitution and were inclined to consider digyny to be the origin of triploidy in these species. TAKAGI [1970] noted a high incidence of triploidy in mouse eggs after hormone-treated superovulation; 16 triploids in 51 blastocysts and 8 in 25 implanted embryos. Quite contrary to our deduction with the rat, he concluded, on the basis of the number of specially marked chromosomes of male origin, that every case of triploidy had resulted from digyny [TAKAGI, 1971]. McFEELY [1967] has described the occurrence of XYY triploidy in the pig to support diandry origin. In any event, the true incidences of triploid variants and the mechanism involving the production of the anomalies should be determined at the 1-cell stage. In our study, death of triploid embryos was extensive during the short period between the 1-cell and blastocyst stages. Determination of the sex chromosome constitution of these triploids is under investigation to determine whether there is any specific tendency of the 3 sex variants, XXX, XXY, and XYY, toward early death.

In man, triploidy occurs in 1–2% of all diagnosed pregnancies [BOUÉ and BOUÉ, 1972; CARR, 1971]. The majority of these are aborted before midgestation [BOUÉ and BOUÉ, 1970; CARR, 1971]; on rare occasions they may reach term [SCHINDLER and MIKAMO, 1970]. Diandry has been suggested as the origin of human triploidy on the basis of compiled cytogenetic studies of spontaneous abortion from many sources [SCHINDLER and MIKAMO, 1970]. The proportion of the three sex chromosome variants showed an approximate ratio of 5:10:1 in 170 collected cases [MIKAMO, 1971]. The occurrence of XYY variant establishes diandry as a cause of human triploidy. Its low incidence may reflect poor viability, since the ratio of 1:2 between the XXX and XXY types suggests that diandry is the major mechanism in its production. However, analyses of heteromorphic banding patterns in both parents and their triploid offspring in recent studies suggest that both diandry and digyny are involved in the causal mechanism [JONASSON et al., 1972; UCHIDA and LIN, 1972].

Overall incidence of chromosome anomalies was significantly increased following delayed ovulation in the rat in both BUTCHER and FUGO's [1967] experiment and ours. However, when the anomalies were classified into polyploidy, aneuploidy, and mosaic according to the specific effects of overripeness acting individually on the fertilization, meiotic, and cleavage divisions, the incidence of aneuploids in our delayed group showed only an inconclusive tendency, because of our limited material. However, it is highly significant that the pentobarbital-induced delayed ovulation elicits these chromosomal anomalies when our result is pooled with that of BUTCHER and FUGO [1967]: 11 aneuploids in 627 cases of the 6-day cycle group; none in the 640 of the control group (p < 0.005).

There may be ways to improve the method of chromosomal analysis other than the simple increase of the case numbers to obtain a statistically reliable result. As shown by DONAHUE [1972], TARKOWSKY [1966] and our study, the first cleavage division is chromosomally analyzable and the techniques seem to be improvable. Our experience has proved that chromosome constitution of nearly all blastomeres of the 2nd and 3rd cleavage division is analyzable with accuracy by modifying and adapting the time of egg collection, by timing *in vitro* culture and colcemid treatment, and by fixing and drying the preparations. Incidence of aneuploids and mosaics can thus be obtained with accuracy. Such methodological improvement may contribute to the investigation of various possible causes for chromosome anomalies as well.

The increased incidence of mosaic in the pentobarbital induced 6-day cycle group is also highly significant compared with only the 4- or 5-day cycle group when the data of our study and those of BUTCHER and FUGO [1967] are again pooled: 19 in 627 cases in the 6-day cycle and 4 in 640 in the 4- or 5-day cycle (p <0.005). However, as mentioned before, the effect of pentobarbital is suspect in these materials. It is of a medical importance to pursue the investigation of the effect of this chemical since it is a generally used anesthetic.

Preovulatory overripeness of the ovum is very likely to be a cause of chromosomal anomalies. It acts upon not only the chromosomes but also the embryonic development, as emphasized by WITSCHI [1952, 1969, 1971] and by others [BUTCHER *et al.*, 1969; BUTCHER and FUGO, 1967; FUGO and BUTCHER, 1966; MIKAMO, 1961, 1968 b, 1970] in discussing the etiologic factors of human teratogenic development. Retrospective studies with human materials supply evidence to support the concept that preovulatory overripeness occurs in human reproduction most frequently as a result of pathological pregnancies [HERTIG, 1967; IFFY, 1962, 1963, 1965; IFFY *et al.*, 1972, 1973; JONGBLOET, 1969]. The recent electron microscopic studies by SZOLLOSI [1971] with postovulatory overripe mouse eggs and by PELUSO and BUTCHER [1973] with preovulatory overripe rat eggs are important in elucidating the process of aging in the ovum and the mechanism by which teratogenic development comes about.

Acknowledgments

We acknowledge Mr. T. PASSANTINO for his skillful technical assistance, Prof. M. SASAKI, for permitting us to use his laboratory accommodations, Drs. S. MATSUI and M. OSHIMURA for their help in preparing photographs. The work was supported by the Biomedical Division of the Population Council, the Rockefeller University.

References

AUSTIN, C.R.: Anomalies of fertilization leading to triploidy. J. cell. comp. Physiol. *56:* suppl. 1, p. 1 (1960).

AUSTIN, C.R.: Chromosome deterioration in aging eggs of the rabbit. Nature, Lond. *213:* 1018 (1967).

AUSTIN, C.R.: Aging and reproduction. Post-ovulatory deterioration of the egg. J. Reprod. Fertil. Suppl. *12:* 39 (1970).

BOUÉ, J.G. et BOUÉ, A.: Les aberrations chromosomiques dans les avortements spontanés humains. Presse méd. *78:* 635 (1970).

BOUÉ, J.G. and BOUÉ, A.: Personal commun. (1972).

BUTCHER, R.L.; BLUE, J.D., and FUGO, N.W.: Overripeness and the mammalian ova. III. Fetal development at midgestation and at term. Fertil. Steril. *20:* 223 (1969).

BUTCHER, R.L. and FUGO, N.W.: Overripeness and mammalian ova. II. Delayed ovulation and chromosome anomalies. Fertil. Steril. *18:* 297 (1967).

CARR, D.H.: Chromosome studies in selected spontaneous abortions. Polyploidy in man. J. med. Genet. *8:* 164 (1971).

DONAHUE, R.P.: Cytogenetic analysis of the first cleavage division in mouse embryos. Proc. nat. Acad. Sci., Wash. *69:* 74 (1972).

EVERETT, J.W. and SAWYER, C.H.: A 24-hour periodicity in the 'LH-release apparatus' of female rats, disclosed by barbiturate sedation. Endocrinology *47:* 198 (1950).

FREEMAN, M.E.; BUTCHER, R.L., and FUGO, N.W.: Alteration of oocytes and follicles by delayed ovulation. Biol. Reprod. *2:* 209 (1970).

FUGO, N.W. and BUTCHER, R.L.: Overripeness and the mammalian ova. I. Overripeness and early embryonic development. Fertil. Steril. *17:* 804 (1966).

FUGO, N.W. and BUTCHER, R.L.: Effects of prolonged estrous cycles on reproduction in aged rats. Fertil. Steril. *22:* 98 (1971).

HERTIG, A.T.: The overall problem in man; in BENIRSCHKE Comparative aspects of reproductive failure, p. 11 (Springer, Berlin 1967).

IFFY, L.: Contribution to the aetiology of placenta previa. Amer. J. Obstet. Gynec. *83:* 969 (1962).

IFFY, L.: The time of conception in pathological gestations. Proc. roy. Soc. Med. *56:* 1098 (1963).

IFFY, L.: Embryologic studies of time of conception in ectopic pregnancy and first trimester abortion. Obstet. Gynec. *26:* 490 (1965).

IFFY, L.; CHATTERTON, R.T., jr., and JAKOBOVITS, A.: The 'high weight for dates' fetus. Amer. J. Obstet. Gynec. *115:* 238 (1973).

IFFY, L.; WINGATE, M.B., and JAKOBOVITS, A.: Postconception 'menstrual' bleeding. Int. J. Gynaec. Obstet. *10:* 41 (1972).

JONASSON, J.; THERKELSEN, A.J.; LAURISTEN, J.G., and LINDSTEN, J.: Origin of triploidy in human abortuses. Hereditas *71:* 168 (1972).

JONGBLOET, P.H.: The intriguing phenomenon of gametopathy and its disastrous effects on the human progeny. Maandschr. Kindergeneesk. *37:* 261 (1969).

JONGBLOET, P.H.: An investigation into the occurrence of overripeness ovopathy in the normal population. Maandschr. Kindergeneesk. *38:* 228 (1970).

LANMAN, J.T.: Delays during reproduction and their effects on the embryo and fetus. II. Aging of eggs. New Engl. J. Med. *278:* 1047 (1968).

MCFEELY, R.A.: Chromosome abnormalities in early embryos of the pig. J. Reprod. Fertil. *13:* 579 (1967).

MIKAMO, K.: Overripeness of the egg in *Xenopus laevis* Daudin; D. Sci. thesis, Hokkaido Univ. (1961).

MIKAMO, K.: Mechanism of non-disjunction of meiotic chromosomes and degeneration of maturation spindles in eggs affected by intrafollicular overripeness. Experientia *24:* 75 (1968a).

MIKAMO, K.: Intrafollicular overripeness and teratogenic development. Cytogenetics *7:* 212 (1968b).

MIKAMO, K.: Anatomic and chromosomal anomalies in spontaneous abortion. Possible correlation with overripeness of oocytes. Amer. J. Obstet. Gynec. *106:* 243 (1970).

MIKAMO, K.: Cytogenetic studies on the possible teratogenecity of contraceptive steroids. 7th Int. Congr. Fertil. Steril., Tokyo and Kyoto 1971.

PELUSO, J.J. and BUTCHER, R.L.: Personal commun. (1973).

RODMAN, T.C.: Chromatid disjunction in unfertilized aging oocytes. Nature, Lond. *233:* 191 (1971).

SCHINDLER, A.M. and MIKAMO, K.: Triploidy in man. Report of a case and a discussion on etiology. Cytogenetics *9:* 116 (1970).

SHAVER, E.L. and CARR, D.H.: Chromosome abnormalities in rabbit blastocysts following delayed fertilization. J. Reprod. Fertil. *14:* 415 (1967).

SHAVER, E.L. and CARR, D.H.: The chromosome complement of rabbit blastocysts in relation to the time of mating and ovulation. Canad. J. Genet. Cytol. *11:* 287 (1969).

SZOLLOSI, D.: Morphological changes in mouse eggs due to aging in the fallopian tube. Amer. J. Anat. *130:* 209 (1971).

TAKAGI, N.: High incidence of triploid embryos associated with artificial polyovulation in mice. Chrom. Inf. Serv. *11:* 32 (1970).

TAKAGI, N.: Superovulation and chromosomal fetal karyotype in mice (in Japanese). Jap. J. Genet. *46:* 443 (1971).

TARKOWSKI, A.K.: An air-drying method for chromosome preparations from mouse eggs. Cytogenetics *5:* 394 (1966).

TOYODA, Y. and CHANG, M.C.: Delayed ovulation and embryonic development in the rat treated with pentobarbital sodium. Endocrinology *84:* 1456 (1969).

UCHIDA, I.A. and LIN, C.C.: Identification of triploid genome by fluorescence microscopy. Science *176:* 304 (1972).

VICKERS, A.D.: Delayed fertilization and chromosomal anomalies in mouse embryos. J. Reprod. Fertil. *20:* 69 (1969).

WITSCHI, E.: Overripeness of the eggs as a cause of twinning and teratogenesis. A review. Cancer Res. *12:* 763 (1952).

WITSCHI, E.: Teratogenic effects from overripeness of the egg; in Congenital malformations, Proc. 3rd Int. Conf., The Hague 1969, p. 157 (Excerpta Medica, Amsterdam 1969).

WITSCHI, E.: Developmental causes of malformation. Experientia *27:* 1245 (1971).

WITSCHI, E. and LAGUENS, R.: Chromosomal aberrations in embryos from overripe eggs. Develop. Biol. *7:* 605 (1963).

YAMAMOTO, M. and INGALLS, T.H.: Delayed fertilization and chromosome anomalies in the hamster embryo. Science *176:* 518 (1972).

Authors' address: Dr. KAZUYA MIKAMO and Dr. HIDEO HAMAGUCHI, Department of Biological Science, Asahikawa Medical College, *Asahikawa* (Japan)

Aging Gametes. Int. Symp., Seattle 1973, pp. 98–121 (Karger, Basel 1975)

Mammalian Eggs Aging in the Fallopian Tubes

DANIEL SZOLLOSI

Department of Biological Structure, University of Washington, Seattle, Wash.

Various developmental anomalies in mammals, including humans, have been ascribed to changes in the ovum that are due to its aging in the fallopian tube [AUSTIN, 1970; BOUÉ and BOUÉ, 1966; BLANDAU, 1952; CHANG, 1952 a, b; HAMMOND, 1934; IFFY and WINGATE, 1970; SCHINDLER and MIKAMO, 1970; SHAVER and CARR, 1967; THIBAULT, 1967; WITSCHI and LAGUENS, 1963]. These were expressed often by chromosomal irregularities such as triploidy, mosaics, mixoploidy, monosomy, and trisomy. In experimental animals the relationships between the length of delay of insemination and a decrease in fertility [ADAMS and CHANG, 1962; BRADEN, 1959; HAMMOND, 1934], and/or an increase in abnormal development, and embryonic mortality have been convincingly demonstrated [ADAMS and CHANG, 1962; AUSTIN, 1970; BLANDAU and JORDAN, 1941; BLANDAU and YOUNG, 1939; CHANG, 1952 a; PIKO and BOMSEL-HELMREICH, 1960; SHAVER and CARR, 1967]. The lifetime of ovulated mammalian eggs was put at a matter of hours. Similar chromosomal abnormalities and developmental failure have been observed in amphibia [MIKAMO, 1968; WITSCHI and LAGUENS, 1963] when eggs were retained in the uterus before ovulation for 3–5 days before expected ovulation. In fish, the rate of development decreases only 15–21 days after the eggs are retained in the coelomic cavity (although only at low temperatures) [PETIT *et al.*, personal commun., 1973].

Fig. 1. Mouse eggs aged for 20 h in the oviduct. The cortical granules (CG) have migrated centripetally. Two granules are slightly swollen. × 28,500.

Fig. 2. Rat egg aged 22 h. The CG remain at the same distance from the cell membrane as in freshly ovulated eggs. × 23,500.

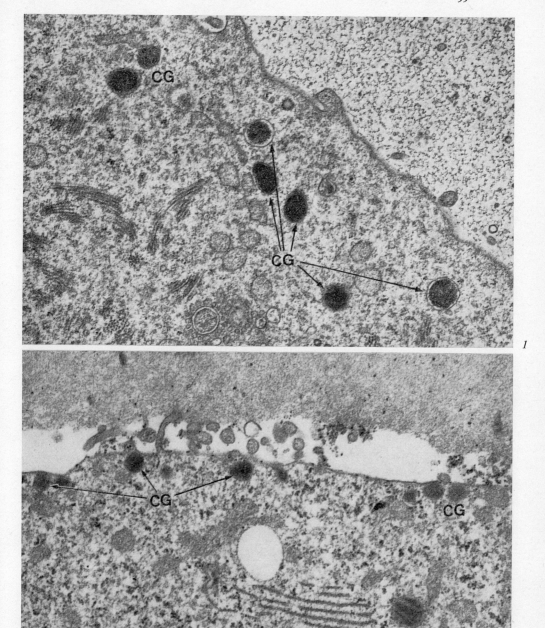

Morphologically the degeneration and full or partial dispersion of the spindle have been reported [AUSTIN, 1967; BLANDAU, 1952; CHANG, 1952; LONGO, 1973 a; SZOLLOSI, 1971; VICKERS, 1969]. In the cytoplasmic cortex a disappearance of the cortical granules was the most significant parallel structural change [AUSTIN, 1970; SZOLLOSI, 1971; YANAGIMACHI and CHANG, 1961]. It is very important to understand the morphological basis underlying the developmental anomalies. In the mouse a light and electron microscopic study demonstrated that the meiotic spindle assumed a radial rather than a paratangential position, and the spindle made a centripetal migration until it assumed again a central position in the ovum followed by an occasional reconstitution of a large central nucleus. This nucleus is identical morphologically in all respects to pronuclei. In the cytoplasm of mouse eggs the cortical granules had migrated centrally also and were swollen.

In this electron microscope study new observations on aging rat and rabbit eggs are described and compared with earlier studies on mouse eggs. Particularly polyspermy, digyny, and spindle instability are discussed. Attempts are made to correlate the observed developmental problems with morphological changes. Other recent studies on mammalian eggs are drawn upon to permit a more general discussion and interpretation as to the possible cytological basis of some of the observed developmental problems.

I. Polyspermy

One of the consistent findings in aged eggs is triploidy, some of which could be reliably identified as having been caused by the entrance of 2 spermatozoa [AUSTIN and BRADEN, 1953; BRADEN, 1959; HANCOCK, 1959; HUNTER, 1967; PIKO, 1958; PIKO and BOMSEL-HELMREICH, 1960; THIBAULT, 1959]. Originally it was thought unlikely that the occurrence of cortical granules in hamster eggs played a possible role in blocking polyspermy [AUSTIN, 1956]. Later, when it was found that the cortical granules that are general constituents of the mammalian egg cortex were absent shortly after sperm pe-

---

Fig. 3. Rabbit egg aged 24 h. The CG remain in an unaltered position in close proximity to the cell membrane. The perivitelline space is filled with an electron-dense material of unknown nature. × 14,000.

Fig. 4. Rabbit egg aged 26 h. In addition to the peripheral CGs, there are many other CGs 5–10 μm from the cell membrane (arrowheads). Their density is similar to that at the periphery of the egg. × 10,000.

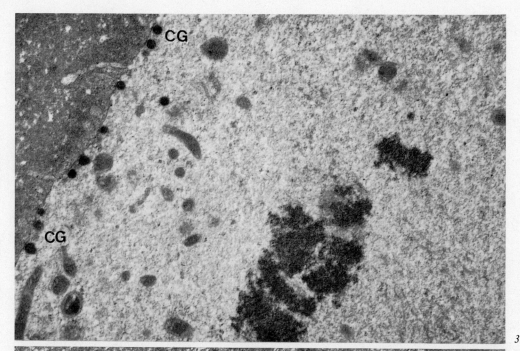

3

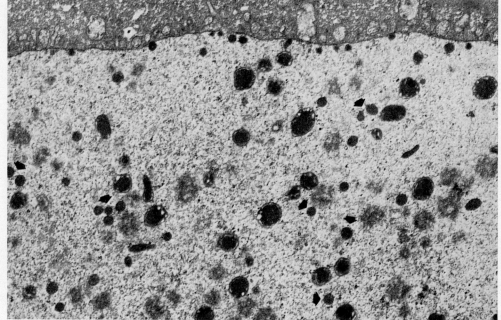

4

netration,the possible involvement of the cortical granules in the block to polyspermy was proposed [SZOLLOSI, 1962, 1967]. More recently the correct-
ness of this working hypothesis was experimentally demonstrated [BARROS
and YANAGIMACHI, 1971]. In mouse eggs the cortical granules do not remain
at the egg cortex during aging but migrate centripetally while they swell
(fig. 1) [SZOLLOSI, 1971]. The content of the granules, which originally are
uniformly electron dense, become more dispersed and show occasionally a
periodic content. In aging rabbit eggs larger, less compact cortical granules
can be found 1.0–1.5 µm from the cell membrane than in its immediate vicinity [GULYAS, personal commun.].

In an experimental series of aging rat and rabbit eggs[1], however, the frequency of cortical granules near the cell surface was unaltered until 23 h after
ovulation (fig. 2, 3). The distance between the membrane limiting the cortical
granules and the cell membrane apparently had not changed. Some granules,
to be sure, were found farther in the cytoplasm in most mammalian eggs
since they originate in the Golgi apparatus [SZOLLOSI, 1967], which is scattered throughout the egg, but they were not obviously swollen (fig. 4). In rabbit eggs, LONGO [1973 a] found that during the early stages of aging the cortical granules located in the subcortical cytoplasm migrate close to the egg cell
membrane where they accumulate in clusters. In aged pig eggs [FLECHON and
HUNTER, personal commun.] the cortical granules also remain at the cortex
with apparently unaltered disposition.

Polyspermy after delayed mating has been often enough reported to give
credence to the likelihood that even though the cortical granules remain at
the egg cortex they cannot fuse any longer with the cell membrane to empty
their contents into the perivitelline space. It is possible that the fusion reaction may be considerably slowed down as a consequence of aging. Delayed
but fertilized eggs were not studied in this series of experiments. In 7 sponta-

---

1   Ovulation in rats was estimated from the time of demonstration of behavioral
estrus by pudendal stimulation [BLANDAU et al., 1941]. Only rats were used that had
previously had at least 2 normal 4-day cycles and that were accustomed to handling.
Eggs were flushed from the oviduct with medium 199 at the estimated time of ovulation
and 10, 15, and 24 h after ovulation and immediately fixed in 1.5% glutaraldehyde in
0.075 M cacodylate buffer. After postosmication the eggs were dehydrated and embedded
in Epon 812. In some cases both fixatives contained 1 part/1,000 ruthenium red [LUFT, 1971].
Rabbits were mated with vasectomized males and the eggs were flushed with Lock's
solution 24 and 36 h thereafter. The fixative contained 1.25% glutaraldehyde, 0.25%
paraformaldehyde in 0.05 M cacodylate buffer [GULYAS, 1972]. The eggs were then dehydrated and embedded as above.

neously occurring polyspermic rabbit eggs the cortical granules remained unextruded near the surface of the eggs [GULYAS, 1973], signaling that the fusion reaction was inhibited. A further alternative, that the cortical granule material became inactivated even though liberated at time of sperm penetration, cannot be excluded but appears unlikely.

During aging of the egg in the hamster the cortical granule material is reportedly extruded, a phenomenon that could, with time, render the eggs unfertilizable [YANAGIMACHI and CHANG, 1961]. Even though in these experiments a PAS positive material was demonstrated in the perivitelline space, its origin could not be traced directly to the cortical granules. Extrusion of the cytoplasmic blebs containing intact cortical granules was reported by LONGO [1973 a, b] in *in vivo* aging rabbit and hamster eggs. The extrusion of cortical granule material by dehiscence, which generally occurs after sperm attachment, was not observed, however [SZOLLOSI, 1967]. Thus the contents of the cortical granules are not truly free in the perivitelline space to participate in blocking reaction.

In my own studies on aging rat and rabbit eggs the cortical granules remained intact and in the proximity of the egg cell membrane. A material that gave metachromatic reaction with toluidine blue on semi-thin sections often accumulated in the perivitelline space of such eggs (fig. 7, 10). The same material reacts positively with ruthenium red [LUFT, 1971; SZUBINSKA and LUFT, 1971] in electron microscopic preparations, from which it can be inferred that it may be an acidic glycoprotein. Even cell remnants (vesicles, on occasion even containing mitochondria-like inclusions) could be found in the perivitelline space of rabbit eggs indicating that they may originate either from the egg or from the bulbous terminations of follicle cell processes (fig. 3, 4). The latter are frequently found in rabbit eggs [FLECHON, personal commun.; LONGO, 1973 a] but rarely in rat eggs. An analysis of human triploidy suggests that aging may result in dispermy [SCHINDLER and MIKAMO, 1970] implicating again the failure of the cortical reaction.

Changes of the egg surface may be at the root of various altered reactions in the cell cortex in aging eggs. The most obvious morphological changes in rabbit eggs involve the microvilli, which apparently swell and become irregular as the internal core-filaments disappear. The frequency of microvilli is reduced on the surface of rat eggs as some of those remaining increase in diameter. In mouse eggs the surface changes are minimal. Microvilli are, however, very sensitive to changes in the environment and, before making any valid conclusion, the nature of the flushing fluid, handling, and fixative must be known and carefully evaluated. With advanced aging the apparent budding off of the egg's cortical cytoplasm is enhanced [Longo, 1973 a, b]. More subtle changes, which do not find morphological expression, may change the behavior of the cell membranes between the egg and spermatozoa and the membrane surrounding the cortical granules.

II. Digyny

A large percentage of mammalian eggs becomes digynic after delayed mating. In the rat [Blandau, 1952] and mouse [Szollosi, 1971] the second polar body is often not extruded. In the mouse the rotation of the originally paratangentially oriented meiotic spindle takes a radial orientation followed by centripetal migration. The spindle rotation was sometimes observed in rat eggs after 15 h in the oviduct (fig. 5). In some eggs after 24 h the spindle had migrated at least partially toward the center even though reconstitution of the nucleus did not follow. In other rat eggs the intact spindle remained at a peripheral position in a somewhat enlarged, ooplasmic elevation (fig. 6). In the rabbit, when the aging eggs were allowed to remain 14 h in the duct, the spindle was peripherally located with a radial position (fig. 7–9). Because in this strain of rabbit the spindle is paratangentially oriented in freshly ovulated eggs – Gulyas [personal commun.] finds the same, as opposed to the report of Longo [1973 a] – the radial orientation of the spindle means that the spindle rotates [Chang, 1952 b]. Judging by the sectioned material the integrity of the spindle was not obviously affected structurally. The dispersion of the spindle and chromosomes in flattened eggs [Austin, 1967] could reflect the loss of their structural rigidity after 7 h in the duct. But, to achieve this lability, external forces must be applied (flattening by the coverslip) to displace the chromosomes.

When rabbit eggs were aged 26 h in the fallopian tube the spindle was still intact and in general maintained the same morphology it had shortly after ovulation. The entire spindle has moved, however, centripetally (fig. 10–12). Neither the completion of the division nor the reconstitution of a nucleus was observed. Longo [1973 a] saw a nucleus only in fragmenting

---

Fig. 5. The spindle assumed a radial position in rat eggs aged 15 h. × 6,000.

Fig. 6. After rotation, the spindle often migrates centrally in rat eggs aged from 15 to 24 h. The spindle microtubules are embedded in a matrix of medium electron density. This material forms a large mass at the spindle pole, apparently representing an aggregation of the microtubule foci (MFs) in one large mass. × 9,000.

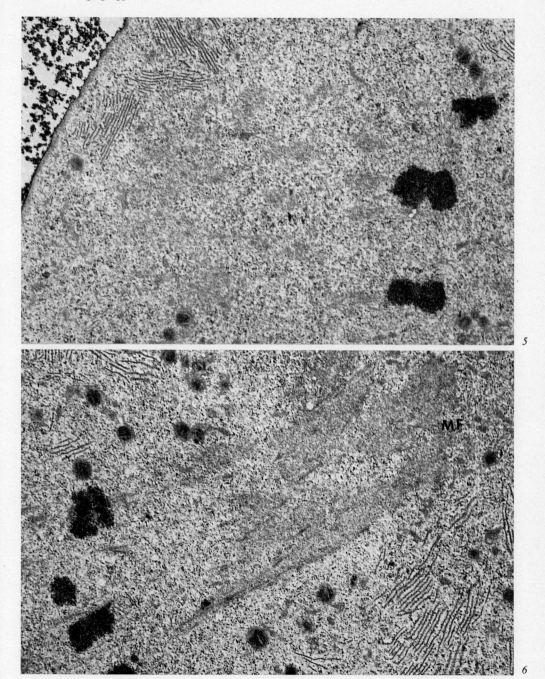

5

6

eggs. A nucleus was never seen in rat eggs. In contrast large nuclei are frequently found in both intact and fragmenting mouse eggs [Szollosi, 1971]. Such nuclei are identical to pronuclei in all respects: the nucleoli are exclusively of filamentous nature, and peripherally nuclear blebbing (called extrusion of 'tertiary nucleoli' in the rat) also occurs [Szollosi, 1965, 1971]. Potentially the displaced spindle could complete mitosis without cytokinesis producing 2 daughter nuclei in the same cytoplasm. Trinucleated rabbit eggs with a single polar body were interpreted in such a manner [Adams and Chang, 1962; Austin, 1967; Thibault, 1967]. The nuclei must be reconstituted before DNA synthesis can take place; subsequently digynic (or polyspermic) development can proceed to any extent.

More extensive chromosomal changes due to aging were observed in rabbit eggs by Chang [1952 b], Longo [1973 a], and Gulyas [personal commun.]. After 4 h in the duct the integrity of the metaphase plate of the second maturation division already seemed to be affected, and dispersion was initiated. In several cases the orientation of the spindle had also changed. After a longer delay (10–60 h in the duct) the microtubule bundles became disorganized, and cytoplasmic organelles invaded the spindle area. In some eggs aged 20–30 h the chromosomes became scattered in the ooplasm, and later on a few annulate lamellae took up a proximal alignment with the chromosome. Microtubules were often associated with the scattered chromosomes. In other regions annulate lamellae were rare although they developed profusely in fertilized eggs [Gulyas, 1972]. In the proximity of all male pronuclei in polyspermic eggs some annulate lamellae also developed in rabbit [Gulyas, 1973] and pig eggs [Szollosi and Hunter, 1973].

When rabbit eggs were cooled to 10°C and aged for 24 h *in vitro* and after they were reimplanted in the oviduct it was found that the spindle broke down and that the chromosomal group began to migrate centrally. Such eggs were called 'activated' [Chang, 1954]. The instability of the spindle at suboptimal temperatures could be expected according to our current knowl-

---

Fig. 7, 8. Light micrographs of rat eggs aged 15 and 22 h, respectively. The spindle remained in both of these cases at the periphery. In figure 7 the perivitelline space shows a strong metachromatic reaction with toluidine blue (large arrowhead). In figure 8 the section passes through the region of the spindle pole (small arrowhead). Four degenerating cells are in the proximity of the egg. × 800.

Fig. 9. A parallel thin section to figure 8. At the spindle pole, a large aggregation of material with medium electron density represents a fused MF. A material of similar electron density apparently embeds the microtubules. × 5,500.

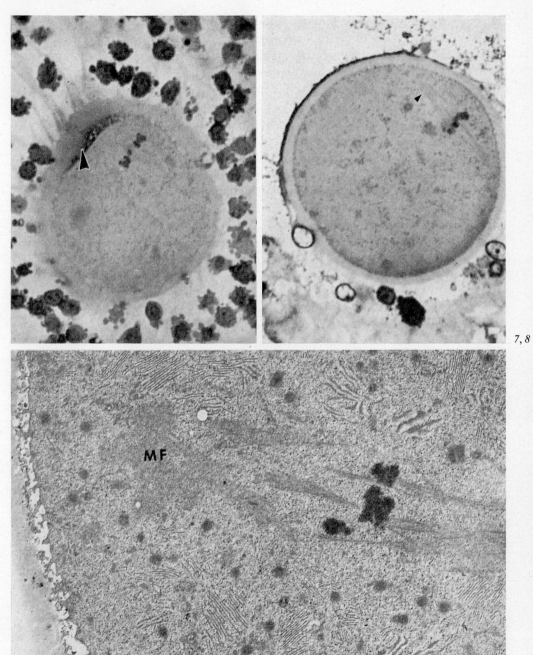

7, 8

9

edge of microtubule behavior at low temperatures. Either the spindle degenerated as the dispersed chromosomes formed several micronuclei or it reconstituted a large central 'pronucleus'; in either case it was followed by chromosome condensation and cleavage [CHANG, 1954; CHALMEL, 1962]. The 'activated' eggs could be penetrated by spermatozoa *in vitro* and *in vivo* and were able to retain their normal reaction in defense of polyspermy. They produced a large number of triploid conditions. The sperm nucleus occasionally remained compact, and the paternal chromosomes did not participate in the cleavage division [CHALMEL, 1962].

In 90% of aging eggs spontaneous activation was observed [LONGO, 1973 b]. Activation included spindle rotation, the migration of the spindle into a central position of the ovum, and in some eggs the reconstitution of a pronucleus. In 10% of the eggs a '2-cell stage' was found. It is not known whether the 2-cell stage was due to completion of the division of the meiotic spindle or whether the cleavage division was induced after the reconstitution of a nucleus.

Spindle rotation and the centripetal migration appear to be a uniform feature of the aged mammalian eggs thus far studied whereas reconstitution of a large nucleus seems to be frequent in some species and rare or absent in others. The mechanism of migration is, however, not known.

III. Spindle Instability

Insemination and development of aging eggs often result in formation of subnuclei [BLANDAU, 1952; CHANG, 1954]. A similar condition could be induced experimentally by treating the female with colcemid close to the expected time of the second meiotic division [EDWARDS, 1961]. It may be proposed that spindle stability in aging may have the same effect as colcemid and cold treatment, that is, an attack on the integrity of microtubules.

Fig. 10, 11. Rabbit eggs aged in the fallopian tube 14 and 25 h, respectively. In figure 10 the spindle is still peripheral but with a radial orientation. The perivitelline space is filled with a material that strongly stains metachromatically with toluidine blue (arrowhead). In figure 11 the spindle has migrated partially centripetally. × 800.

Fig. 12. An electron micrograph of the 2nd meiotic spindle that has migrated centripetally in a parallel section to figure 11. Cortical granules, mitochondria have penetrated the spindle in places. × 5,000.

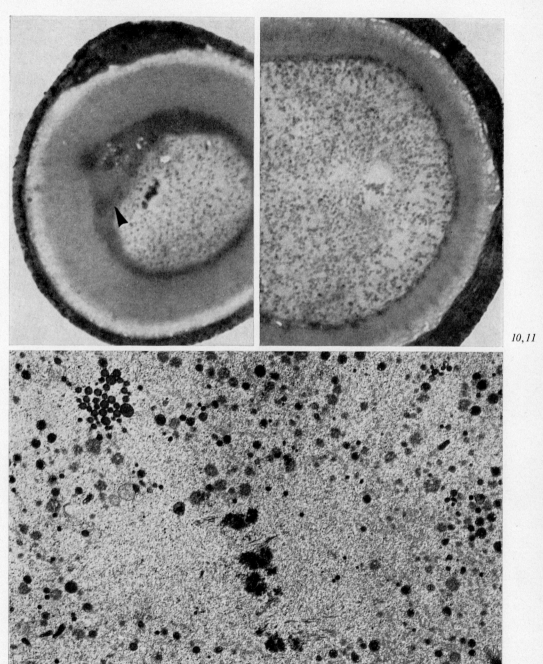

10,11

12

The detailed studies on the structure of meiotic spindles in the mouse egg [SZOLLOSI *et al.*, 1972] provide, however, a different explanation based on the morphology of the maturation spindles. A reconstruction of the spindle from serial thin sections by the conventional transmission electron microscope (fig. 13) and the study of 0.5- to 1.0-μm sections at 1,000,000 V (fig. 14) demonstrated the absence of centrioles from the spindle poles at meiosis and from the first and second cleavage divisions. In the first meiotic division the centriole is replaced by a ring of electron-dense material composed of thin filaments, referred to as microtubule foci (MFs), from which microtubules radiate in an astral form but apparently preferentially toward the chromosomes. The MFs thus correspond to microasters. No obvious interconnection or morphological link was found between the individual MFs in analysis of serial thin sections of the first meiotic spindle. At the pole of the second meiotic spindle and of the first cleavage spindles one or more large fibrillar masses represent the aggregation of the MFs. In thick sections, observed with the high voltage microscope, the MFs appear, however, to form a caplike dense structure at the spindle poles (fig. 14). The proximity of MFs may mimic a spatial overlap and more uniform and continuous structure.

My earlier unpublished studies on rat eggs and particularly the more systematic and thorough studies on aging rat and rabbit eggs, included as a part of this communication, as well as the most recent studies of LONGO [1973 a] and GULYAS [personal commun.], support the hypothesis that centrioles may be absent in general from early stages of mammalian development (fig. 15, 16). Cleavage spindles have not been regularly studied in detail in mammals other than the mouse.

The absence of centrioles from the meiotic spindle and early development may serve as a starting point in attempting to understand some of the chromosomal anomalies found in aging eggs rather than artificial destruction of the spindle by low temperature or chemical agents. Because of the less firm polar anchoring, possibly resulting from the absence of centrioles, the chromosomes may disperse with their respective microtubules, possibly even

---

Fig. 13. At the spindle pole of mouse eggs of the first cleavage division, the MFs migrate close to each other and fuse in one or a few large filamentous masses. Many small vesicles are always present at the MFs. × 7,500.

Fig. 14. A high voltage electron micrograph of the 2nd meiotic metaphase. A 1-μm thick section shows a cap-like structure to which microtubules radiate (small arrowheads). In the thickness of the section the adjacent filamentous aggregations mimic a nearly fused, continuous structure. × 4,500.

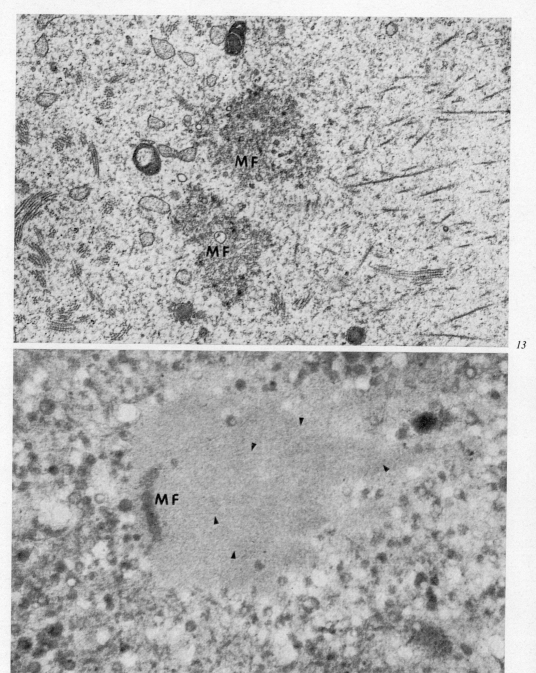

13

14

carrying along the MFs (fig. 17). The dispersion of the second meiotic spindle of the rabbit [Austin, 1967; Chang, 1952 b; Longo, 1973 a] and the mouse [Szollosi, 1971] could be so interpreted. In mouse eggs the chromosome displacement was considered a migration of one metaphase chromosome with all its associated structures. If such an egg was fertilized at that phase the remaining chromosomal group could complete the meiotic division as usual. The separated chromosome (or chromosomes) would form a micronucleus (nuclei) and the bulk of the maternal chromosomes would reconstitute a female pronucleus. Each nuclear fraction supposedly completes its individual DNA synthesis. At the time of synkaryon formation all nuclei fuse into one metaphase plate giving rise to one (or more) extra chromosomes and provide the basis for nondisjunction. The fusion of all micronuclei produced by colcemid treatment into one metaphase plate in mouse eggs was clearly demonstrated [Edwards, 1961].

Whatever else the general function of centrioles may be in the division apparatus of most animal cells they may provide the spindle with a firm structural center. The spindle with MFs – these structures were called satellites or pericentriolar bodies in the earlier literature [Szollosi, 1964] – are also equivalent to MTOCs [Pickett-Heaps, 1971] and are therefore more labile, and errors during division occur more easily.

Dispersion of chromosomes and degeneration of the second meiotic spindle are some of the observed morphological events in eggs of *Xenopus laevis* also [Mikamo, 1968]. In frogs the aging of eggs for 3–5 days in the uterus was described as the major cause of meiotic and mitotic nondisjunction [Witschi and Laguens, 1963]. The spindle of amphibian eggs was not yet examined by electron microscopic means to determine whether they might also lack centrioles. The spindle of *Xenopus* is barrel-shaped as judged from light microscopy [Mikamo, 1968], i.e., the spindle does not seem to focus in a well-defined center, and it is possible that centrioles are absent in this family of vertebrates. If this assumption is correct and is confirmed in future studies, the spindle and chromosomal anomalies occurring in meiosis and early cleavage stages may be compared favorably to those described above in the mouse.

Fig. 15, 16. The spindle pole of the 2nd meiotic spindle of the rat and rabbit eggs respectively aged for 20–25 h in the fallopian tube. A large filamentous, electron-dense mass represents in both cases a fused MF. The spindle microtubules are embedded in the rat egg in a matrix material morphologically similar to the material of the MF (fig. 15). This is not the case in rabbit eggs (fig. 16). × 14,500.

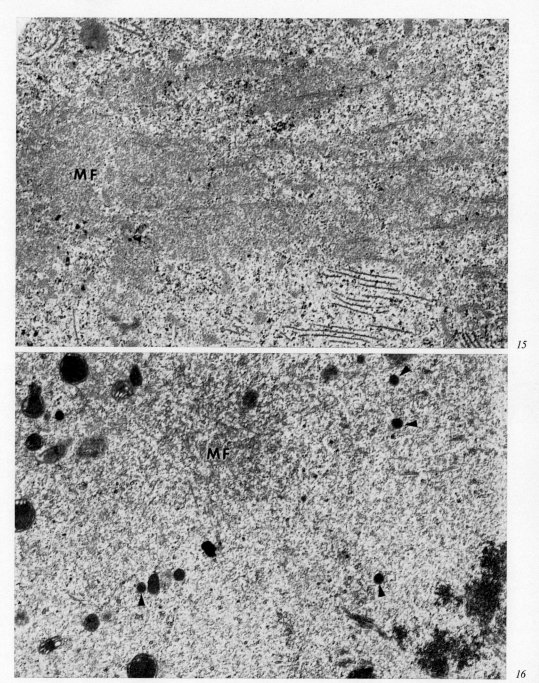

15

16

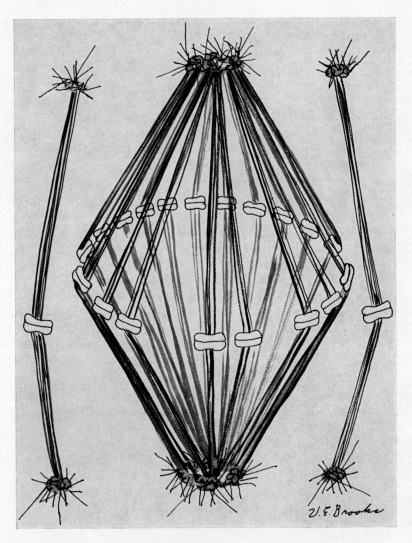

Fig. 17. A schematic representation of the disintegration of the 2nd meiotic spindle.
Two metaphase chromosomes and their microtubules and MFs are shown having migrated
out of the spindle.

The structure of chromosomes was unaltered in all but one case when the metaphase plates were studied. They consisted of highly condensed thin filaments. The kinetochores with their associated microtubules were apparently similar to the kinetochores of higher organisms (fig. 18) [CALARCO, 1972]. The chromosomal microtubules diverge indicating that they may project from one kinetochore to different MFs. In the one exception observed the chromosomes partially loosened and their borders became indistinct and the fibers interdigitated. This may be an example of 'sticky' chromosomes.

The spindle usually remained intact in the rat and, interestingly, the microtubules of the spindle were embedded in a matrix material. This material was particularly noticeable in the pole region and may account for its higher stability.

IV. Other Cytoplasmic Changes

In some aged eggs no cytoplasmic changes were noticeable, other than the rotation and displacement of the spindle. Undoubtedly these movements must bring about more extensive streaming in the ooplasm, but because of the usual random dispersion of the organelles it is not recognizable. During the movements of the spindle some organelles penetrate its territory (fig. 12, 16) [SZOLLOSI, 1971; LONGO, 1973 a]. In rat and mouse eggs the yolk-like material with its characteristic alignment and periodicity occupies the largest portion of the ooplasm. Although it is difficult to make any quantitative assessment, it appears particularly in the rat that its organization becomes less rigid. Occasionally some regions are irregularly arranged and are of lower electron density in aging eggs.

Multivesiculate bodies occur with high frequency in most mammalian eggs. They appear to be unchanged throughout the aging process. In rat eggs, in which multivesiculate bodies occurred more frequently than in all other eggs studied, they may aggregate into large clusters (fig. 19). Aggregation or clumping, very prominent in rabbit eggs [LONGO, 1973 a] in the late stages, may be a general sign of degeneration.

Questions have to be raised: Should the high mortality rate, abnormal development, and the cytological changes discussed above be ascribed directly to malfunction due to aging? Could some of these alterations be secondary in nature owing to changes in the environment? Unfertilized eggs tend to remain in the cumulus or in a viscous fluid formed by the mixture of the liquor folliculi, secretions of the oviduct, and degeneration of the follicle cells. The

passage of the eggs from the ampulla into the isthmus of the oviduct is delayed. The most clearcut indications that the environment may play an important role in affecting the eggs was seen in the rat. The specimen recovered
15 and 24 h after ovulation showed with increasing frequency clusters of degenerating epithelial cells lining the oviduct in the immediate vicinity of the
ova (fig. 8, 20). Even though the defoliation and degeneration of the oviductal epithelium were not studied in detail, drastic pH changes and the presence of lytic enzymes may be assumed. It can be argued that some of the anomalies that cannot be defined may be the consequence of the rapid and increasing environmental changes. The rat ampulla is invaded by increasing
numbers of mast cells (fig. 21). Macrophages and leucocytes are not found in
the oviduct as they are in the uterus where they already may have initiated
phagocytosis of spermatozoa in case the animal has been mated [SOUPART,
1970; FLECHON, 1973]. The change of the cell population surrounding the
eggs may be another important parameter to consider in discussion of the aging phenomenon.

An efficient mechanism to bring about sudden, drastic degeneration of
those eggs not penetrated by a spermatozoon within a certain number of
hours in the oviduct could eliminate some developmental anomalies. Rabbit,
pig, and hamster eggs degenerate more rapidly than eggs of the ewe and cow
[THIBAULT, 1967]. Many eggs degenerate in the rat within the first 24 h. The
recovery of eggs at 24 h was significantly lower than the recovery at the approximate time of ovulation (4–7 eggs in contrast to 10–14). In addition to
the harmful environmental change discussed above, autophagic activity of
the egg itself may lead to self-destruction. Large, electron-dense structures in
the egg cytoplasm were interpreted as autophagosomes (or lysosomelike
structures) in the mouse [SZOLLOSI, 1971] and rabbit [LONGO, 1973 a].

Those eggs that may survive in spite of cellular or chromosomal abnormalities may be rejected at various points of development as indicated by
studies of abortuses [IFFY and WINGATE, 1970; SCHINDLER and MIKAMO,
1970] and by the general decrease in fertility [ADAMS and CHANG, 1962].
Some abnormal embryos may be rejected at the time of implantation owing
to competition with their normal siblings. In humans, where such competi-

---

Fig. 18. In this rat egg aged 22 h the kinetochores (k) have not changed structurally.
Two microtubules project clearly at an angle of about 25°. The microtubules are
embedded in the dense matrix material close to the chromosomes. × 14,500.

Fig. 19. In aging rat eggs the multivesiculated bodies aggregate in large masses.
× 7,500.

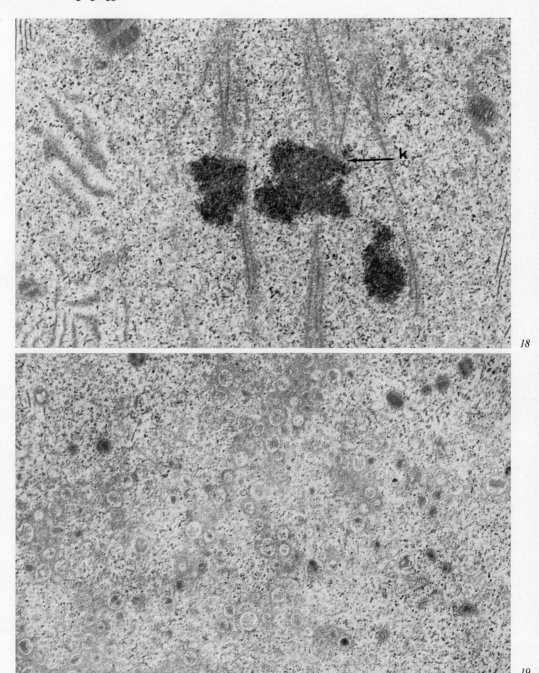

18

19

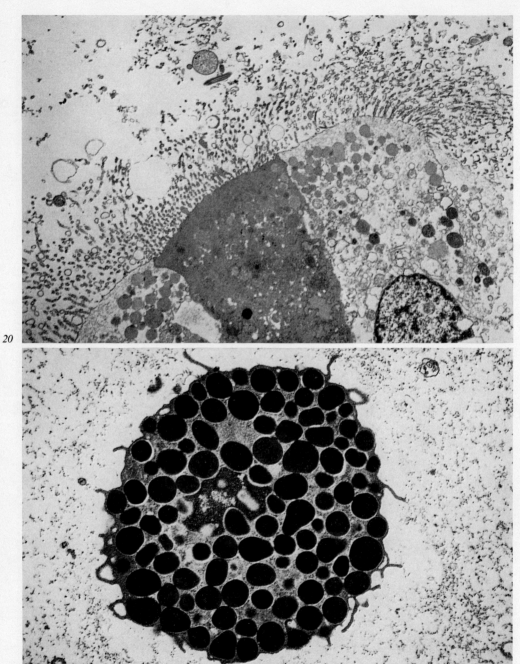

tion is rare, embryos with various degrees of abnormality may survive giving rise to the well-known defects of Down's, Kleinfelter's, and triple X syndromes.

Acknowledgments

Many thanks are due to Dr. B. J. GULYAS for electron micrographs and permission to cite some of his unpublished observations. Dr. F. J. LONGO very kindly forwarded to me a preprint of his studies on aging rabbit and hamster eggs. Discussions with Prof. C. THIBAULT and Dr. O. BOMSEL-HELMREICH were very helpful during the writing of the manuscript. The kind cooperation of Dr. BOLING and his students at Linfield College in securing well-timed ovulations in rats is gratefully acknowledged. The experimental work was supported by grant No. HDO3752 from the NIH. Some parts of this work were completed in Prof. THIBAULT's Laboratory, Station Centrale de Physiologie animale, Jouy-en-Josas (France).

The work with the high voltage microscope was carried out in collaboration with Dr. J. LAIDLER at the Westinghouse Hanford Company, Richland, Wash.

References

ADAMS, C.E. and CHANG, M.C.: The effect of delayed mating on fertilization in the rabbit. J. exp. Zool. *151:* 155–158 (1962).

AUSTIN, C.R.: Cortical granules in hamster eggs. Exp. Cell Res. *10:* 533–540 (1956).

AUSTIN, C.R.: Chromosome deterioration in aging eggs of the rabbit. Nature, Lond. *213:* 1018–1019 (1967).

AUSTIN, C.R.: Aging and reproduction: postovulatory deterioration of the egg. J. Reprod. Fertil. Suppl. *12:* 39–53 (1970).

AUSTIN, C.R. and BRADEN, A.W.H.: An investigation of polyspermy in the rat and rabbit. Austr. J. Biol. Sci. *6:* 674 (1953).

AUSTIN, C.R. and BRADEN, A.W.H.: Time relations and their significance in the ovulation and penetration of eggs in rats and the rabbit. Austr. J. Biol. Sci. *7:* 179 (1954).

BARROS, C. and YANAGIMACHI, R.: Induction of zona reaction in golden hamster eggs by cortical granule material. Nature, Lond. *233:* 268–269 (1971).

BLANDAU, R.J.: The female factor in fertility. I. Effects of delayed fertilization on the development of the pronuclei in rat ova. Fertil. Steril. *3:* 349–365 (1952).

Fig. 20. Defoliating and degenerating epithelial cells of the fallopian tube are frequently found near eggs when flushed 22 h after ovulation. In this case 3 adjacent secretory cells are shown. × 11,000.

Fig. 21. The ampulla of the fallopian tube is invaded by a number of mast cells 15–22 h after ovulation. × 10,000.

BLANDAU, R.J.; BOLING, J.L., and YOUNG, W.C.: The length of heat in the albino rat as determined by the copulatory response. Anat. Rec. *79:* 453 (1941).

BLANDAU, R.J. and JORDAN, E.S.: The effect of delayed fertilization on the development of the rat ovum. Amer. J. Anat. *64:* 275–291 (1941).

BLANDAU, R.J. and YOUNG, W.C.: The effects of delayed fertilization on the development of the guinea pig ovum. Amer. J. Anat. *64:* 303 (1939).

BOUÉ, J.G. et BOUÉ, A.: Les aberrations chromosomiques dans les avortements spontanés humains. C.R. Acad. Sci. *263:* 2054–2058 (1966).

BRADEN, A.W.H.: Are nongenic defects of the gametes important in the etiology of prenatal mortality? Fertil. Steril. *10:* 285–298 (1959).

BRADEN, A.W.H. and AUSTIN, C.R.: Fertilization of the mouse egg and the effect of delayed coitus and of heat shock treatment. Austr. J. Biol. Sci. *7:* 552–565 (1954).

CALARCO, P.G.: The kinetochore in oocyte maturation; in BIGGERS and SCHUETZ Oogenesis, chapt. 4 (University Park Press, Baltimore 1972).

CHALMEL, M.C.: Possibilité de fécondation des œufs de lapine activés parthénogénétiquement. Ann. Biol. anim. Biochem. Biophys. *2:* 279–297 (1962).

CHANG, M.C.: Effects of delayed fertilization on segmenting ova, blastocysts, and fetuses in rabbit. Fed. Proc. *11:* 24 (1952a).

CHANG, M.C.: Fertilizability of rabbit ova and the effects of temperature *in vitro* on their subsequent fertilization and activation *in vivo*. J. exp. Zool. *121:* 351–382 (1952b).

CHANG, M.C.: Development of parthenogenetic rabbit blastocysts induced by low temperature storage of unfertilized eggs. J. exp. Zool. *125:* 127 (1954).

EDWARDS, R.G.: Induced heteroploidy in mice: effect of deacetyl-methyl colchicine on eggs at fertilization. Exp. Cell Res. *24:* 615–617 (1961).

FLECHON, J.E.: Etude cytochimique ultrastructurale de la phagocytose de spermatozoïdes dans la lumière utérine chez la lapine (submitted for publication, 1973).

GULYAS, B.J.: The rabbit zygote. III. Formation of the blastomere nucleus. J. Cell Biol. *55:* 533–541 (1972).

GULYAS, B.J.: Spontaneous polyspermy in the rabbit zygote. Anat. Rec. *175:* 335 (1973).

HAMMOND, J.: The fertilization of rabbit ova in relation to time: a method of controlling litter size, the duration of pregnancy and the weight of young at birth. J. exp. Biol. *11:* 140–161 (1934).

HANCOCK, J.L.: Polyspermy of pig ova. Vet. Rec. *70:* 1200 (1959).

HUNTER, R.H.F.: The effects of delayed insemination on fertilization and early cleavage in the pig. J. Reprod. Fertil. *13:* 133–147 (1967).

IFFY, L. and WINGATE, M.B.: Risks of rhythm method of birth control. J. Reprod. Med. *5:* 11 (1970).

LONGO, F.J.: Ultrastructural changes in rabbit eggs aged *in vivo*. Biol. Reprod. (submitted, 1973 a).

LONGO, F.J.: Spontaneous activation of the hamster egg *in vivo*. Abstr. to be presented and published. Biol. Reprod. (1973b).

LUFT, J.H.: Ruthenium red and violet. I. Chemistry, purification, method of use for electron microscopy and mechanism of action. Anat. Rec. *171:* 347 (1971).

MIKAMO, K.I.: Intrafollicular overripeness and teratologic development. Cytogenetics *7:* 212 (1968).

PICKETT-HEAPS, J.: The autonomy of the centriole: fact or fallacy? Cytobios *3:* 205–214 (1971).

PIKO, L.: Etude de la polyspermie chez le rat. C.R. Acad. Soc. Biol. *152:* 1356–1358 (1958).

PIKO, L. and BOMSEL-HELMREICH, O.: Triploid and rat embryos and other deviants after colchicine treatment and polyspermy. Nature, Lond. *186:* 737 (1960).

SCHINDLER, A.M. and MIKAMO, K.: Triploidy in man. Cytogenetics *9:* 116 (1970).

SHAVER, E.L. and CARR, D.H.: Chromosome abnormalities in rabbit blastocysts following delayed fertilization. J. Reprod. Fertil. *14:* 415 (1967).

SOUPART, P.: Leucocytes and sperm capacitation in the rabbit uterus. Fertil. Steril. *21:* 724 (1970).

SZOLLOSI, D.: Cortical granules: a general feature of mammalian eggs. J. Reprod. Fertil. *4:* 223 (1962).

SZOLLOSI, D.: Structure and function of centrioles and their satellites from the jelly fish, *Phialidium gregarium.* J. Cell Biol. *21:* 465 (1964).

SZOLLOSI, D.: Extrusion of nucleoli from pronuclei of the rat. J. Cell Biol. *25:* 545 (1965).

SZOLLOSI, D.: Development of cortical granules and the cortical reaction in rat and hamster eggs. Anat. Rec. *159:* 431 (1967).

SZOLLOSI, D.: Morphological changes in mouse eggs due to aging in the fallopian tube. Amer. J. Anat. *130:* 209 (1971).

SZOLLOSI, D.; CALARCO, P., and DONAHUE, R.P.: Absence of centrioles in the first and second meiotic spindles of mouse oocytes. J. Cell Sci. *11:* 521 (1972).

SZOLLOSI, D. and HUNTER, R.H.F.: Ultrastructural aspects of fertilization in the domestic pig: sperm penetration and pronucleus formation. J. Anat. (in press, 1973).

SZUBINSKA, B. and LUFT, J.H.: Ruthenium red and violet. III. Fine structure of the plasma membrane and extraneous coats in Amoeba *(A. proteus* and *Chaos chaos).* Anat. Rec. *171:* 417 (1971).

THIBAULT, C.: Analyse de la fécondation de l'œuf de la truie après accouplement ou insémination artificielle. Ann. Zootech. Suppl. *8:* 165 (1959).

THIBAULT, C.: Analyse comparée de la fécondation et de ses anomalies chez la brebis, la vache et la lapine. Ann. Biol. anim. Biochem. Biophys. *7:* 5 (1967).

VICKERS, A.D.: Delayed fertilization and chromosomal anomalies in mouse embryos. J. Reprod. Fertil. *20:* 69 (1969).

WITSCHI, E. and LAGUENS, R.: Chromosomal aberrations in embryos from overripe eggs. Develop. Biol. *7:* 605 (1963).

YANAGIMACHI, R. and CHANG, M.C.: Fertilizable life of golden hamster ova and their morphological changes at the time of losing fertilizability. J. exp. Zool. *148:* 185 (1961).

Author's address: Dr. DANIEL SZOLLOSI, Institut National de la Recherche Agronomique, Station de Recherches de Physiologie Animale, *F-78350 Jouy-en-Josas* (France)

Aging Gametes. Int. Symp., Seattle 1973, pp. 122–150 (Karger, Basel 1975)

Biochemical Aspects of Aging in Spermatozoa in Relation to Motility and Fertilizing Ability

THADDEUS MANN and CECILIA LUTWAK-MANN

Agricultural Research Council's Unit of Reproductive Physiology and Biochemistry, University of Cambridge, Cambridge

Aging represents a sequence of events of great complexity, the biology of which can be studied at various levels. At the so-called supracellular level, i.e., in the entire organism, the aging process can be equated with a general and progressive loss of vigor, an irreversible state of decrepitude advancing on a broad front, and a rapidly increasing probability of death. A process of this kind need not necessarily reflect aging changes that occur at the cellular level, i.e., in individual cells, such as the male or female gametes. As a matter of fact, it is still a matter of dispute among gerontologists to what extent generalized aging of man or animal is directly related to senescence changes in the various types of cells. In man, some of the evidence for the existence of a direct relationship between the supracellular and cellular aspects of aging derives from experiments on diploid cells that have been shown to survive in cultures better when obtained from younger than from older donors [HAYFLICK, 1965; MARTIN et al., 1970]. Similar conclusions have been drawn from observations on tissue explants transferred from rats or chickens to culture media, where the duration of the so-called latent period, defined as the time required for cells to migrate from the explants, was shown to be directly proportional to the donors' age [CRISTOFALO, 1972; SOUKUPOVÁ et al., 1970]. As these observations have been made with cells that grow and multiply mitotically, conclusions drawn from them need not necessarily apply to spermatozoa, which are haploid, nongrowing, and mitotically inactive cells.

Certain other current theories of cellular aging and death, based on studies of polyploid cells, also fail to impress the gametologist when he is told that accelerated aging of cells is due in a large measure to a 'chaotic, senseless, slow continuation of morphogenesis' [MEDVEDEV, 1964], or to an 'error catastrophy' in the regulatory mechanism of intracellular synthesis of

RNA and protein, precipitated by defects in genetic programming of differentiation, and consequent mistranslation, i.e., faulty action of so-called informational macromolecules [ORGEL, 1963; STREHLER, 1967; VON HAHN, 1971]. Spermatozoa, unlike polyploid cells, are incapable of differentiating, and notoriously deficient in RNA and protein-synthesizing ability; it is therefore difficult to see how sperm senescence could arise from this type of biological incompetence. For example, in a bovine spermatozoon there is, on the average, 3.25×10^{-12}g DNA in the nucleus [SANDRITTER et al., 1960] and 1.24×10^{-15}g DNA in the 72 mitochondria of the middle-piece [BAHR and ENGLER, 1970], but the RNA accounts for no more than 0.02% of the total DNA content [ABRAHAM and BHARGAVA, 1963]. Moreover, the little evidence there is indicates that this exceedingly small amount of RNA is synthesized wholly on the mitochondrial and not the nuclear DNA-template and that the minute amount of protein synthesized by bovine spermatozoa on incubation with labelled amino acids is entirely of mitochondrial and not nuclear origin [PREMKUMAR and BHARGAVA, 1972].

Notwithstanding the reservations that one may have about the relevance to spermatozoa of some of the currently fashionable theories of aging, the spermatozoon represents an excellent object for gerontological study because it is a cell capable of surviving for extended periods of time, under conditions in vitro as well as in vivo, and at the same time endowed with two remarkable cellular functions, namely motility and fertilizing ability, that depend on highly specific biochemical and metabolic characteristics. These properties provide the investigator with a wide range of valuable criteria for assessing the cellular viability, longevity, and death of the spermatozoa. Another experimental asset is that spermatozoa neither grow nor multiply, so that the analytical results can be expressed in terms of constant and quantitatively defined cell numbers.

The biochemical processes that cause a spermatozoon to age consist of a sequence of events that on the whole fits into the general pattern of aging at the so-called cellular level. In some ways certain biochemical aspects of sperm aging resemble more the situation prevailing in so-called resting bacteria, which become nonviable upon cessation of their growth and differentiation, than the changes that occur in cells of animal tissues that are mitotically active and strictly dependent on blood and lymph supply. The situation in resting, that is, in nondividing microorganisms, was ascribed by HINSHELWOOD [1951] to 'an actual waxing and waning of individual parts of the cell machinery'. To quote HINSHELWOOD, 'in the resting state of the cell, the various enzyme activities gradually decay, and eventually the cells become nonviable', probably by following rules 'mathematically analogous to those which must govern the law of decay of the atoms of a radioactive element'. But sperm aging, which we would like to define as a gradual decay in structural, mechanochemical, and fertilizing properties of mature spermatozoa, is a phenomenon of far greater complexity than the changes that occur in resting bacteria. The rate and extent of aging changes in spermatozoa are, moreover, much more intimately related to their extracellular environment.

I. Effect of Environment on Aging Spermatozoa

There are three distinct environmental situations in which sperm aging has been studied, namely the male reproductive tract, i.e., prior to ejaculation of semen; the female reproductive tract, i.e., after semen deposition in either the vagina, cervix, or uterus; and under conditions *in vitro*.

In the male reproductive tract interest centers mainly upon the fate of spermatozoa in the epididymis, the vas deferens and the ampulla of the vas. It is particularly difficult to define the aging changes in the epididymis, as this requires a clear-cut demarcation line to be drawn between epididymal maturation and aging proper. This vexing problem of how to disentangle developmental from purely degenerative phenomena is by no means limited to the spermatozoa; it applies equally to other cells. In fact, there is much to be said for the concept that in spermatozoa the aging process constitutes an inevitable but physiologically normal continuation of maturation. Seen in that context, sperm maturation and aging represent two distinct phases of the same process.

When considering spermatozoa that have undergone aging in the male reproductive tract, we are faced with yet another dilemma, namely that of determining to what extent changes that occur during the passage in the epididymis and vas are influenced by the age of the individual. No one doubts that male fertility declines with advancing age, but by and large it appears that, in man at any rate, viable spermatozoa are produced over a remarkably long period of years. Otherwise it would be difficult to accept as genuine the frequent reports in both the medical and lay press about men who became fathers at the age of 70, 80, or even 90 [AMELAR, 1966; SEYMOUR *et al.*, 1935]. As regards bulls, we can vouch for the existence at the Animal Research Station, Cambridge, of an animal aged 22 years that, though experiencing some difficulty in mounting a cow, has repeatedly been shown to yield ejaculates containing motile and fertile spermatozoa. Considering the fact that spermatozoa first appear in the semen of a bull at the age of 8 or 9 months, a 22-year span provides an impressive record of male fertility in the bovine species.

But in old bulls as in old men, the overall quality of semen, as assessed by combined morphological, functional, and biochemical criteria, is distinctly inferior to that of younger and sexually more active individuals. This can be attributed partly to a deterioration with age in the quality of the spermatozoa as such, but to some extent it is the result of those retrograde changes in the endocrine status of the aging male that bring about a decline in the testosterone-dependent activity of male accessory organs concerned with the formation and secretion of seminal plasma.

In man, the blood-plasma levels of testosterone seem to remain within the same range from adolescence until the age of 50 years, or possibly even longer [HUDSON et al.,1967], but thereafter the testosterone levels fall [VERMEULEN et al., 1972], and this, together with a decreasing excretion of testosterone and marked alterations in the rates of steroid conversion, may account, to some extent at any rate, for the age-dependent changes in the chemistry of human seminal plasma. One such chemical change is the decline in the amount of seminal fructose secreted by the seminal vesicles of aging men [GRAYHACK, 1961; KUEHNAU and NOWAKOWSKI, 1960; NOWAKOWSKI and SCHMIDT, 1958; SCHIRREN, 1963]. Next there is the diminishing output by the aging human prostate of acid phosphatase and probably also of other enzymes, e.g., lactate dehydrogenase [GRAYHACK and KROPP, 1964; KIRK, 1948, 1949]. Up to a point these changes are undoubtedly due to falling levels of circulating androgens, but there are probably other contributing factors, including vascular changes leading to diminished supply of blood and nutrients to the testes and male accessory organs of aging men, progressive tubular fibrosis, focal hyalinization of seminiferous tubules, and a reduced number of capillaries, all features commonly encountered in the testes of aging men [SUORANTA, 1971]. Experimental observations in animals support these assumptions. In the ram, ischemia lasting only a few minutes interferes with the flow of spermatozoa from isolated and perfused testes [LINZELL and SETCHELL, 1968], and in the dog, a relationship has been shown to exist between the testicular blood flow and the gonadotrophin-stimulated secretion of testosterone [EIK-NES, 1964].

As yet there is no convincing evidence that the secretion of testicular fluid, as opposed to sperm output, is also affected by old age. In men, no changes were noted to occur with advancing age in either the production rate or the protein pattern of seminiferous tubular fluid [KOSKISMIES et al., 1973], and similarly in rats, no decrease in the secretion of the rete testis fluid was observed under conditions of suppressed spermatogenesis [SETCHELL and WAITES, 1972], suggesting that testicular fluid secretion occurs independently of spermatogenesis. On the other hand, there is much evidence to indicate that the flow and chemical composition of the male accessory fluids are seriously affected when the blood supply to the accessory organs is curtailed. This follows clearly from experiments on rats, in which ischemia resulting from arterial interruption of blood supply to the coagulating glands was shown to inhibit the process of fructose secretion; this inhibition was overcome as soon as a collateral circulation was formed [CLEGG, 1954].

In bulls, the decrease in semen quality accompanying advancing age is reflected in the well-documented fall in breeding efficiency [COLLINS et al., 1962; CZAUDERNA, 1971; ROTTENSTEN, 1972; RZEZNIK, 1971]. The age-dependent fall in the fertility of bulls is associated with a number of changes in seminal characteristics, as shown for instance by FOOTE et al., [1971] who scrutinized the performance records of a large number of bulls used for artificial insemination. They found that the semen quality of bulls aged 2–6 years was markedly superior to that of animals that were more than 6 years old in respect to fertility, assessed by the so-called nonreturn rate, the percentage of viable and morphologically normal spermatozoa in semen, and the ability of spermatozoa to survive a prolonged period of storage in the frozen state.

Less is known about the age-dependent changes in bovine seminal plasma, which so far have been studied mainly with reference to fructose and citric acid, both of which are secreted in the bull by the seminal vesicles [MANN, 1946]. The determination of either fructose or citric acid provides an index of the testosterone-dependent secretory activity in the bovine seminal vesicles, and is indirectly a good marker of the bull's androgenic status [LINDNER and MANN, 1960; MANN, 1967]. But when interpreting the concentration values for seminal fructose or citric acid as indicators of a declining hormonal status in an aging animal, one must not forget that similar changes can be brought about by other events, such as, for example, a short period of underfeeding or malnutrition [BARONOS et al., 1969; DAVIES et al., 1957; MANN et al., 1960, 1967]. It is easy to ascribe a wrong meaning to seminal plasma analysis if one fails to take into account the marked seasonal variations in the composition of bovine semen. Seasonal influence is a factor that has often been neglected in past studies concerning variability in semen quality, and yet this is of paramount importance in farm animals, such as the bull and stallion [LEIDL, 1958; MANN et al., 1956], and even more so in wild-living seasonal breeders, such as the deer [SHORT and MANN, 1966]. Seasonal changes in the composition of semen are moreover by no means restricted to the accessory secretions and seminal plasma but occur in the spermatozoa as well. For instance in the male goat, sperm glycerol kinase, an enzyme that catalyses the phosphorylation of glycerol by ATP, has an activity several times lower during the summer months than at other times of the year [MOHRI et al., 1970].

The structural and functional alterations in spermatozoa, set in motion in the epididymis as part of the sperm maturation process, do not stop at ejaculation but continue upon semen deposition in the female tract, where the survival potential of spermatozoa rapidly diminishes. In the rabbit, for example, spermatozoa remain viable in the epididymis for as long as 40 days, but in the female genital tract deterioration of their fertilizing ability begins as soon as 20 h, and is virtually complete at 32 h; yet at the same time, rabbit spermatozoa must spend at least a few hours in the female genital tract before they acquire the capacity to fertilize [CHANG and PINCUS, 1964; HAMMOND and ASDELL, 1926; NOYES and THIBAULT, 1962; TESH and GLOVER, 1969]. It is obviously difficult to distinguish with precision between capacitation and aging of rabbit spermatozoa in the female tract, and one might even be inclined to consider these two phenomena as successive phases of the same physiological process.

Of the biochemical changes that the spermatozoa undergo in the uterus of the rabbit doe, the most striking are increased respiration and aerobic glycolysis [FOLEY and WILLIAMS, 1967; HAMNER and WILLIAMS, 1963; MOUNIB and CHANG, 1964; MURDOCH and WHITE, 1967]. Washing uterine spermatozoa with saline solution does not deprive them of their enhanced metabolic activity. Therefore, the above-mentioned metabolic rises are presumably due not so much to the nutrient effect of the uterine secretion as to changes that have taken place within the sperm cells, perhaps as part of the capacitation process. Whether or not these particular metabolic changes can be regarded as an indispensible part of capacitation is by no means certain.

We also lack at present precise information about effects that the age of the female exerts on the life span and metabolic performance of spermatozoa within her own reproductive tract. But the existence of such effects is highly probable, not only owing to changes that occur in the hormonal status of the aging female, but also to the alterations in the chemistry of the aging uterus as such. The collagen content of the uterus, for example, is known to increase with age, even irrespective of pregnancy, as demonstrated by experiments on mice [FINN et al., 1963]. Certain uterine enzymes, including some that participate in carbohydrate metabolism, become less active with age; this is probably due partly to declining hormone levels and partly to a diminishing response of dying tissues to hormonal stimulation [ADELMAN, 1972; SINGHAL, 1967].

Another environmental situation, also linked up with changes due to aging, arises in spermatozoa maintained under conditions *in vitro* in various diluents and media, including those in which semen is routinely stored, either fresh or frozen, for the purpose of artificial insemination. As yet it is unknown whether sperm aging *in vitro* is caused by the same processes as sperm aging *in vivo*. Again, this is a set of problems by no means restricted to the spermatozoa. These problems complicate all research on cellular aging and especially those investigations in which cell cultures are used as model systems [CRISTOFALO, 1972].

From the biological viewpoint the most important consequence of sperm aging *in vitro* is decreased fertility and increased incidence of embryonic mortality. This has been repeatedly demonstrated by artificial insemination of animals such as cattle [SALISBURY, 1967; SALISBURY and FLERCHINGER, 1967], pigs [FIRST *et al.*, 1963], and rabbits [KOEFOED-JOHNSEN *et al.*, 1971] and is best documented in the case of the bovine species. The extensive literature on this subject has been reviewed by SALISBURY and HART [1970], whose article provides a valuable source of information on changes that take place in bull semen stored either for a few days at 4–5°C, or for prolonged periods of time at much lower temperatures, such as that of solid carbon dioxide (−79°C) or liquid nitrogen (−196°C). Among the many intriguing but poorly understood aspects of sperm aging *in vitro* discussed in that review are reports that semen that had been collected from bulls during the summer maintained its fertilizing ability *in vitro* less well than semen collected during the colder part of the year. There are also reports that when bull semen is stored at 4°C an improvement in its fertilizing potential can occur on the first day of storage, followed later by a decline. According to SALISBURY and HART [1970] the probable cause of this peculiar phenomenon is that whereas in freshly ejaculated semen: 'Spermatozoa containing aberrant chromatin, or those which are otherwise abnormal, may compete effectively with normal sperm for fertilization sites, later they are unable to do so and a higher proportion of the available ova are then fertilized by more normal spermatozoa, resulting in higher fertility in the relatively brief time span which occurs before aging supervenes.'

We need more information on whether changes similar to those that occur in semen stored at 4° C also take place in deep-frozen semen, though presumably at a greatly reduced rate. There are at present available for artificial insemination specimens of glycerol-frozen bovine semen that have been cold-stored for more than 20 years, and undoubtedly their fertilizing potential, assessed quantitatively by the so-called 'nonreturn rates' of inseminated cattle, has somewhat declined over the years. At the same time, over the last 20 years the techniques of handling frozen semen have greatly improved, and so it is uncertain to what extent the poor results obtained with frozen-thawed semen by the early investigators were due simply to inept handling. Of special significance in this respect is the report by FOOTE [1972] who collected semen from 15 bulls and stored it under strictly controlled conditions in ampules immersed in liquid nitrogen for 1–25 months prior to artificial insemination. He observed no progressive decline in fertility during that period, and the actual nonreturn rates for 3,222 inseminations with semen stored for 18–25 months were not significantly different from values recorded for 17,820 inseminations with semen stored 1–12 months. However under less rigidly controlled conditions of storage, deleterious changes soon become apparent in bull spermatozoa, particularly in the sperm nuclei [PAUFLER and FOOTE, 1967].

II. Nuclear Instability as a Factor in Sperm Senescence

The notion that sperm aging, *in vivo* and *in vitro*, is the outcome of chemical changes in the chromatin and deoxyribonucleic acid of the sperm nucleus had many advocates among the early investigators of spermatozoa, and, although less fashionable nowadays, it still survives in a somewhat modified form. The two methods routinely used for measuring the DNA content of individual sperm nuclei involve microspectrophotometric procedures in which the amount of light absorbed by a sperm nucleus is determined either in unstained microscopic preparations by utilizing the absorption of ultraviolet light by nucleic acid at 257 nm, or by first staining the spermatozoa with the Feulgen reagent and then measuring the light absorption in the visible region, usually at 546 nm. The considerable literature concerning these two methods has been reviewed and critically evaluated on several occasions, and the pitfalls inherent in the uncritical use of 'Feulgen stainability' as a quantitative measure of sperm DNA have often been stressed [MANN, 1964, 1968, 1970; SANDRITTER, 1966]. In contrast to methods based on measuring of nucleic acid in ultraviolet light, 'Feulgen stainability', i.e., the intensity of the color reaction given by the Schiff's fuchsin-sulfurous acid reagent, is not a reliable test of the DNA content in sperm nuclei. This is because the ability of spermatozoa to take up Feulgen stain can be altered by a variety of factors, including permeability of the individual sperm heads to the stain and the physico-chemical properties of the deoxyribonucleoprotein complex as a whole. Therefore, alterations in Feulgen stainability, such as have been reported to accompany spermateliosis in the testis, sperm maturation in the epididymis, capacitation in the female tract, sperm aging *in vitro*, etc., need not necessarily reflect true changes in the content of DNA as such, but are probably the outcome of more intricate changes in the properties of the deoxyribonucleoprotein complex as a whole, for instance, in its state of polymerization, the number of phosphate groups available for binding of histochemical stains or the basicity of nuclear proteins that can influence markedly electrostatic binding of nuclear protein to the nucleic acid [GLEDHILL, 1966; GLEDHILL *et al.*, 1966]. The physical and chemical changes that occur in the deoxyribonucleoprotein complex during spermateliosis and sperm maturation are probably also responsible for the observed reduction in the capacity of spermatozoa to bind tritium-labelled actinomycin D and the progressively increasing resistance of sperm DNA to heat denaturation (so-called melting profile), as demonstrated by both ultraviolet microspectrophotometry and acridine orange microfluorimetry [GLEDHILL, 1971].

With these reservations in mind, Feulgen stainability can nevertheless serve occasionally as a useful, though rather imprecise, indicator of changes that occur in aging spermatozoa. In ejaculated bovine semen, for example, the differences in response of individual spermatozoa to the Feulgen stain are most likely due to a varying percentage of fully viable and less viable sperm cells. This probably applies also to observations made in rabbits where it was shown that ampullary spermatozoa yield significantly lower 'Feulgen-DNA' values than epididymal spermatozoa and that ligation of the vas deferens results in a significant decrease in Feulgen stainability of epididymal spermatozoa [BOUTERS *et al.*, 1967]. All these and other similar findings agree with the concept that sperm aging *in vivo* does affect the sperm nucleus but has no influence on its DNA content as such.

There is at present no satisfactory evidence that the DNA content of spermatozoa changes *in vivo* between the stage of spermateliosis and fertilization. During the passage of spermatozoa in the epididymis there occurs a significant reduction in Feulgen stainability, and following ejaculation, during the sojourn in the female genital tract, individual spermatozoa may even be able to show once more an intensified Feulgen reaction but without a concomitant variation in the amount of true DNA as determined by ultraviolet absorption. Changes of this sort may stem from the variable character of nuclear proteins. Recent work by ESNAULT [1973] indicates that if ram spermatozoa have lost some of the Feulgen stainability during epididymal passage, it can be restored by treatment with dithiothreitol, a reagent that reduces S-S to SH groups. This suggests that the disulfide bonds in the nuclear proteins play a role in the Feulgen reaction of spermatozoa.

Contrary to what at one time we were made to believe [SALISBURY et al., 1961], it is now becoming increasingly evident that there is no significant change in the content of DNA in spermatozoa stored in vitro. It was not possible to demonstrate any such change in the rabbit [MILLER and BLACKSHAW, 1968]; nor has it been possible to detect any appreciable loss of radioactivity in rabbit spermatozoa labelled in vivo with tritiated thymidine and stored in vitro for 10 days after ejaculation [KOEFOED-JOHNSEN et al., 1968]. Similarly, no significant changes in either DNA or histone content could be demonstrated in bovine semen diluted with the egg-yolk citrate diluent and stored in the presence of antibiotics at 5°C for periods of up to 9 days [BLACKSHAW and SALISBURY, 1972]. It is also clear now that the DNA content of human spermatozoa remains unchanged following storage for either 1 week at 6°C, or 2–75 weeks in a deep-frozen state [ACKERMAN and SOD-MORIAH, 1968], though the conception rate in women is definitely lower after insemination with frozen-thawed spermatozoa than with fresh human semen [BEHRMAN, 1971; CARLBORG, 1971].

All these findings do not rule out the possibility that, in spite of unchanged DNA content, some other more subtle changes may occur during sperm aging in vitro in the deoxyribonucleoprotein as a whole. It has been said, for example, that the DNA-protein complex extracted from aged bovine spermatozoa differs antigenically from that prepared from fresh spermatozoa [TODOROVIC et al., 1969]. There remains also the fact that both spermatozoa and mammalian seminal plasma are rich in nucleolytic as well as proteolytic enzymes [MANN, 1964, 1972], and one wonders whether powerful hydrolytic enzymes such as these play a role in sperm aging, either in vitro or in vivo, or alternatively, whether they are perhaps engaged in the disposal at various stages of aged or dead spermatozoa.

III. Defects in the Cellular Membranes and Acrosome, and Increased Permeability of the Aging Spermatozoon

Age-dependent alterations in the nucleus are only one, not very dependable, indicator of the physico-chemical changes that affect senescent spermatozoa. Several other sperm organelles, and especially the sperm membranes and acrosomes, are also implicated in the aging process. What is perhaps most impressive and encouraging in recent biochemical investigations concerning these organelles is the emphasis increasingly placed on obtaining meaningful correlation of chemical findings with observations on the function and ultrastructure of aging spermatozoa.

Efforts to comprehend and link up the morphological and functional changes associated with sperm aging have been particularly evident in those studies that relate the breakage of the plasma membrane and outer acrosomal membrane to osmotic changes, loss of acrosomal material, and increase of cellular permeability, all of which occur when spermatozoa become less viable [DREVIUS, 1972; JONES, 1973 a, b]. As a result of such comparative studies it has become quite clear that the actosome must be considered as a modified and specialized lysosome and that acrosomal enzymes, in particular some of the proteinases, have an essential part to play in various physiological phenomena connected with normal sperm function, such as the acrosomal reaction, 'zona lysis' and fertilization [ALLISON and HARTREE, 1968, 1970; STAMBAUGH et al., 1969; ZANEVELD et al., 1971].

We also appreciate now more fully than hitherto, the importance of the sperm membranes and the acrosome in the process of increased permeability in spermatozoa that are degenerating, not only as a result of aging, but also as a result of faulty handling, mechanical injury, osmotic damage, cold shock, freezing and thawing, spermicidal agents, etc.

In a simple and at the same time convenient form one can demonstrate differences in permeability to extracellular substances, which are evident respectively in viable, partially viable, and nonviable spermatozoa, by determining the degree of uptake of so-called live-dead or differential stains such as eosin. The usefulness of this method in the study of sperm aging is illustrated in figure 1, showing smears of bull and ram spermatozoa that had been treated with a nigrosin-eosin mixture in order to distinguish between noneosinophilic, partially eosinophilic, and strongly eosinophilic spermatozoa. This technique has proved to be of considerable practical value, enabling even under field conditions a quick evaluation of 'live' (noneosinophilic) and 'dead' (eosinophilic) spermatozoa in semen specimens collected from farm animals and examined fresh or after storage [CAMPBELL et al., 1956; DOTT, 1956].

Differential live-dead stains have been also applied successfully in the assessment of effects of freezing and thawing on sperm permeability and viability and in demonstrating the rise in permeability that occurs in spermatozoa subjected to cold shock, a treatment which involves sudden cooling from body temperature to a few degrees above 0°C and renders ram or bull sper-

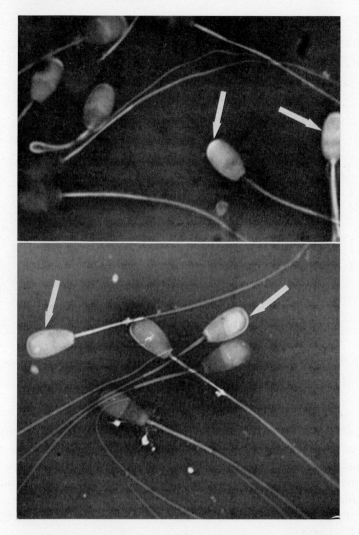

Fig. 1. Spermatozoa of ram (top) and bull (bottom) exposed to the live-dead dif-ferential nigrosin-eosin stain; the noneosinophilic (live) spermatozoa are indicated by arrows.

matozoa completely and irreversibly immotile and thus nonviable. Cold shock, which must not be confused with the effect of freezing to temperatures below 0°C, was first described by MILOVANOV [1934]. MILOVANOV also takes the credit for the observation that, provided that cooling of bull spermatozoa

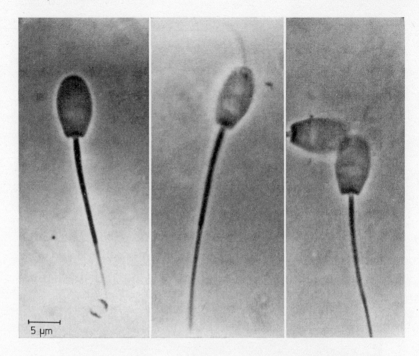

Fig. 2. Three ram spermatozoa from the same ejaculate (phase contrast phot.): normal (left); dead (middle), and treated with 50 mM sodium deoxycholate (right).

to a temperature slightly above 0°C is done very slowly, motility is not lost and can be restored by bringing the temperature of the spermatozoa up to body temperature. We now also know that, under such conditions of slow cooling, spermatozoa are not rendered eosinophilic and their metabolic ability is not affected as much as in cold-shocked spermatozoa [Bishop and Hancock, 1951; Chang and Walton, 1940; Lasley *et al.*, 1942; Mann and Lutwak-Mann, 1955].

The rapid and irreversible immobilization and increased permeability due to cold shock coincide with certain characteristic structural changes in spermatozoa, including a pronounced 'swelling' of the acrosome. This type of swelling is often observed in degenerating spermatozoa, such as are commonly encountered in normal ejaculated semen. Figure 2 shows three ram spermatozoa, all from the same ejaculate. Two were present in a sample of semen that was fixed immediately after ejaculation, and of these two, one shows all the characteristic features of a normal sperm cell, but the other,

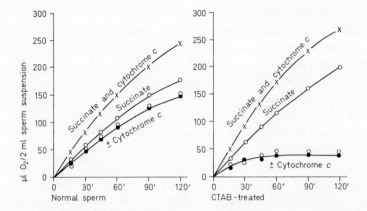

Fig. 3. Effect of sodium succinate on the oxygen consumption of ram spermatozoa, in the presence (+) or absence (–) of cytochrome c; left, normal spermatozoa; right, spermatozoa which have been treated with 2 mM cetyltrimethylammonium bromide (CTAB) and then CTAB removed by washing [KOEFOED-JOHNSEN and MANN, 1954].

with its characteristically swollen head, is obviously degenerating and can be pronounced dead. The third spermatozoon comes from another sample of the same ejaculate, treated prior to fixation by a surface-active spermicidal agent. It exhibits swelling changes similar to those of the dead spermatozoon present in fresh semen.

The increased permeability of moribund spermatozoa is reflected not only in their reaction to stains such as eosin but also to other extracellular substances such as succinate, for example [KOEFOED-JOHNSEN and MANN, 1954; MANN, 1958; MANN and LUTWAK-MANN, 1955]. Upon the addition of succinate to fresh semen or once-washed ram spermatozoa, the rate of oxygen uptake increases only slightly. But a much larger increase occurs when succinate alone or with cytochrome c is added to a sperm suspension in which the percentage of deteriorating cells has gone up as a result of either prolonged storage *in vitro*, cold shock, or treatment with a spermicidal detergent such as cetyltrimethylammonium bromide (CTAB). The respiratory response of CTAB-treated spermatozoa to succinate is shown in figure 3. The curves on the left represent the behavior of a suspension of normal, motile ram spermatozoa, which react with only a small increase in O_2 uptake to the addition of succinate alone; the rate is slightly enhanced in the presence of succinate + cytochrome c. The curves on the right illustrate the behavior of spermatozoa that have first been rendered irreversibly immotile by preincubation with

2 mM CTAB and were then washed to remove the excess of detergent; such spermatozoa can be seen to consume very little oxygen, but their O_2 uptake is markedly increased by succinate, particularly if added with cytochrome c. These experiments show that an increase in oxygen consumption of spermatozoa *per se* does not necessarily indicate an improvement, or even the maintenance, of sperm cell viability. On the contrary, an enhanced respiratory rate may be the result of cellular disorganization and impending death.

The increased permeability of spermatozoa that had been rendered nonviable by prolonged storage, cold shock, spermicidal agents, or mechanical injury, such as centrifugation and excessive washing, not only speeds up the entry of extracellular substances into the sperm cells but at the same time causes leakage of important intracellular sperm constituents into the external medium. The primary biochemical lesion responsible for such leakage is probably due to a change in the state of surface lipoproteins that protect the sperm cells. One of the earliest symptoms of leakage is an upset in the normal progress of ionic exchange reactions leading to a rapid loss of potassium and certain other ions. Cold shock in particular causes a rapid loss of potassium and magnesium ions from spermatozoa and at the same time an influx of sodium and calcium, but by adding lecithin, casein, or ethylenediaminetetracetate one can at least partly protect spermatozoa against cold shock, probably because of the calcium-binding properties of these substances [BLACKSHAW and SALISBURY, 1957; QUINN and WHITE, 1966, 1968]. It seems that the passage of calcium into the interior of the sperm cell in some way provokes disorganization of the protoplasm, but the exact mechanism of that effect and of the calcium-membrane interactions in spermatozoa needs to be more fully explored.

Another consequence of sperm damage and senescence is the loss of vital coenzymes. Using ram semen we have shown that following cold shock spermatozoa not only lost much of their ATP but were incapable of resynthesizing it [MANN and LUTWAK-MANN, 1955]. More recently it has been possible to extend similar observations to the cyclic form of adenosine monophosphate (cyclic AMP). This nucleotide leaks out at a remarkably high rate from bull, boar or ram spermatozoa as a result of even minor damage [TASH and MANN, 1973]. In the future it should be possible to utilize the determination of intracellular cyclic AMP as a very sensitive criterion of aging and other degenerative processes in spermatozoa.

Yet another sperm coenzyme that has been studied in aging spermatozoa is nicotinamide adenine dinucleotide (NAD). Analyses have shown that, unlike cyclic AMP, the NAD content of ram spermatozoa remains practical-

ly unchanged during 2 days of storage *in vitro* at 14°C, and even after 3 days it
still accounts for about 50% of the original value [BROOKS and MANN, 1972].
The difference in the behavior of cyclic AMP and NAD is probably due to the
fact that as a rule these two nucleotides occur in different cell organelles. The
formation of cyclic AMP from ATP requires the presence of adenyl cyclase,
an enzyme that is known to be associated with cell surfaces and membranes;
this presumably accounts for the loss of cyclic AMP from spermatozoa, the
surface of which had been damaged. On the other hand, NAD is located in
the mitochondrial sheath, largely in a bound form, and thus it is less susceptible to leakage.

IV. Enzyme Leakage from Moribund Spermatozoa

The leakage of intracellular substances from moribund spermatozoa is
by no means restricted to small-molecular substances, such as ions or nucleotides, but affects also large-molecular constituents, such as cytochrome *c*, lipoproteins, and a wide range of enzymes, some of them of vital importance
to the metabolic performance of spermatozoa. The leakage of cytochrome *c*
in aging or damaged animal or human spermatozoa was convincingly demonstrated by the liquid-air spectroscopic technique of KEILIN and HARTREE
[1950], which greatly intensifies the absorption spectra of intracellular hema-
tin compounds [MANN, 1951].

Of the various enzymes that pass readily from spermatozoa into the extracellular environment, hyaluronidase provides the oldest known and probably most studied example of an acrosomal (lysosomal) enzyme. The rate of
hyaluronidase release is so high that in the past this phenomenon was
thought to be a secretory function of normal spermatozoa until it became
clear that it characterizes a dying-off cell population. It is nevertheless true
that hyaluronidase can also be released by viable spermatozoa. In freshly collected bull semen incubated at 20°C, the release of the enzyme follows the
course of a first-order reaction and occurs at a high rate [MASAKI and HAR-
TREE, 1962]; to quote an example, when spermatozoa were separated from
bull semen 30 min after ejaculation, they contained 560 turbidity units of hy-
aluronidase/ml semen, but when they were separated 90 min after ejaculation, the activity decreased to 170 units/ml.

Glycolytic enzymes, such as hexokinase, glucose phosphate isomerase,
and lactate dehydrogenase, also leak from spermatozoa into the extracellular
media under the influence of hypoosmotic shock, cold shock, or freezing.

This has been well described by HARRISON and WHITE [1972] whose study provides some interesting information on the differences in the release rates of these three enzymes, due most likely to spatial differentiation in their distribution within the sperm structure. The high release rate of hexokinase, for example, could be explained by the association of this enzyme with membrane structures. The rapid leakage of both glucose phosphate isomerase and lactate dehydrogenase from the cytoplasmic droplets as compared with the leakage of the dehydrogenase, slower than the isomerase, from the droplet-free spermatozoa, agrees with the assumption that whereas in the droplets a soluble form of lactate dehydrogenase is compartmented with the isomerase, the droplet-free spermatozoa contain some bound lactate dehydrogenase in the interior of the sperm tail and glucose phosphate isomerase somewhere toward the exterior portion of the tail.

Other enzymes that diffuse from aging spermatozoa into seminal plasma and storage media are certain transaminases [CRABO et al., 1971; FLIPSE, 1960; GRAHAM and PACE, 1967; GREGOIRE et al., 1961; POVOA and VILLELA, 1960; VAN DER HORST et al., 1972]. The enzymes studied in this group were mainly glutamic oxaloacetic transaminase and phenylalanine ketoglutaric transaminase. Dilution and storage of semen from farm animals can lead to release of sperm transaminases at a high rate, even though such spermatozoa still retain good fertilizing capacity. In some experiments, e.g. with boar semen samples stored at 5°C, the release of transaminase was negatively correlated with motility, but in other cases such a relationship could not be established. These findings have been interpreted to indicate that extracellular transaminase activity provides a measure of injury to sperm membranes, but not to those parts of the structure that are directly associated with motility.

V. Lipid Redistribution and Peroxide Reactions

Brief reference has been made earlier to the loss of lipid in the form of lipoprotein, which occurs in damaged spermatozoa as a result of increased permeability [MASAKI and TOMIZUKA, 1966; PICKETT and KOMAREK, 1967]. Lipoproteins are well known to be readily denatured by freezing and thawing of biological material, and some of them have been shown to release their lipid components as a result of such treatment. LOVELOCK [1957], whose studies have greatly contributed to a fuller understanding of the response of cells and lipoproteins to freezing, pointed out that the lipoproteins of cellular membranes are particularly susceptible to denaturation by freeze-thawing; our own studies on spermatozoa have provided additional support for that view [MANN, 1964; MANN and LUTWAK-MANN, 1955]. The preserving influence that glycerol exerts on frozen spermatozoa is probably due, in part at least, to the ability of this substance to protect lipoproteins from denaturation. But it is remarkable how differently spermatozoa of different animal species react to either freeze-thawing or cold shock, or even to such relatively mild treatments as dilution and washing. Species differ widely in respect to the total amount of sperm phospholipid released as well as to the percentage content of individual phospholipid components. For example, ram spermatozoa contain much less phospholipid than those of the boar, but they release a much higher percentage of total phospholipid after either freeze-thawing or cold shock, and the material released from ram and boar spermatozoa respectively contains different percentages of phosphatidyl choline and phosphatidyl ethanolamine [DARIN et al., 1973]. Presumably variations of this kind stem from species-specific differences in sperm lipids, but to some extent they may also reflect the different sensitivity to adverse treatment of the individual lipoproteins, particularly those that are located in sperm membranes and acrosomes. Species differences of this kind also probably explain the variable rate of success that has been achieved with glycerol and other protective agents in the practice of semen preservation by deep freezing. As is well known, artificial insemination of glycerol-frozen bull semen has been much more successful in practice than that of either ram or boar semen [POLGE et al., 1970]. One of the puzzling aspects of this problem is that, unlike bovine, the frozen spermatozoa of either ram or boar recover their motility on thawing much better than their fertilizing ability.

The changes that affect the concentration and distribution of sperm phospholipids in vivo are even more complicated than those in vitro because, as has been said before, it is difficult to draw a demarcation line between sperm aging and phenomena such as maturation, capacitation, and disposal of excess spermatozoa in either the male or the female reproductive tract. Moreover, we have as yet no definite answers to the following questions: (1) How much chemical interchange is there between the lipids and their metabolites belonging to spermatozoa and those present in the secretions of the male or female reproductive tract? (2) Can sperm lipids serve as an energy source for spermatozoa equally in vivo and in vitro, and to what extent does depletion of this lipid reserve shorten the life of spermatozoa in vivo [HARTREE and MANN, 1961]? (3) How much is sperm survival and metabolism in vivo controlled by hormonal factors, in particular testosterone [JONES and GLOVER, 1973]? All these questions, and especially the problem of distinguishing between sperm maturation and aging proper in the epididymis, could perhaps be solved if techniques were worked out for studying these processes in organ cultures. One hopes that recent efforts made along these lines [ORGEBIN-CRIST and TICHENOR, 1972] will speed up developments in that area.

As a result of a great many comparative studies on the lipid composition of ejaculated, epididymal, and testicular spermatozoa, we know that *in vivo*, particularly in the epididymis, profound changes take place in the major phospholipid components of spermatozoa [DAWSON and SCOTT, 1964; POULOS *et al.*, 1973; QUINN and WHITE, 1967; SCOTT *et al.*, 1967]. The present position can best be summarized by stating that the content of most sperm phospholipids, and also of nonesterified cholesterol, decreases markedly during the epididymal passage. It may be that this decrease, which presumably reflects a diminishing content of protein-bound lipids, is responsible for the greater susceptibility of ejaculated spermatozoa to cold shock than epididymal spermatozoa. This may also provide at least a partial explanation for the increased resistance to cold shock of ejaculated semen following the addition of phospholipids such as lecithin [BLACKSHAW and SALISBURY, 1957; KAMPSCHMIDT *et al.*, 1953; LASLEY and BOGART, 1944; LASLEY and MAYER, 1944; QUINN and WHITE, 1967; WHITE and WALES, 1960, 1961]. The loss of phospholipids during epididymal passage does not affect all lipid constituents to the same degree. In bovine spermatozoa, for example, by far the greatest loss occurs in the palmitic acid fraction, but at the same time there is no significant loss of docosahexenoic acid, which is the principal fatty acid component of phospholipids in bovine spermatozoa.

In many biological materials stored aerobically oxidative lipid metabolism is known to be frequently associated with the appearance of toxic metabolites in the form of organic lipid peroxides. Surprisingly, the possibility that spermatozoa, either live or dead, may give rise to such products has hitherto received very little attention, in spite of the known harmful action on spermatozoa of hydrogen peroxide [MANN, 1964; MROTEK *et al.*, 1966], and the equally well-established fact that hydrogen peroxide can actually be produced by spermatozoa, for instance, during the oxidative deamination of certain amino acids [TOSIC and WALTON, 1950]. If one could demonstrate the formation of organic peroxides in spermatozoa and link it up causally with the aging process, it would materially strengthen the so-called free radical theory of cellular aging, namely the concept that lipid oxidation and the free radical reactions associated with it are a major cause of the swelling and degeneration of cellular membranes, particularly those that normally encapsulate the lysosomes; deteriorative changes in such membranes could subsequently lead to release of lysosomal enzymes and ultimately autodigestion of the cell [PACKER et al., 1967]. At the same time, the demonstration that organic peroxide can be formed by spermatozoa would revive the now almost defunct theory of 'auto-intoxication' [GRAY, 1930]. According to GRAY's theory, the irreversible senile decay of spermatozoa and the concomitant structural deterioration are largely the outcome of auto-intoxication in the sense that 'the products of activity inhibit the essential reactions of life'. This view is in line with the more general concept that certain processes in normal cells 'that are steadily progressing, turn out to be harmful to the system involved' [KOHN, 1971].

Accordingly, an attempt was recently made to find out whether spermatozoa are in fact capable of producing organic peroxides and, if so, whether sperm aging or damage can enhance the rate of peroxide formation [JONES and MANN, 1973]. The chemical procedure employed for that purpose was the thiobarbituric acid method, which depends on measuring the red-coloured reaction product formed by thiobarbituric acid (TBA) with lipid peroxides; in this way one can determine quantitatively the so-called 'lipid peroxidation potential' of tissues and tissue extracts [BARBER and BERNHEIM, 1967; BERNHEIM, 1963; BERNHEIM et al., 1948; KOHN and LIVERSEDGE, 1944].

Experiments showed that, in suspensions of ram spermatozoa incubated aerobically for 2 h at 37°C or subjected to cold shock, a strong TBA reaction develops and that, furthermore, the TBA reactant is released by the cold-shocked spermatozoa into the extracellular medium; predictably, catalase added to the sperm suspensions did not interfere with the formation of the organic peroxide nor did it alter the course of the TBA reaction [JONES and MANN, 1973]. This study, aimed at elucidating the chemical nature of the organic peroxide, and at discovering the identity of the fatty acid that is undergoing peroxidation, is still in progress. But even the results at hand strongly suggest that peroxidation plays an important part in the process of sperm aging and degeneration, at any rate under conditions in vitro.

VI. Concluding Remarks

Sperm aging, broadly defined as a gradual and irreversible decay in the structural, mechanochemical, and fertilizing properties of mature spermatozoa, is a phenomenon of great complexity. It consists of a sequence of events that fit into the general pattern of aging at the so-called cellular level. The prevailing trend in research at present is to study aging not only in whole sperm cells but in separated organelles as well, i.e., at the subcellular level.

Many of the biochemical events operative in spermatozoa as part of the aging process have been investigated with reference to changes that can be either induced or accelerated by artificial means such as cold shock, freezing and thawing, dilution and washing, treatment with spermiostatic and spermicidal substances, and by prolonged storage *in vitro*. These researches have provided insight into the biochemical aspects of sperm senescence under conditions *in vitro*. It is still an open question to what extent it is justifiable to equate the aging process *in vitro*, either in its entirety or in part, with the events that take place in the living organism under the influence of factors operative at the supracellular level, such as hormones, secretory products of the male and female reproductive tract, and various agents emanating from the environment.

There are indications that the early stages of sperm senescence *in vitro* and *in vivo* have certain features in common. Biochemical investigations indicate that the initial defect that triggers off the degenerative changes in spermatozoa occurs in the sperm membranes and the acrosome. An early sign of degeneration is the swelling of the acrosome and structural abnormalities evident in the acrosomal and plasma membranes. This causes an increase in cellular permeability followed by an accelerated penetration of extracellular substances and loss through leakage from spermatozoa of essential intracellular constituents. Some of the compounds lost in this way are in the form of small molecular material such as potassium ions or nucleotide coenzymes. In addition, large molecular material passes from spermatozoa into the extracellular environment in the form of various proteins, particularly lipoproteins and enzymes.

Some of the enzymes released by degenerating spermatozoa are of lysosomal nature and stem from the various components of the acrosomal complex, but others, for example certain glycolytic enzymes, and also cytochrome *c*, are derived from other organelles, including mitochondria. These losses of vital enzymes and coenzymes result in exhaustion of energy sources, deficiency in the mechanism that controls energy transfer and utilization, disturbances in metabolism such as a rapidly falling rate of glycolysis, alterations in the oxidation state of sulphydryl compounds and phospholipids, and the recently discovered formation of organic peroxide.

Nuclear instability is another factor implicated in sperm aging. The mature spermatozoon is a nongrowing, nonmultiplying, and mitotically inert cell, and its ability to synthesize either RNA or protein is very limited. Moreover, what little evidence there is indicates that the minute amount of RNA that the spermatozoa contain is synthesized on the mitochondrial and not the nuclear DNA template. As regards the DNA of the sperm nucleus, the notion that its content changes during sperm aging *in vivo* or *in vitro* is no longer tenable. It is now clear that variations in the so-called Feulgen stainability of aging spermatozoa are due not to alterations in the DNA content *per se* but are probably a reflection of changes in the deoxyribonucleoprotein as a whole.

In investigations with mammalian semen, particularly with spermatozoa stored *in vitro* or surviving in the female reproductive tract, it has been noticed repeatedly that the fertilizing ability of spermatozoa can be lost before cessation of motility and metabolic activity. A similar phenomenon has been described in semen subjected to short-wave irradiation. These observations show how much the definition of sperm aging depends on the choice of criteria applied in the evaluation of sperm viability.

Acknowledgments

We are greatly indebted to Dr. H. M. DOTT and Mr. R. PATMAN for providing the photomicrographs of spermatozoa, and to the Editors of the Biochemical Journal for the permission to reproduce figure 3.

References

ABRAHAM, K. A. and BHARGAVA, P. M.: Nucleic acid metabolism of mammalian spermatozoa. Biochem. J. *86:* 298 (1963).
ACKERMAN, D. R. and SOD-MORIAH, U. A.: DNA content of human spermatozoa after storage at low temperatures. J. Reprod. Fertil. *17:* 1 (1968).
ADELMAN, R. C.: Age-dependent control of enzyme adaptation. Adv. Gerontol. Res. *4:* 1 (1972).
ALLISON, A. C. and HARTREE, E. F.: Lysosomal nature of the acrosomes of ram spermatozoa. Biochem. J. *111:* 35 P (1968).
ALLISON, A. C. and HARTREE, E. F.: Lysosomal enzymes in the acrosome and the possible role in fertilization. J. Reprod. Fertil. *21:* 501 (1970).
AMELAR, R. D.: Infertility in men. (Davis, Philadelphia 1966).
BAHR, G. F. and ENGLER, W. F.: Considerations of volume, mass, DNA, and arrangement of mitochondria in the midpiece of bull spermatozoa. Exp. Cell Res. *60:* 338 (1970).
BARBER, A. A. and BERNHEIM, F.: Lipid peroxidation: its measurement, occurrence and significance in animal tissues. Adv. Gerontol. Res. *2:* 355 (1967).

BARONOS, S.; MANN, T.; ROWSON, L.E.A., and SKINNER, J.D.: The effect of nutrition and androgens on the composition of bovine blood plasma and seminal plasma at puberty. Brit. J. Nutr. *23:* 191 (1969).

BEHRMAN, S.J.: Preservation of human sperm by liquid nitrogen vapour freezing; in INGELMAN-SUNDBERG and LUNELL Current problems in fertility, p. 10 (Plenum Publishing, New York 1971).

BERNHEIM, F.: Biochemical implications of pro-oxidants and antioxidants. Radiat. Res. Suppl. *3:* 17 (1963).

BERNHEIM, F.; BERNHEIM, M.L.C., and WILBUR, K.M.: The reaction between thiobarbituric acid and the oxidation products of certain lipids. J. biol. Chem. *174:* 257 (1948).

BISHOP, M.W.H. and HANCOCK, J.L.: Unpublished observations (1951). cf HANCOCK, J.L.: The morphology of bull spermatozoa, J. exp. Biol. *29:* 445 (1952).

BLACKSHAW, A.W. and SALISBURY, G.W.: Factors influencing metabolic activity of bull spermatozoa. Cold shock and its prevention. J. Dairy Sci. *40:* 1099 (1957).

BLACKSHAW, A.W. and SALISBURY, G.W.: The effect of storage *in vitro* on the DNA content of bull spermatozoa. Austr. J. Biol. Sci. *25:* 175 (1972).

BOUTERS, R.; ESNAULT, C.; SALISBURY, G.W., and ORTAVANT, R.: Discrepancies in analyses of deoxyribonucleic acid in rabbit spermatozoa, involving Feulgen staining (Feulgen-DNA) and ultraviolet light absorption (UV-DNA) measurements. J. Reprod. Fertil. *14:* 355 (1967).

BROOKS, D.E. and MANN, T.: Relation between the oxidation state of nicotinamide-adenine dinucleotide and the metabolism of spermatozoa. Biochem. J. *129:* 1023 (1972).

CAMPBELL, R.C.; DOTT, H.M., and GLOVER, T.D.: Nigrosin eosin as a stain for differentiating live and dead spermatozoa. J. agric. Sci. *48:* 1 (1956).

CARLBORG, L.: Some problems involved in freezing and insemination with human sperm; in INGELMAN-SUNDBERG and LUNELL, Current problems in fertility, p. 23 (Plenum Publishing, New York 1971).

CHANG, M.C. and PINCUS, G.: Fertilizable life of rabbit sperm deposited into different parts of the female tract. Proc. 5th Int. Congr. Anim. Reprod., Trento 1964, vol. 4, p. 377.

CHANG, M.C. and WALTON, A.: The effects of low temperature and acclimatization on the respiratory activity and survival of ram spermatozoa. Proc. roy. Soc. B *129:* 517 (1940).

CLEGG, E.J.: The effect of arterial interruption on the fructose content of the rat coagulating gland. Proc. Soc. Study Fertil. *6:* 7 (1954).

COLLINS, W.E.; INSKEEP, E.K.; DREHER, W.H.; TYLER, W.J., and CASIDA, L.E.: Effect of age on fertility of bulls in artificial insemination. J. Dairy Sci. *45:* 1015 (1962).

CRABO, B.G.; BOWER, R.E.; BROWN, K.I.; GRAHAM, E.F., and PACE, M.M.: Extracellular glutamic-oxaloacetic transaminase as a measure on membrane injury in spermatozoa during treatment; in INGELMAN-SUNDBERG and LUNELL, Current problems in fertility, p. 33 (Plenum Publishing, New York 1971).

CRISTOFALO, V.J.: Animal cell cultures as a model system for the study of aging. Adv. Gerontol. Res. *4:* 45 (1972).

CZAUDERNA, A.: Jakosc nasienia buhajow aukcyjnych trzech ras w wojewodztwie krakowskim, ze szczegolnym uwzglednieniem wplywu wieku na parametry jakosciowe nasienia. Zeszyty problemowe postepów nauk rolniezych *124:* 157 (1971).

DARIN, A.C.; POULOS, A., and WHITE, I.G.: Phospholipids released by ram, bull and boar spermatozoa after cold-shocking and freezing. J. Reprod. Fertil. *32:* 312 (1973).

DAVIES, D.V.; MANN, T., and ROWSON, L.E.A.: Effect of nutrition on the onset of male sex hormone activity and sperm formation in monozygous bull-calves. Proc. roy. Soc. B *147:* 332 (1957).

DAWSON, R.M.C. and SCOTT, T.W.: Phospholipid composition of epididymal spermatozoa prepared by density gradient centrifugation. Nature, Lond. *202:* 292 (1964).

DOTT, H.M.: Partial staining of spermatozoa in the nigrosin-eosin stain. Proc. 3rd Int. Congr. Anim. Reprod., Cambridge 1956, vol. 3, p. 42.

DREVIUS, L.-O.: Bull spermatozoa as osmometers. J. Reprod. Fertil. *28:* 29 (1972).

EIK-NES, K.B.: On the relationship between testicular blood flow and secretion of testosterone in anaethetized dogs stimulated with human chorionic gonadotrophin. Canad. J. Physiol. Pharmacol. *42:* 671 (1964).

ESNAULT, C.: Reactivation of the Feulgen reaction of ram spermatozoa by dithiothreitol. J. Reprod. Fertil. *32:* 153 (1973).

FINN, C.A.; FITCH, S.M., and HARKNESS, R.D.: Collagen content of barren and previously pregnant uterine horns in old mice. J. Reprod. Fertil. *6:* 405 (1963).

FIRST, N.L.; STRATMAN, F.W., and CASIDA, L.E.: Effect of sperm age on embryo survival in swine. J. anim. Sci. *22:* 135 (1963).

FLIPSE, R.J.: Metabolism of bovine semen. IX. Glutamic-oxaloacetic and glutamic-pyruvic transaminase activities. J. Dairy Sci. *43:* 773 (1960).

FOLEY, C.W. and WILLIAMS, W.L.: Effect of bicarbonate and oviduct fluid on respiration of spermatozoa. Proc. Soc. exp. Biol. Med. *126:* 634 (1967).

FOOTE, R.H.: Aging of spermatozoa during storage in liquid nitrogen. Proc. 4th Tech. Conf. Animal Reproduction and Artificial Insemination, Nat. Ass. Animal Breeders (1972).

FOOTE, R.H.; LARSON, L.L., and HAHN, J.: Can fertility of sires used in artificial insemination be improved. A.I. Digest *20:* 1 (1971).

GLEDHILL, B.L.: Studies on the DNA content, dry mass and optical area of ejaculated spermatozoal heads from bulls with normal and lowered fertility. Acta vet. scand. *7:* 1 (1966).

GLEDHILL, B.L.: Changes in deoxyribonucleoprotein in relation to spermateliosis and the epididymal maturation of spermatozoa. J. Reprod. Fertil. Suppl. *13:* 77 (1971).

GLEDHILL, B.L.; GLEDHILL, M.P.; RIGLER, R., jr., and RINGERTZ, N.R.: Changes in deoxyribonucleoprotein during spermiogenesis in the bull. Exp. Cell Res. *41:* 652 (1966).

GRAHAM, E.F. and PACE, M.M.: Some biochemical changes in spermatozoa due to freezing. Cryobiology *4:* 75 (1967).

GRAY, J.: The senescence of spermatozoa. II. J. exp. Biol. *8:* 202 (1930).

GRAYHACK, J.T.: Changes with aging in human seminal vesicle fluid fructose concentration and seminal vesicle weight. J. Urol., Baltimore *86:* 142 (1961).

GRAYHACK, J.T. and KROPP, K.: Changes with aging in prostatic fluid: citric acid, acid phosphatase and lactic dehydrogenase concentration in man. Trans. amer. Ass. gen.-urin. Surg. *56:* 6 (1964).

GREGOIRE, A.T.; RAKOFF, A.E., and WARD, K.: Glutamic-oxaloacetic transaminase in semen of human, bull and rabbit seminal plasma. Int. J. Fertil. *6:* 73 (1961).

HAHN, H.P. VON: Failures of regulation mechanisms as causes of cellular aging. Adv. Gerontol. Res. *3:* 1 (1971).

HAMNER, C.E. and WILLIAMS, W.L.: Effect of the female reproductive tract on sperm metabolism in the rabbit and fowl. J. Reprod. Fertil. *5:* 143 (1963).

HAMMOND, J. and ASDELL, S.A.: The vitality of the spermatozoa in the male and female reproductive tracts. J. exp. Biol. *4:* 155 (1926).

HARRISON, R.A.P. and WHITE, I.G.: Glycolytic enzymes in the spermatozoa and cytoplasmic droplets of bull, boar and ram, and their leakage after shock. J. Reprod. Fertil. *30:* 105 (1972).

HARTREE, E.F. and MANN, T.: Phospholipids in ram semen: metabolism of plasmalogen and fatty acids. Biochem. J. *80:* 464 (1961).

HAYFLICK, L.: The limited *in vitro* lifetime of human diploid cell strains. Exp. Cell Res. *37:* 614 (1965).

HINSHELWOOD, C.: Decline and death of bacterial populations. Nature, Lond. *167:* 666 (1951).

HORST, C.J.G. VAN DER; HENDRIKSE, J., and GEMERT, W. VAN: Determination of phenylalanine-α-ketoglutarate transaminase in boar semen as a criterion of dilution without loss of fertilizing capacity. Netherl. J. vet. Sci. *5:* 3 (1972).

HUDSON, B.; COGHLAN, J.P., and DULMANIS, A.: Testicular function in man; in Ciba Found. Collog. Endocrinology of the Testis, p. 140 (Churchill, London 1967).

JONES, R. and GLOVER, T.D.: The effects of castration on the composition of epididymal plasma. J. Reprod. Fertil. (in press, 1973).

JONES, R. and MANN, T.: The formation of organic peroxide by ram spermatozoa. Proc. roy. Soc. B (in press, 1973).

JONES, R.C.: Changes occurring in the head of boar spermatozoa: vesiculation or vacuolation of the acrosome? J. Reprod. Fertil. *33:* 113 (1973a).

JONES, R.C.: The plasma membrane of ram, boar and bull spermatozoa. J. Reprod. Fertil. *33:* 179 (1973b).

KAMPSCHMIDT, R.F.; MAYER, D.T., and HERMAN, H.A.: Viability of bull spermatozoa as influenced by various sugars and electrolytes in the storage medium. Res. Bull. Mo. agric. Exp. Stn No. 519 (1953).

KEILIN, D. and HARTREE, E.F.: Further observations on absorption spectra at low temperatures. Nature, Lond. *165:* 504 (1950).

KIRK, E.: The acid phosphatase concentration of prostatic fluid in young, middle-aged, and old individuals. J. Gerontol. *3:* 98 (1948).

KIRK, E.: The effect of testosterone administration on acid phosphatase concentration of the prostatic exprimate in old men. Urol. Cutan. Rev. *53:* 683 (1949).

KOEFOED-JOHNSEN, H.H.; FULKA, J., and KOPECNY, V.: Stability of thymine in spermatozoal DNA during storage *in vitro.* Proc. 4th Int. Congr. Anim. Reprod. and Artif. Insem., Paris 1968, vol. 2, p. 1263.

KOEFOED-JOHNSEN, H.H. and MANN, T.: Studies on the metabolism of semen. IX. Effect of surface active agents with special reference to the oxidation of succinate by spermatozoa. Biochem. J. *57:* 406 (1954).

KOEFOED-JOHNSEN, H.H.; PAVLOK, A., and FULKA, J.: The influence of the ageing of rabbit spermatozoa *in vitro* on fertilizing capacity and embryonic mortality. J. Reprod. Fertil. *26:* 351 (1971).

KOHN, H.I. and LIVERSEDGE, M.: A new aerobic metabolite whose production by brain is inhibited by apomorphine, emetine, ergotomine, epinephrine and menadione. J. Pharmacol. exp. Ther. *62:* 292 (1944).

KOHN, R.R.: Principles of mammalian aging, p. 9 (Prentice Hall, Englewood Cliffs 1971).

KOSKISMIES, A.I.; KORMANO, M., and ALFTHAN, O.: Proteins of the seminiferous tubule fluid in man – evidence for a blood-testis barrier. J. Reprod. Fertil. *32:* 79 (1973).

KUEHNAU, J., jr. und NOWAKOWSKI, H.: Untersuchungen über Ejakulatzitronensäure beim Menschen. Endokrinologie, Lpz. *40:* 1 (1960).

LASLEY, J.F. and BOGART, R.: Some factors affecting the resistance of ejaculated and epididymal spermatozoa of the boar to different environmental conditions. Amer. J. Physiol. *141:* 619 (1944).

LASLEY, J.F.; EASLEY, G.T., and MCKENZIE, F.F.: A staining method for the differentiation of live and dead spermatozoa. Anat. Rec. *82:* 167 (1942).

LASLEY, J.F. and MAYER, D.T.: A variable physiological factor necessary for the survival of bull spermatozoa. J. amer. Sci. *3:* 129 (1944).

LEIDL, W.: Klima und Sexualfunktion männlicher Haustiere. (Schaper, Hannover 1958).

LINDNER, H.R. and MANN, T.: Relationship between the content of androgenic steroids in the testes and the secretory activity of the seminal vesicles in the bull. J. Endocrin. *21:* 341 (1960).

LINZELL, J.L. and SETCHELL, B.P.: The output of spermatozoa and fluid by, and the metabolism of, the isolated perfused testis of the ram. J. Physiol., Lond. *195:* 25 (1968).

LOVELOCK, J.E.: The denaturation of lipid-protein complexes as a cause of damage by freezing. Proc. roy. Soc. *147:* 427 (1957).

MANN, T.: Studies on the metabolism of semen. III. Fructose as a normal constituent of seminal plasma. Site of formation and function of fructose in semen. Biochem. J. *40:* 481 (1946).

MANN, T.: Studies on the metabolism of semen. VII. Cytochrome in human spermatozoa. Biochem. J. *48:* 386 (1951).

MANN, T.: Biochemical basis of spermicidal activity. Proc. Soc. Study Fertil. *9:* 3 (1958).

MANN, T.: The biochemistry of semen and of the male reproductive tract; 2nd. ed. (Methuen, London 1964).

MANN, T.: Appraisal of endocrine testicular activity by chemical analysis of semen and male accessory secretions. Ciba Found. Colloq. Endocrin. *16:* 233 (1967).

MANN, T.: Biochemical aspects of gamete survival in the male and female genital tract. 6th Congr. Int. Reprod. Anim. Insem. Artif., Paris 1968, vol. 1.

MANN, T.: Chemical analysis of semen as a diagnostic aid in reproductive failure. Proc. 6th Wld Congr. Fertil. Steril., Tel Aviv 1968 (Israel Academy of Sciences and Humanities, 1970).

MANN, T.: Advances in male reproductive physiology. Fertil. Steril. *23:* 699 (1972).

MANN, T.; LEONE, E., and POLGE, C.: The composition of the stallion's semen. J. Endocrin. *13:* 279 (1956).

MANN, T. and LUTWAK-MANN, C.: Biological changes underlying the phenomenon of cold shock in spermatozoa. Arch. Sci. Biol. *39:* 578 (1955).

MANN, T.; ROWSON, L.E.A., and HAY, M.: Evaluation of androgenic and gonadotrophic activity in male twin-calves by analysis of seminal vesicles and semen. J. Endocrin. *21:* 361 (1960).

MANN, T.; ROWSON, L.E.A.; SHORT, R.V., and SKINNER, J.D.: The relationship between nutrition and androgenic activity in pubescent twin-calves, and the effect of orchitis. J. Endocrin. *38:* 455 (1967).

MARTIN, G.M.; SPRAGUE, C.A., and EPSTEIN, C.J.: Replicative life-span of cultivated human cells. Effects of donor's age, tissue and genotype. Lab. Invest. *23:* 86 (1970).

MASAKI, J. and HARTREE, E.F.: Distribution of metabolic activity, phospholipid and hyaluronidase between the heads and tails of bull spermatozoa. Biochem. J. *84:* 347 (1962).

MASAKI, J. and TOMIZUKA, T.: Change in phospholipid content of spermatozoa during maturation and aging. II. Change in plasmalogen content of bull spermatozoa during storage at 4°C. Bull. nat. Inst. Anim. Ind. *11:* 91 (1966).

MEDVEDEV, Z.A.: The nucleic acids in development and aging. Adv. Gerontol. Res. *1:* 181 (1964).

MILLER, O.C. and BLACKSHAW, A.W.: The DNA of rabbit spermatozoa aged *in vitro* and its relation to fertilization and embryo survival. Proc. 4th Int. Congr. Anim. Reprod. and Artif. Insem., Paris 1968, vol. 2, p. 1275.

MILOVANOV, V.K.: Iskustvennoe osemenenie s.-h. zivotnyh. (Moscow 1934).

MOHRI, H.; HASEGAWA, S., and MASAKI, J.: Seasonal changes in glycerol kinase activity of goat spermatozoa. Biol. Reprod. *2:* 352 (1970).

MOUNIB, M.S. and CHANG, M.C.: Effect of *in utero* incubation on the metabolism of rabbit spermatozoa. Nature, Lond. *201:* 943 (1964).

MROTEK, J.J.; HOEKSTRA, W.G., and FIRST, N.L.: Effect of boar semen senility on per-oxidation of semen lipids. J. anim. Sci. *25:* 688 (1966).

MURDOCH, R.N. and WHITE, I.G.: The metabolism of labelled glucose by the rabbit spermatozoa after incubation *in utero*. J. Reprod. Fertil. *14:* 213 (1967).

NOWAKOWSKI, H. und SCHMIDT, H.: Das Altern der männlichen Keimdrüsen. Symp. dtsch. Ges. Endokrin., vol. 5, p. 207 (1958).

NOYES, R.W. and THIBAULT, C.: Endocrine factors in the survival of spermatozoa in the female reproductive tract. Fertil. Steril. *13:* 346 (1962).

ORGEBIN-CRIST, M.C. and TICHENOR, P.L.: A technique for studying sperm maturation *in vitro*. Nature, Lond. *239:* 227 (1972).

ORGEL, L.E.: The maintenance of the accuracy of protein synthesis and its relevance to ageing. Proc. nat. Acad. Sci., Wash. *49:* 517 (1963).

PACKER, L.; DEAMER, D.W., and HEATH, R.L.: Regulation and deterioration of structures in membranes. Adv. Gerontol. Res. *2:* 77 (1967).

PAUFLER, S.K. and FOOTE, R.H.: Influence of light on nuclear size and deoxyribonucleic acid content of stored bovine spermatozoa. J. Dairy Sci. *50:* 1475 (1967).

PICKETT, B.W. and KOMAREK, R.J.: Effect of cold shock and freezing on loss of lipid from spermatozoa. J. Dairy Sci. *50:* 753 (1967).

POLGE, C.; SALAMON, S., and WILMUT, I.: Fertilizing capacity of frozen boar semen following surgical insemination. Vet. Rec. 424 (1970).

POULOS, A.; VOGLMAYR, J. K., and WHITE, I. G.: Changes in the phospholipid composition of bovine spermatozoa during their passage through the male reproductive tract. J. Reprod. Fertil. *32:* 309 (1973).

POVOA, H. and VILLELA, G. G.: Transaminase in seminal plasma of man. Experientia *16:* 199 (1960).

PREMKUMAR, E. and BHARGAVA, P. M.: Transcription and translation in bovine spermatozoa. Nature, Lond. *240:* 139 (1972).

QUINN, P. J. and WHITE, I. G.: The effect of cold shock and deep-freezing on the concentration of major cations in spermatozoa. J. Reprod. Fertil. *12:* 263 (1966).

QUINN, P. J. and WHITE, I. G.: Phospholipid and cholesterol content of epididymal and ejaculated ram spermatozoa and seminal plasma in relation to cold shock. Austr. J. Biol. Sci. *20:* 1205 (1967).

QUINN, P. J. and WHITE, I. G.: The effect of pH, cations and protective agents on the susceptibility of ram spermatozoa to cold shock. Exp. Cell Res. *49:* 31 (1968).

ROTTENSTEN, K.: Alderens indflydelse pa tyrenes frugtbarhed. Institut for Sterilitetsforskning Aarsberetning (Annual Report), p. 219 (1972).

RZEZNIK, K.: Wplyw wieku, eksploatacji i zywienia na poziom fruktozy w nasieniu buhajów. Zeszyty problemowe postepów nauk rolniczych *124:* 225 (1971).

SALISBURY, G. W.: Aging phenomena in spermatozoa. III. Effect of season and storage at –79°C to –88°C on fertility and prenatal losses. J. Dairy Sci. *50:* 1683 (1967).

SALISBURY, G. W.; BIRGE, W.; TORRE, L. DE LA, and LODGE, J.: Decrease in nuclear Feulgen-positive material (DNA) upon aging *in vitro* storage of bovine spermatozoa. J. biophys. biochem. Cytol. *10:* 353 (1961).

SALISBURY, G. W. and FLERCHINGER, F. H.: Aging phenomena in spermatozoa. I. Fertility and prenatal losses with use of liquid semen. J. Dairy Sci. *50:* 1675 (1967).

SALISBURY, G. W. and HART, R. G.: Gamete aging and its consequences. Biol. Reprod. Suppl. *2:* 1 (1970).

SANDRITTER, W.: Methods and results in quantitative cytochemistry; in WIED Introduction to quantitative cytochemistry, p. 159 (Academic Press, New York 1966).

SANDRITTER, W.; MÜLLER, D. und GENSECKE, O.: Ultraviolettmikrospektrophotometrische Messungen des Nukleinsäuregehaltes von Spermien und diploiden Zellen. Acta histochem. *10:* 139 (1960).

SCHIRREN, C.: Relation between fructose content of semen and fertility in man. J. Reprod. Fertil. *5:* 347 (1963).

SCOTT, T. W.; VOGLMAYR, J. K., and SETCHELL, B. P.: Lipid composition and metabolism in testicular and ejaculated spermatozoa. Biochem. J. *102:* 456 (1967).

SETCHELL, B. P. and WAITES, G. M.: The effects of local heating of the testis on the flow and composition of rete testis fluid in the rat, with some observations on the effects of age and unilateral castration. J. Reprod. Fertil. *30:* 225 (1972).

SEYMOUR, F. I.; DUFFY, C., and KOERNER, A.: A case of authenticated fertility in man of 94. J. amer. med. Ass. *105:* 1423 (1935).

SHORT, R. V. and MANN, T.: The sexual cycle of a seasonally breeding mammal, the roebuck *(Capreolus capreolus)*. J. Reprod. Fertil. *12:* 337 (1966).

SINGHAL, R. L.: Effect of age on the induction of glucose-6-phosphatase and fructose diphosphatase in rat uterus. J. Gerontol. *22:* 77 (1967).

SOUKUPOVÁ, M.; HOLEČKOVÁ, E., and HNEVKOVSKY, P.: in HOLEČKOVÁ and CRISTOFALO Aging in cell and tissue culture, p. 41 (Plenum Publishing, New York 1970).

STAMBAUGH, R.; BRACKETT, B.G., and MASTROIANNI, L.: Inhibition of *in vitro* fertilization of rabbit ova by trypsin inhibitors. Biol. Reprod. *1:* 223 (1969).

STREHLER, B.L.: The nature of cellular age changes; in WOOLHOUSE Aspects of the biology of ageing, p. 149 (Academic Press, New York 1967).

SUORANTA, H.: Changes in the small blood vessels of the adult human testis in relation to age and to some pathological conditions. Virchows Arch. path. Anat. Abt. A *352:* 165 (1971).

TASH, J.S. and MANN, T.: Adenosine 3′:5′-cyclic monophosphate in semen, and its relation to motility, survival and metabolism of spermatozoa. Proc. roy. Soc. B (in press, 1973).

TESH, J.M. and GLOVER, T.D.: Ageing of rabbit spermatozoa in the male tract and its effect on fertility. J. Reprod. Fertil. *20:* 287 (1969).

TODOROVIC, R.A.; GRAVES, C.N., and SALISBURY, G.W.: Aging phenomena in spermatozoa. IV. Immunoserological characterization of the deoxyribonucleic acid-protein extracted from fresh and aged bovine spermatozoa. J. Dairy Sci. *52:* 1415 (1969).

TOSIC, J. and WALTON, A.: Metabolism of spermatozoa. The formation and elimination of hydrogen peroxide by spermatozoa and effects on motility and survival. Biochem. J. *47:* 199 (1950).

VERMEULEN, A.; RUBENS, R., and VERDONCK, L.: Testosterone secretion and metabolism in male senescence. J. clin. Endocrin. Metab. *34:* 730 (1972).

WHITE, I.G. and WALES, R.G.: The susceptibility of spermatozoa to cold shock. Int. J. Fertil. *5:* 195 (1960).

WHITE, I.G. and WALES, R.G.: Comparison of epididymal and ejaculated semen of the ram. J. Reprod. Fertil. *2:* 225 (1961).

ZANEVELD, L. J. D.; ROBERTSON, R. T.; KESSLER, M., and WILLIAMS, W. L.: Inhibition of fertilization *in vivo* by pancreatic and seminal plasma trypsin inhibitors. J. Reprod. Fertil. *25:* 387 (1971).

Authors' address: Dr. THADDEUS MANN and Dr. CECILIA LUTWAK-MANN, Agricultural Research Council's Unit of Reproductive Physiology and Biochemistry, University of Cambridge, *Cambridge CB2 3EZ* (England)

Aging Gametes. Int. Symp., Seattle 1973, pp. 151–165 (Karger, Basel 1975)

Effects of Aging of Sperm in the Female and Male Reproductive Tracts before Fertilization on the Chromosome Complement of the Blastocysts

Evelyn L. Shaver and Patricia A. Martin-DeLeon

Department of Anatomy, University of Western Ontario, London, Ontario

The effect on fertility of the prolonged storage of sperm has been studied in a variety of invertebrate and vertebrate species. Good reviews of the literature have been published by Lanman [1968] and Salisbury and Hart [1970]. Fertility of a mammal depends on three factors, firstly the number of eggs shed at ovulation, secondly the number of these ova that are fertilized, and thirdly the number of fertilized ova that develop and result in viable young. Aging spermatozoa have an effect on the latter two factors of fertility. Spermatozoa may be aged either in the female reproductive tract before ovulation or in the male tract before ejaculation. In either environment, a decline in fertility occurs with increased storage periods.

Although reports have been published of increased preimplantation loss occurring when oocytes are fertilized by aging spermatozoa [Tesh, 1969; Tesh and Glover, 1969], the detailed examination of these early stages has been reported in a few cases only. Maurer et al. [1969] observed reduced cleavage rates in ova recovered from rabbits inseminated 20 h before ovulation. An increased incidence of dispermy was reported by Harper [1970 a] in oocytes fertilized by spermatozoa that had remained 14 h or longer in the female tract of the rabbit. Many chromosome abnormalities result from anomalies of fertilization and early cleavage and result in early embryonic loss. Carr [1971] has estimated that in the human approximately 40% of early fetal wastage may be due to chromosome abnormalities.

This chapter deals firstly with published data concerning the spontaneous incidence and type of chromosome abnormalities in blastocysts from various species. Secondly, the chromosome complement of rabbit blastocysts arising from oocytes that have been fertilized by spermatozoa aged either in the female tract before ovulation or in the male tract before ejaculation is discussed.

I. The Spontaneous Incidence of Chromosome Abnormalities

The blastocyst stage of development provides a sufficient number of cells for cytogenetic analysis, and various methods have been published that provide preparations technically suitable for the accurate counting and karyotyping of the chromosomes [ISSA *et al.*, 1968; MCFEELY, 1966; SHAVER and CARR, 1967; TARKOWSKI, 1966]. Earlier developmental stages have also been studied; however, the number of cells in metaphase is limited and certain chromosome anomalies, particularly when an additional cell line is present, require that more than one or two metaphases be examined from each zygote.

The incidence of chromosome abnormalities in blastocysts recovered before implantation has been reported for the pig, the cow, the rabbit, and the mouse. The various studies that record control data are listed in table I. A reference is included only when the total number of blastocysts analyzed and a description of the chromosome abnormalities were given. The proportion of blastocysts with demonstrable chromosome abnormalities varied between 1 and 12%. This diversity may be due to species, or to genetic or technical variation. The types of chromosome anomalies reported included polyploidy, mixoploidy, aneuploidy, mosaicism, and structural abnormalities.

Polyploidy, or exact multiples of the haploid number of chromosomes, with the exception of diploidy, occurred in 9 of the 35 abnormalities listed in table I. Seven of the polyploids, 4 triploids and 3 tetraploids, were recovered from gilts [MCFEELY, 1967]. Spontaneous triploidy was not found in any of the blastocysts analyzed from rabbits and only in one of 309 blastocysts recovered from mice [VICKERS, 1969]. A species difference, therefore, is apparent in the incidence of spontaneous triploidy. The remaining polyploid blastocyst was a pentaploid recovered from the rabbit [SHAVER and CARR, 1969]. In addition to the polyploids a haploid was recorded among the blastocysts analyzed by VICKERS [1969].

Mixoploidy, evident when a polyploid cell line is associated with a diploid line, occurred in 5 blastocysts. The most common form was the mixoploid that included a tetraploid cell line and was seen in blastocysts recovered from the cow [MCFEELY and RAJAKOSKI, 1968] and the rabbit [MARTIN and SHAVER, 1972; SHAVER and CARR, 1969]. The only mixoploid not containing a tetraploid line was a 2n/3n blastocyst recovered from a gilt [MCFEELY, 1967].

Aneuploidy is represented by chromosome numbers that are not exact multiples of the haploid complement. Trisomy, in which the chromosome complement has one extra chromosome, was present in 3 of the 36 chromo-

Table I. Chromosome abnormalities in blastocysts of pig, cow, rabbit, and mouse

Authors	Animal	Ovulation	Number of blasto-cysts	Chromosomally abnormal		Abnormalities
				number	per-centage	
McFeely [1967]	pig	spontaneous	88	9	10	4 triploid (3n) 3 tetraploid (4n) 1 mixoploid (2n/3n) 1 structural anomaly
McFeely and Rajakoski [1968]	cow	spontaneous	12	1	8.3	1 mixoploid (2n/4n)
Shaver and Carr [1969]	rabbit	spontaneous	58	1	1.7	1 mosaic (45/44)
Shaver and Carr [1969]	rabbit	induced with 25 iu HCG	73	5	6.8	1 pentaploid (5n) 2 mixoploids (2n/4n and 2n/4n/8n) 1 trisomy (45) 1 structural anomaly
Shaver [1970]	rabbit	induced with 75–300 iu HCG	75	2	2.7	1 mosaic (43/44) 1 structural anomaly
Martin and Shaver [1972]	rabbit	induced with 60 iu HCG	105	1	1.0	1 mixoploid (2n/4n)
Hofsaess and Meacham [1971]	rabbit	induced with 50 iu HCG	75	9	12	2 monosomy (43) 4 hypodiploid (42) 2 mosaics (43/45) 1 hyperdiploid mosaic (47/88)
Vickers [1969]	mouse (albino, PDE strain)	superovulated 3 iu PMSG + 3 iu HCG	309	8	2.6	1 triploid (3n) 1 haploid (n) 2 trisomy (41) 1 hypodiploid mosaic (34/37/39) 2 structural anomalies

somally abnormal blastocysts. Two trisomies were found among mouse [VICKERS, 1969] and one among rabbit [SHAVER and CARR, 1969] blastocysts. No blastocysts exhibiting trisomy have been reported for either the pig or the cow, to date. The only report of a blastocyst missing one or more chromosomes from the diploid complement was that of HOFSAESS and MEACHAM [1971] where 6 of the 9 chromosomally abnormal rabbit blastocysts were hypodiploid. With the exception of one 43/44 mosaic, no case of hypodiploidy has been found in our series of 311 rabbit blastocysts. Differences in technique or genetic background may be responsible for this discrepancy.

Chromosome mosaicism is represented when two or more cell lines are present. Five blastocysts recovered from rabbits were chromosome mosaics. HOFSAESS and MEACHAM [1971] reported two 43/45 mosaics and one hyperdiploid blastocyst with a tetraploid cell line together with cells containing 47 chromosomes. SHAVER and CARR [1969] noted a 44/45 and SHAVER [1970] a 43/44 mosaic blastocyst. A complex hypodiploid mosaic (34/37/39) with a structural anomaly consisting of a minute chromosome present in the 37 cell line was recovered in the mouse [VICKERS, 1969].

Blastocysts with a diploid complement but having one or more chromosomes with structural anomalies visible with the microscope were reported in several instances. A deletion of the short arms of submetacentric chromosomes was observed in blastocysts from the pig [McFEELY, 1967] and the rabbit [SHAVER, 1970]. SHAVER and CARR [1969] described a blastocyst with a chromosome complement showing a deletion of the short arms of a metacentric chromosome and a deletion of the long arms of a submetacentric chromosome. VICKERS [1969] reported the greatest number of structural abnormalities in control data for the mouse. She noted an isochromosome, a minute chromosome and a blastocyst that has 2 cell lines, one with a normal diploid complement and the other with an isochromosome.

II. Chromosome Abnormalities Following Aging Spermatozoa in the Female Tract

The length of time spermatozoa may reside in the female reproductive tract and still be capable of fertilizing oocytes varies considerably with the species studied. The early studies based fertility on the number of live births recorded after various sperm aging periods. A progressive decline in litter size was noted with increasing storage times [LANMAN, 1968; SALISBURY and HART, 1970].

In the rabbit, HAMMOND and ASDELL [1926] noted a marked decrease in litter size when insemination occurred between 26 and 30 h before ovulation. More recently, TESH [1969] studied the effect on fertilization and postimplantation development when spermatozoa were aged in does by varying the time between artificial insemination and the injection of luteinizing hormone. At the 29-hour storage period a significant decrease in the number of ova fertilized and an increase in postimplantation loss were observed.

Detailed examination of the preimplantation stages following fertilization of oocytes by aged spermatozoa was made by MAURER et al. [1969]. Aging sperm for 20 h in the female reproductive tract of the rabbit before ovulation reduced fertilization and cleavage rates. In addition, fewer of the cleaved ova developed into blastocysts in vitro in comparison with ova from control animals.

The chromosome complement of blastocysts recovered from rabbits in which ova were fertilized by aged spermatozoa was studied by MARTIN and SHAVER [1972]. Does were artifically inseminated, then injected with human chorionic gonadotropin (HCG) at various times ranging from 0–21 h postinsemination. Ovulation was presumed to occur 10 h after injection. Therefore spermatozoa remained 10–31 h in the female tract before ovulation. A count of corpora lutea was made at autopsy 6 days after injection to give an indication of the number of ova released.

A graph depicting the percentage of ova recovered as blastocysts following the various sperm storage periods is shown in figure 1. The greatest percentage recovery, 94%, occurred after spermatozoa had resided in the female tract 18 h before ovulation. After this period of aging, the recovery rate decreased until no blastocysts were found at the 31-hour interval. This limit of the fertilizable life of the rabbit spermatozoon is in close agreement with that recorded by HAMMOND and ASDELL [1926] and TESH [1969]. The increase in the percentage of blastocysts recovered at the 18-hour aging period may be due to a greater number of oocytes having been fertilized. BRADEN [1953] noted an increased number of spermatozoa at the site of fertilization about 20 h after mating. HARPER [1970 b] suggested that a newly ovulated oocyte had a better chance of being fertilized at this time.

In the study by MARTIN and SHAVER [1972], cytogenetic analysis of blastocysts revealed 14 chromosome abnormalities. This included one chromosome anomaly, a 2n/4n mixoploid, which was recovered among 105 blastocysts examined in the control series. This gave an incidence of 1% compared with 9.7% reported for the 134 blastocysts obtained from females in the experimental series. The difference was found to be statistically significant. The

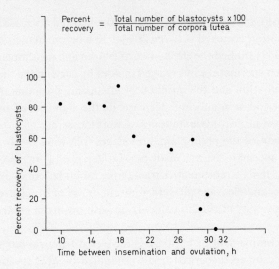

$$\text{Percent recovery} = \frac{\text{Total number of blastocysts} \times 100}{\text{Total number of corpora lutea}}$$

Fig. 1. The effect of aging rabbit spermatozoa in the female reproductive tract on the recovery of blastocysts.

Table II. Chromosome abnormalities and sex ratio of rabbit blastocysts recovered after sperm aging *in utero*

Aging period[1], h	Number of blastocysts karyotyped	Sex[2] ♂	♀	Abnormalities
10 (control)	105/109	51	54	1 mixoploid (2n/4n)
14	24/24	13	10	1 chimera, 2 mosaics (43/44 and 44/45)
16	21/25	12	9	1 mosaic (43/44)
18	30/30	21	9	1 mosaic (43/44), 2 mixoploids (2n/4n and 2n/4n/8n)
20	12/14	3	9	1 mosaic (44/45)
22	11/11	7	3	1 chimera
25	12/13	7	5	
28	18/19	14	3	1 chimera, 2 mixoploids (2n/4n and 2n-1/2n/4n)
29	1/1		1	
30	5/5	3	2	

1 Time between insemination and ovulation.
2 Chimeric blastocysts not included.
Data from MARTIN and SHAVER [1972].

remaining 13 chromosomally anomalous blastocysts were distributed throughout the various aging periods and included mixoploidy, mosaicism, and chimerism (table II).

The mixoploids and mosaic blastocysts would have probably arisen through errors of the early cleavage divisions and therefore are formed of cells derived from a single zygote. The chimeras, however, have cells containing two different sex chromosome complements, XX and XY, and would be derived from two distinct zygote lineages.

Three of the mosaics had a cell line with one chromosome missing (43/44). This was one of the large metacentric chromosomes in two cases and a small acrocentric, perhaps the Y chromosome, in the remainder. The two mosaics with a trisomic cell line had an additional large acrocentric chromosome in one case and a small acrocentric in the other. Errors at the first cleavage division were postulated as probably giving rise to the mosaic blastocysts through chromosomal nondisjunction or lagging at anaphase [MARTIN and SHAVER,1972]. In addition, a blastocyst was found to contain three cell lines, 43/44/88, with the missing chromosome being a medium-sized submetacentric. This blastocyst, because of the tetraploid population was classed as a mixoploid.

The most interesting chromosome abnormality found among the blastocysts was chimerism. The three chimeric blastocysts contained about equal numbers of cells with an XY (fig. 2) and an XX (fig. 3) sex chromosome complement. Chimerism as detected by chromosome analysis has not been reported among blastocysts in any other series. The origin of chimerism was thought to be through dispermy involving the ovum pronucleus and the second polar body [MARTIN and SHAVER, 1972].

III. Chromosome Abnormalities Following Aging Spermatozoa in the Male Tract

Spermatozoa may be aged in the male reproductive tract experimentally by means of bilateral ligation of the corpus epididymis. Thus fresh spermatozoa are prevented from entering the cauda epididymis, vas deferens and, subsequently, the ejaculate. Early studies concerned the loss of fertility, as judged by litter size, of females inseminated with spermatozoa aged in the male tract for varying periods of time. Complete infertility resulted 38 days after surgical ligation of the epididymis in the rabbit [HAMMOND and ASDELL, 1926], 20–35 days in the guinea pig [YOUNG, 1929] and 21 days in the rat

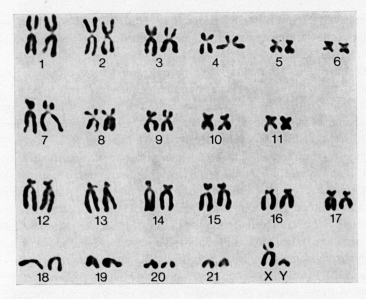

Fig. 2. Karyotype of cell from XY population of a chimeric blastocyst. By permission from MARTIN and SHAVER [1972].

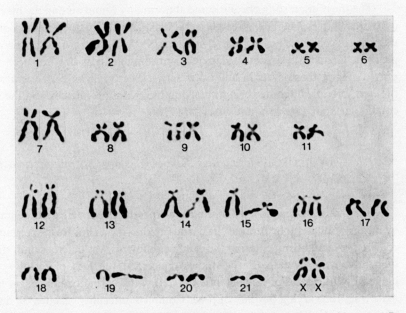

Fig. 3. Karyotype of cell from XX population in the same chimeric blastocyst. By permission from MARTIN and SHAVER [1972].

[WHITE, 1933]. Increased pre- and postimplantation loss and a number of congenital defects were noted in the rabbit [TESH and GLOVER, 1969] and the guinea pig [YOUNG, 1931] with increasing spermatozoal age. IGBOELI and FOOTE [1969] noted a decrease in cleavage of ova and also in litter size when rabbit spermatozoa had aged in the cauda epididymis 28–35 days.

Chromosome analysis of blastocysts recovered from female rabbits inseminated with aged sperm has been reported by MARTIN-DELEON et al. [1973]. In this study, the corpus epididymis was bilaterally ligated in 8 males, and a sham operation performed on 2 males. Ejaculates were collected from each male before operation and at varying intervals afterwards. Females were inseminated with sperm aged at intervals varying from 7–35 days postligation. Other does served as controls, being inseminated with ejaculates obtained from each male 2–4 days before operation and from 6 additional males that did not undergo epididymal ligation. Semen collected 21–35 days after ligation contained a large number of nonmotile spermatozoa. Anomalous forms were found among spermatozoa aged 14 days, including decapitated spermatozoa and a number with head cap and tail defects. At 7 days postligation, head cap abnormalities were the main anomalies seen in smears.

A decrease in the recovery rate of blastocysts was first observed at the 19- to 21-day interval. No blastocysts were obtained from 3 females inseminated with 35-day-old sperm (table III). This result agreed closely with that of HAMMOND and ASDELL [1926] in which litter size decreased at the 20 days aging interval with complete infertility noted at 38 days.

The incidence of chromosome abnormalities in the experimental group was significantly greater than that in the control group. Eight of 72, or 11%, of the blastocysts recovered from females inseminated with spermatozoa aged 7–27 days were chromosomally abnormal compared with 1/125, or 0.8%, for the controls (table III). One triploid (66, XXY) and two mixoploid blastocysts were recovered after spermatozoa had aged 7 days. Oocytes fertilized by spermatozoa aged 12 days or longer gave rise to 5 blastocysts with chromosome abnormalities. Trisomy was the most frequent anomaly with 3 of the blastocysts having an extra chromosome in all cells and one mosaic blastocyst containing a trisomic as well as a diploid cell line. The remaining chromosome abnormality was a structural anomaly, in which a deletion of the short arm of a homologue of chromosome 5 had occurred.

A preliminary study of the influence of prolonged periods of sexual rest on fertilization and early cleavage that may lead to chromosomally anomalous blastocysts has been initiated [SHAVER, unpublished]. To date four males, rested for periods of 28, 42, 49 and 56 days, were mated to females. The fe-

Table III. Chromosome abnormalities and sex ratio of rabbit blastocysts recovered after sperm aging in male tract[1]

Aging period, days	Number of females	Number of blastocysts karyotyped	Sex		Abnormalities
			♂	♀	
0[2]	2	20/24	10	10	
0[3]	13	105/109	51	54	1 mixoploid (2n/4n)
7	3	23/24	15[4]	8	2 mixoploids (2n/4n)
					1 triploid, XXY
12–15	4	32/32	16	16	1 trisomy
					1 mosaic (44/45)
					1 structural anomaly
19–21	2	8/9	3	5	2 trisomies
27	1	9/9	2	7	
35	3				

1 Corpus epididymis ligated bilaterally.
2 Sham operation.
3 Controls.
4 Triploid included.
Data from MARTIN-DELEON *et al.* [1973].

males were killed 6 days later; the blastocysts were recovered and examined chromosomally. A normal recovery rate was observed throughout the various aging periods with a total of 42 blastocysts recovered from the four females. Forty of the blastocysts could be examined chromosomally. Two abnormalities, a trisomy and a 43/44 mosaic, were recovered from females mated to males rested for periods of 42 and 49 days, respectively. A preponderance of the XX sex chromosome complement was noted, with 25 of the 40 blastocysts having the XX and 15 the XY complex.

In a study of the influence of infrequent collection of rabbit spermatozoa on fertility and embryonic mortality, MILLER *et al.* [1970] could detect no statistically significant difference in semen quality, fertilization rate, or embryonic mortality. Obviously, more data needs to be collected on the incidence of chromosome abnormalities in blastocysts recovered from does mated with sexually rested males. However, it is of interest that a trisomic blastocyst was found in the series and that trisomy was also increased among blastocysts arising from oocytes fertilized by spermatozoa aged in the male reproductive tract following ligation of the corpus epididymis.

IV. Discussion

Aging of the male gamete *in vivo* appears to lead to an increased incidence of chromosomally anomalous embryos in the rabbit. Of considerable interest is the type of chromosome abnormalities found in blastocysts arising from oocytes fertilized by spermatozoa aged in the two different environments as compared with the number and type of spontaneous anomalies recorded.

Chimerism was the most interesting chromosome anomaly that appeared when spermatozoa were aged in the female reproductive tract. FORD [1969] reviewed the mechanisms that lead to chimerism. The two main routes postulated were through two separate acts of syngamy or contributions from two independent zygotes. Chimeras have been produced experimentally in mice by the fusion of two separate morulae after removal of the zona pellucida [MINTZ, 1962; TARKOWSKI, 1961]. However, spontaneous fusion of zygotes would be difficult in the rabbit because of the barrier formed by the thick mucin coat. The more probable origin of chimerism in the rabbit is through two acts of syngamy, such as dispermy with participation of the ovum pronucleus and the second polar body. The retention of the second polar body (digyny) has been reported to occur with increased frequency when rabbit ova were fertilized by aged spermatozoa [THIBAULT, 1967]. Similarly, dispermy has been observed in rabbit eggs when spermatozoa resided in the female tract 14 h or more before ovulation [HARPER, 1970 a]. Recently, HUNTER [1973] noted polyspermic fertilization in pig oocytes after tubal deposition of excessive numbers of spermatozoa and concluded that the incidence of polyspermy was significantly increased when large numbers of capacitated spermatozoa meet newly ovulated eggs.

The chromosome abnormalities detected in blastocysts arising from oocytes fertilized by spermatozoa aged in the male tract may have resulted either from a change in the genetic information contributed by the spermatozoon [SALISBURY and HART, 1970] or from delayed fertilization. Impaired motility of spermatozoa leading to delayed fertilization of an oocyte has been proposed as contributing to the increase in polyploid ova observed after insemination with epididymal spermatozoa [ORGEBIN-CRIST, 1968]. Triploidy has been associated with delayed fertilization in the rabbit [SHAVER and CARR, 1969]. The triploid blastocyst recovered after 7 days aging of sperm [MARTIN-DELEON *et al.*, 1973] could be attributed to postovulatory aging of the oocyte caused by the delayed fertilization that resulted from the aged spermatozoa's impaired progression to the site of fertilization.

Trisomy, the anomaly that occurs most frequently at the longer storage periods, is usually associated with chromosomal nondisjunction or anaphase lagging of chromatids at the second meiotic division. Aged spermatozoa may result in abnormal activation of the egg at the time of fertilization so that the second meiotic division of the ovum does not proceed normally. It is also possible that spermatozoa containing an abnormal genome arising at spermatogenesis would have a greater advantage in competing for fertilization sites because of the lack of fresh spermatozoa in the ejaculates following ligation of the corpus epididymis.

The chromosome anomalies associated with spermatozoa aged in the male tract, such as triploidy and trisomy for large autosomes, are usually lethal during embryonic and fetal development. Mixoploidy, mosaicism, and chimerism, the abnormalities found when spermatozoa were aged in the female, are more compatible with life. The greater postimplantation loss and the larger number of fetal abnormalities reported in the rabbit following fertilization by spermatozoa aged in the male [TESH and GLOVER, 1969] compared with fertilization by spermatozoa aged in the female tract [TESH, 1969] may be associated with the greater lethal effect of the various forms of heteroploidy found among the blastocysts.

The sex ratio of blastocysts resulting from oocytes fertilized by spermatozoa aged in the female tract showed a greater proportion with the XY sex chromosome complex (table II). Although the difference was not significant when compared with the sex ratio of the control series [MARTIN and SHAVER, 1972], it was in agreement with the observation made by HAMMOND and ASDELL [1926] that a slightly greater number of males arose after ova were fertilized by spermatozoa aged in the female tract. On the other hand, the percentage of females in litters born following aging of sperm for 20 days or longer in the male was observed to be markedly increased [HAMMOND and ASDELL, 1926]. From the very limited data available for blastocysts, this same observation can be made. There were twice the number of blastocysts with an XX sex chromosome complement following aging of sperm in the male tract of at least 20 days than blastocysts with an XY complement (table III). Also after periods of sexual rest, the proportion of females appeared to be greater. It may be that the X-bearing spermatozoon remains viable for a longer period following aging in the male reproductive tract. Confirmation of this preliminary observation awaits further research.

Additional studies should be done to determine the incidence and types of chromosome abnormalities that may arise following fertilization of oocytes by aged spermatozoa. Pre- and postimplantation embryos of a variety of species should be investigated. The effect of *in vitro* storage of spermatozoa on the chromosome complement of resulting embryos would be a most interesting study. From the preliminary efforts described in this chapter, it appears that aging of the male gamete may be an important factor in causing chromosomally abnormal zygotes and embryos.

Summary

1. The chromosome complement of blastocysts has been reported for the pig, cow, rabbit, and mouse. Polyploidy, mixoploidy, aneuploidy, mosaics, and structural anomalies have been described.

2. The incidence of chromosome anomalies following sperm aged in the female reproductive tract of the rabbit was 9.7% and included chimerism, mixoploidy, and mosaics. The origin of the chimeric blastocysts was attributed to dispermy involving the ovum pronucleus and the second polar body. The limit of the fertilizable life of the rabbit spermatozoon is approximately 30 h in the female tract.

3. The chromosome complement of rabbit blastocysts arising from oocytes fertilized by spermatozoa aged in the male tract following bilateral ligation of the corpus epididymis was examined. The incidence of chromosome abnormalities was 11% and included triploidy, mixoploidy, and trisomy. The limit of the fertilizable life of the spermatozoon was approximately 4 weeks.

Acknowledgments

We wish to acknowledge the technical assistance of Miss ISOBEL MORRISON. This work was supported by a grant from the Medical Research Council of Canada.

References

BRADEN, A.W.H.: Distribution of sperms in the genital tract of the female rabbit after coitus. Austr. J. Biol. Sci. *6:* 693 (1953).

CARR, D.H.: Chromosome studies in selected spontaneous abortions. III. Early pregnancy loss. Obstet. Gynec. *37:* 750 (1971).

FORD, C.E.: Mosaics and chimaeras. Brit. med. Bull. *25:* 104 (1969).

HAMMOND, J. and ASDELL, S.A.: The vitality of the sperm in the male and female reproductive tracts. J. exp. Biol. *4:* 155 (1926).

HARPER, M.J.K.: Cytological observations on sperm penetration of rabbit eggs. J. exp. Zool. *174:* 141 (1970a).

HARPER, M.J.K.: Factors influencing sperm penetration of rabbit eggs *in vivo.* J. exp. Zool. *173:* 47 (1970b).

Hofsaess, F.R. and Meacham, T.N.: Chromosome abnormalities of early rabbit embryos. J. exp. Zool. *177:* 9 (1971).

Hunter, R.H.F.: Polyspermic fertilization in pigs after tubal deposition of excessive numbers of spermatozoa. J. exp. Zool. *183:* 57 (1973).

Igboeli, G. and Foote, R.H.: Maturation and aging changes in rabbit spermatozoa isolated by ligatures at different levels of the epididymis. Fertil. Steril. *20:* 506 (1969).

Issa, M.; Atherton, G.W., and Blank, C.E.: Chromosomes of the domestic rabbit *Oryctolagus cuniculus*. Cytogenetics *7:* 361 (1968).

Lanman, J.T.: Delays during reproduction and their effects on the embryo and fetus. I. Aging of sperm. New Engl. J. Med. *278:* 993 (1968).

Martin, P.A. and Shaver, E.L.: Sperm aging *in utero* and chromosomal anomalies in rabbit blastocysts. Develop. Biol. *28:* 480 (1972).

Martin-DeLeon, P.A.; Shaver, E.L., and Gammal, E.B.: Chromosome abnormalities in rabbit blastocysts resulting from spermatozoa aged in the male tract. Fertil. Steril. *24:* 212 (1973).

Maurer, R.R.; Whitener, R.H., and Foote, R.H.: Relationship of *in vivo* gamete aging and exogenous hormones to early embryo development in rabbits. Proc. Soc. exp. Biol. Med. *131:* 882 (1969).

McFeely, R.A.: A direct method for the display of chromosomes from early pig embryos. J. Reprod. Fertil. *11:* 161 (1966).

McFeely, R.A.: Chromosome abnormalities in early embryos of the pig. J. Reprod. Fertil. *13:* 579 (1967).

McFeely, R.A. and Rajakoski, E.: Chromosome studies on early embryos of the cow. Proc. 6th Int. Congr. Anim. Reprod., Paris 1968, vol. 2, p. 905.

Miller, O.C.; Graves, C.N., and Lodge, J.R.: Influence of *in vivo* aging of rabbit spermatozoa caused by infrequent collection on fertility and embryonic mortality. J. anim. Sci. *30:* 549 (1970).

Mintz, B.: Formation of genotypically mosaic mouse embryos. Amer. Zool. *2:* 432 (1962).

Orgebin-Crist, M.C.: Maturation of spermatozoa in the rabbit epididymis: delayed fertilization in does inseminated with epididymal spermatozoa. J. Reprod. Fertil. *16:* 29 (1968).

Salisbury, G.W. and Hart, R.G.: Gamete aging and its consequences. Biol. Reprod. *1:* suppl. 2 (1970).

Shaver, E.L.: The chromosome complement of blastocysts from rabbits injected with various doses of HCG before ovulation. J. Reprod. Fertil. *23:* 335 (1970).

Shaver, E.L. and Carr, D.H.: Chromosome abnormalities in rabbit blastocysts following delayed fertilization. J. Reprod. Fertil. *14:* 415 (1967).

Shaver, E.L. and Carr, D.H.: The chromosome complement of rabbit blastocysts in relation to the time of mating and ovulation. Canad. J. Genet. Cytol. *11:* 287 (1969).

Tarkowski, A.K.: Mouse chimaeras developed from fused eggs. Nature, Lond. *190:* 857 (1961).

Tarkowski, A.K.: An air-drying method for chromosome preparations from mouse eggs. Cytogenetics *5:* 394 (1966).

Tesh, J.M.: Effects of the ageing of rabbit spermatozoa *in utero* on fertilisation and prenatal development. J. Reprod. Fertil. *20:* 299 (1969).

TESH, J.M. and GLOVER, T.D.: Ageing of rabbit spermatozoa in the male tract and its effect on fertility. J. Reprod. Fertil. *20:* 287 (1969).

THIBAULT, C.: Analyse comparée de la fécondation et de ses anomalies chez la brebis, la vache et la lapine. Ann. Biol. anim. Biochim. Biophys. *7:* 5 (1967).

VICKERS, A.D.: Delayed fertilization and chromosomal anomalies in mouse embryos. J. Reprod. Fertil. *20:* 69 (1969).

WHITE, W.E.: The duration of fertility and the histological changes in the reproductive organs after ligation of the vasa efferentia in the rat. Proc. roy. Soc. B *113:* 544 (1933).

YOUNG, W.C.: A study of the function of the epididymis. II. The importance of an ageing process in sperm for the length of the period during which fertilizing capacity is retained by sperm isolated in the epididymis of the guinea pig. J. Morphol. Physiol. *48:* 475 (1929).

YOUNG, W.C.: A study of the function of the epididymis. III. Functional changes undergone by spermatozoa during their passage through the epididymis and vas deferens of the guinea pig. J. exp. Biol. *8:* 151 (1931).

Authors' address: Dr. EVELYN L. SHAVER and Dr. PATRICIA A. MARTIN-DELEON, Department of Anatomy, University of Western Ontario, *London, Ontario* (Canada)

Aging Gametes. Int. Symp., Seattle 1973, pp. 166–178 (Karger, Basel 1975)

Fertilizing Capacity of Spermatozoa and Fertilizable Life of Eggs from Immature and Mature Rabbits and Rats

M.C. Chang, K. Niwa and Dorothy M. Hunt

Worcester Foundation for Experimental Biology, Shrewsbury, Mass.

The term puberty is commonly used to denote the early stage of reproductive maturity, but the age of puberty, as we all know, varies a great deal depending on species, nutrition and time of birth. According to Asdell [1964], there is very little information on the puberty of the rabbit. The age of puberty in the female rabbit may vary from $5\frac{1}{2}$ (about 23 weeks) to $8\frac{1}{2}$ months (about 36 weeks). In the white rat the age and weight at the time of vaginal opening also varies for different strains from 41 to 77 days and from 88 to 127 g [cf. Asdell, 1964]. Since the attainment of puberty involves many anatomical and physiological developments and is not a sudden event, the age at which puberty occurs is ill-defined. As we are not aware of any systematic studies on the fertilizing capacity of spermatozoa and the fertilizable life of eggs in immature rabbits and rats, we have examined the number and motility of spermatozoa in the epididymis and induced ovulation by administration of gonadotrophin in these animals at different ages.

I. Animals and Methods

New Zealand white rabbits of relatively pure strain were purchased from a local farm. Adult animals more than 24 weeks old and immature animals with a known date of birth were kept in the laboratory for at least 3 weeks before use.

Immature male rabbits, at least two in each age group, were killed. The caput, corpus, and the cauda of epididymis and the vas deferens were separated and placed in a watch glass. The vas and cauda were flushed with TC

199 (Difco) by means of a 21-gauge needle connected to a syringe, and the caput and corpus were chopped up in saline. The number of spermatozoa in each watch glass and their mobility were then determined. For the study of the fertilizing capacity, only spermatozoa recovered from the cauda were used, and only those samples containing about one million spermatozoa were inseminated in a mature female rabbit.

For the study of ovulation, egg recovery, and fertilization in immature rabbits, at least two young females in each age group were intravaginally inseminated with sperm (20–100 million/rabbit) collected from adult male rabbits by means of an artificial vagina. Soon after insemination the mature and immature rabbits were intravenously injected with 40 iu of HCG (Follutein, Squibb) to induce ovulation. To study the span of the fertilizable life of eggs, 14- to 17-week-old female rabbits were intravenously injected with HCG, and they were either inseminated or twice mated at 8–14 h after injection of HCG.

The mature and immature rabbits were killed about 1 day after insemination or injection of HCG. The ovulation spots or corpora lutea (CL) in the ovaries were counted. Their Fallopian tubes and uteri were flushed with saline for the recovery of eggs. The recovered eggs were mounted on a slide, stained, and examined for evidences of fertilization [Chang, 1952].

White rats of CD strain, descended from Sprague-Dawley rats, were purchased from the Charles River Breeding Laboratories. Their age and weight were known when they arrived at the laboratory. They were kept in constant temperature (23–25°C) under artificial light from 07.00 to 19.00 h. To determine the estrus of mature rats 82–137 days old, vaginal smears were taken every morning. The rats were inseminated at various times before ovulation, at 10.00–11.00, 15.00–16.00, 20.00–21.00 h on the day of proestrus and at 01.00–02.00 h on the day of estrus to determine the length of fertilizing life of spermatozoa. For the determination of the fertilizable life of eggs, female rats were inseminated at various times after ovulation, at 04.00–05.00, 08.00–09.00, or 12.00–13.00 h on the day of estrus.

To study the fertilizing life of sperm in immature rats, we induced superovulation in the 22- to 26-day-old rats by a subcutaneous injection of 10 iu of PMS (Sigma). They were then injected intraperitoneally with 10 iu of HCG 48–52 h later. They were inseminated at either 7–8 or 2–3 h before the injection of HCG or 2–3 or 7–8 h after it. To determine the fertilizable life of eggs in immature rats, 22- to 25-day old rats were superovulated by the same means; however, the HCG was injected 39–40 h after injection of PMS. They were inseminated at 2–13, 16–17, or 20–21 h after the injection of HCG.

Table I. Spermatozoa in the epididymis of immature and mature New Zealand white rabbits

Ages of males, weeks	Number of rabbits examined	Body weight, kg	Weight of testicles, g	Spermatozoa in the epididymis (caput, corpus, cauda, vas)[1]	Total number of sperm in the epididymis (in million)
4,5,6,8,12	10	0.385–3.10	0.3–1.29	0	0
13,14,15	8	2.7–3.8	1.44–3.21	0 →+++ 0 (NM → PM)	0–1.25
16,17,18	11	3.2–4.4	3.9–5.38	0 →++++ (AM → PM)	0–494
19,20,21	9	3.6–4.9	3.4–7.2	++++ (AM → PM)	101–900
22,23	5	4.0–5.2	4.2–7.1	++++ (AM → PM)	140–1,565

Number of spermatozoa (in million) in the epididymes of 22- and 23-week-old rabbits:

Caput	83 (27–153)	9 %
Corpus	71 (4–152)	8 %
Cauda	713 (110–1,376)	80 %
Vas	31 (0.2–73)	4 %
		101 %

1 NM = no motility, AM = active motility, PM = progressive motility.

Table II. Fertilizing capacity of spermatozoa from the cauda and vas of immature rabbits inseminated to mature females

Ages of males, weeks	Number of males used	Number mature females inseminated	Number of sperm/female (in million)	Total number of corpora lutea	Total number of eggs recovered (%)	Total number of eggs fertilized (%)
16, 17, 18	5	13	0.9–77	130	130 (100)	123 (95)
19, 20, 21	7	21	14–104	230	221 (96)	192 (87)
22, 23	4	12	28–189	131	121 (92)	111 (92)

Spermatozoa were obtained by pressing the cauda epididymis of male rats at various ages, and the sperm mass was suspended in a medium without bovine serum albumin [TOYODA and CHANG, 1974]. Intra-uterine insemination was performed in immature and mature female rats by injecting 0.05 and 0.1 ml of sperm suspension ($0.75–2.36 \times 10^6$ sperm), respectively, into each uterine horn by means of a 30-gauge needle attached to a tuberculin syringe. In order to avoid the leakage of sperm the uterine cervix was ligated before insemination for those rats inseminated 8–9 h after ovulation, and the muscle and skin were sutured.

Mature and immature female rats were killed 1–2 days after insemination. Eggs were flushed from the oviducts by means of a 30-gauge needle attached to a syringe, mounted *in toto* [CHANG, 1952], and stained and examined for evidence of fertilization. The cleaved and pronuclear eggs with fertilizing sperm tail were considered as fertilized. Eggs with sperm in the perivitelline space were not considered as fertilized.

II. Results

The epididymis of 43 New Zealand albino rabbits, age of 4–23 weeks, were examined (table I). Although their body weight increased from 0.385 to 3.10 kg, and the weight of both testicles increased from $0.3 \pm$ to 1.29 g, spermatozoa were not found in any part of the epididymis of the rabbits of 4–12 weeks. At the age of 13–15 weeks, body weight increased only about 1 kg, and their testicular weight doubled. Some animals had no sperm; others had a few immotile or motile sperm in the caput, corpus and cauda of the epididymis. Only a few rabbits had sperm in their vas deferentia. At the age of 16–18 weeks, only one animal had no sperm; all the others had sperm (a total of 2.5 to 494 million) throughout their male tracts. The total number of sperm in the epididymis and vas deferentia increased from 100 to 1,565 million between the ages of 19 and 23 weeks.

Since the number of sperm recovered from rabbits 13–15 weeks old was insufficient for insemination, sperm recovered from the cauda epididymis of rabbits 16–23 weeks old were used for insemination of mature rabbits. From the results presented in table II it is clear that there is no difference in the number of eggs fertilized whether sperm were from 16- or 23-week-old males. It seems that as long as there were sufficient numbers of sperm in the cauda, the fertilizing capacity of spermatozoa from animals of different ages was very much the same.

Table III. Ovulation, fertilization and the recovery of eggs from the immature rabbits following insemination and injection of HCG

Ages of females, weeks	Number of rabbits inseminated	Body weight, kg	Total number of CL (range)	Total number of eggs recovered (range)	Total number of eggs fertilized (range)
4, 5, 8	6	0.48–2.2	0	0	0
10, 12, 13	12	2.24–3.05	75 (1–10)	12[1] (0–4) (16%)	0
14, 15	10[2]	3.1–3.45	101 (1–18)	73[1] (0–10) (73%)	19 (0–10) (26%)
16, 17, 18	11[2]	3.45–4.1	102 (4–13)	79[1] (0–13) (78%)	58 (0–12) (74%)
19, 20	9[2]	3.3–4.7	98 (8–15)	96 (7–14) (98%)	74 (0–14) (77%)

1 A few eggs recovered from the uterus 1 day after injection of HCG.
2 Seven of 30 animals had old corpora lutea.

When 6 immature female rabbits from 4 to 8 weeks old were injected intravenously with 40 iu of HCG, ovulation was not induced in all of them, and no follicles were seen in their ovaries. At the age of 10–13 weeks when their body weights increased from 2.24 to 3.05 kg, ovulation was induced by the administration of HCG in all 12 young rabbits although from 75 ovulations only 16% of eggs were recovered including a few eggs recovered from the uterus. Most of these 12 rabbits were inseminated with sperm collected from mature bucks, but not one of the recovered eggs was fertilized. At the age of 14–15 weeks, the number of eggs shed per animal increased. Most of the eggs (73%) were recovered but only 26% of them were fertilized. The recovery rate (78–98%) and fertilization rate (74–77%) reached the normal level at the age of 16–20 weeks (table III). It thus seems that reproductive maturity occurred earlier in the females than in the males (fig. 1) and that the proper development of the female reproductive tract is important for transport and fertilization of eggs.

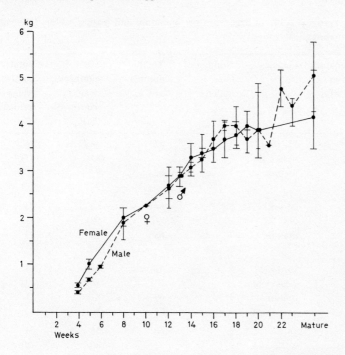

Fig. 1. Production of gametes (♂, ♀) in relation to the age and body weight of New Zealand white rabbits.

Table IV. Fertilizable life of eggs from the immature and mature rabbits following delayed insemination

Time of insemination (hours after injection of HCG)	Females	Number of females inseminated	Total number of CL	Total number of eggs recovered (%)	Total number of eggs fertilized (%)
8	14, 17, 18 weeks old	8	78	67 (86)	59 (88)
	mature	9	108	103 (93)	88 (86)
13	14, 18 weeks old	8	77	71 (92)	12 (17)
	mature	9	100	87 (87)	0 (0)

Table V. Fertilizable life of eggs from the immature and mature rabbits following delayed matings

Time of mating (hours after injection of HCG)	Females[1]	Number of females mated	Total number of CL	Total number of eggs recovered (%)	Total number of eggs fertilized (%)
11	15, 16, 17 weeks old	4	42	34 (81)	16 (47)
	mature	7	82	77 (94)	40 (52)
12	16 weeks old	6	68	63 (93)	23 (37)
	mature	7	68	68 (100)	43 (63)
13	15, 16, 17 weeks old	5	41	31 (76)	4 (13)
	mature	7	69	61 (89)	21 (34)
13.5	16, 17 weeks old	6	64	55 (86)	5 (9)
	mature	7	67	61 (91)	11 (18)
14	16 weeks old	6	67	63 (94)	4 (6)
	mature	7	72	68 (95)	0 (0)

1 Data of mature animals were derived from ADAMS and CHANG [1962].

To determine the fertilizable life of eggs following delayed insemination, immature female rabbits 14–18 weeks old were inseminated with sperm collected from mature males at 8 and 13 h after intravenous injection of HCG. Results presented in table IV indicate that fertilizable life of eggs from immature animals may be slightly longer. In the immature rabbits 17% of the eggs were fertilized but none was fertilized in the mature rabbits when they were inseminated with the same sperm samples 13 h after injection of HCG. Immature rabbits of 15–17 weeks were mated twice by fertile mature bucks at various times after injection of HCG (table V). Results were compared with those obtained from a previous experiment under the same conditions. Although fertilization did occur in the immature rabbits inseminated 14 h after

Table VI. Fertilizing life of spermatozoa from old and immature rats in the female tract of mature and immature rats

Age of males	Time of insemination (hours before the expected time of ovulation)[1]	Mature females (82–137 days old)			Immature females (24–28 days old)		
		number of females used	number of eggs examined	number of eggs fertilized (%)	number of females used	number of eggs examined	number of eggs fertilized (%)
About 330–360 days	2–3 (4–5)	10	132	127 (96)	12	295	192 (65)
	7–8 (9–10)	9	128	93 (72)	11	421	147 (35)
	12–13 (14–15)	10	134	43 (32)	13	473	134 (28)
	17–18 (19–20)	9	126	12 (10)	10	346	16 (5)
64–68 days	2–3 (4–5)	9	128	100 (78)	8	161	100 (62)
	7–8 (9–10)	8	108	18 (17)	11	208	31 (15)
	12–13 (14–15)	8	103	13 (13)	10	207	13 (6)
	17–18 (19–20)	8	104	5 (5)	9	314	11 (4)

1 Figures in parentheses in this column denote the expected time of ovulation in immature rats.

injection of HCG, the fertilization rates in mature animals inseminated from 11 to 13.5 hours after injection of HCG appeared to be higher than that in immature animals treated the same way.

   To determine the fertilizing life of spermatozoa in the female tract, mature female rats (82–137 days old) at proestrus and immature female rats (24–28 days old) treated with PMS and HCG were inseminated at various times before ovulation with spermatozoa obtained from the cauda epididymis of old rats (about 330–360 days old) and from immature rats (64–68 days old), some of whom had no sperm and some of whom had sufficient numbers of spermatozoa in their cauda epididymis for insemination). From table VI it can be seen that the fertilizing life of spermatozoa in the female tract lasted

Table VII. Fertilizable life of eggs from mature and immature rats following delayed insemination with spermatozoa from old, mature, and immature rats

Age of males	Time of insemination (hours after the expected time of ovulation)	Mature females (80–98 days old)				Immature females (24–27 days old)			
		number of females used	number of eggs examined	number of fertilized eggs (%)	percent of abnormal fertilization[1]	number of females used	number of eggs examined	number of fertilized eggs (%)	percent of abnormal fertilization[1]
About 330–360	0–1	8	114	59 (52)	39	13	456	228 (50)	43
	4–5	9	118	33 (28)	24	11	352	37 (11)	57
	8–9	8	98	8 (8)	25	9	302	11 (4)	46
99–152 days	0–1	8	101	69 (68)	51	14	389	274 (70)	43
	4–5	8	110	41 (37)	39	10	389	60 (15)	55
	8–9	8	111	17 (15)	41	11	233	36 (16)	61
64–68 days	0–1	8	105	53 (51)	47	9	204	57 (28)	70
	4–5	8	102	14 (14)	36	9	236	4 (2)	75
	8–9	9	131	17 (13)	35	7	161	2 (1)	0

1 The fertilized eggs had supplementary sperm, dispersed nucleus or other abnormalities.

about 18–20 h. Because the interval between insemination and the expected time of ovulation was 1–2 h longer for the immature rats than for the mature rats, the fertilizing life of spermatozoa in the female tract of immature females may be presumed to be about 2 h longer than that in the female tract of mature females. There was no difference between the spermatozoa obtained from the old and young rats as far as their fertilizing life is concerned. The fertilization rates, however, were higher when spermatozoa were deposited in the mature than when they were deposited in the immature females, indicating a better chance of sperm survival in the tract of mature females unless this was not due to a slightly longer interval between insemination and the expected time of ovulation in the immature rats.

Mature female rats (80–90 days old) at estrus and immature female rats (24–27 days old) treated with PMS and HCG were inseminated at various times after ovulation for the determination of the fertilizable life of eggs. From table VII it can be seen that the fertilizable life of rat eggs lasted about

9 h whether the eggs were from mature or immature rats. The fertilization rates, in general, were not much different whether spermatozoa were from old, mature, or immature rats, especially when deposited in mature rats. This indicates that transporting and fertilizing ability are similar among the males, regardless of age. However, the fertilization rates were generally lower when spermatozoa from the immature males were inseminated into the immature rats, showing that the immature female tract is not well adapted to the transport of eggs and the fertilization of eggs.

The fertilization rates were higher when rats were inseminated 2–4 h before ovulation (62–96%, table VI) than at 0–1 h after ovulation (28–70%, table VII). Obviously spermatozoa are better capacitated for fertilization if they reside in the female tract for a longer time. Only a few abnormal fertilizations, such as the presence of supplementary sperm in the egg and the dispersing of the pronucleus, were observed when rats were inseminated before ovulation (table VI). But a large number of abnormal fertilizations, especially eggs with supplementary sperm, were observed when insemination was performed after ovulation (table VII). This points to a fast deterioration of eggs soon after ovulation. Whether or not such fertilized eggs can develop is still to be determined.

III. Discussion

The presence of sperm in the epididymis was first observed in the immature rabbits at the age of 13–15 weeks. The average number of spermatozoa in the epididymis and vas deferentia of 8 young rabbits was only 0.22 (0–1.25) million. At the age of 16 weeks the average number of sperm from 4 young rabbits was 8.2 (2.45–17.60) million and at the age of 17–18 weeks it was 307 (65–494) million from 5 young rabbits; this indicates a rapid increase of sperm production, about 40 times in a 2-week period. At the ages of 19-23 weeks, the average number of sperm of 13 rabbits was 643 (101–1,565) million, and the sperm production was more or less stable. The fertilizing capacity of spermatozoa from rabbits of different ages, however, is very much the same during the period of rapid increase of sperm production as shown in table II. This is probably so in the rats (tables VI and VII) as long as there are sufficient numbers of spermatozoa for fertilization.

The induction of ovulation by administration of HCG in 4- to 8-week old rabbits was unsuccessful, but superovulation of rats (3 times the normal number of eggs) at 24–26 days old was regularly achieved by administration of PMS followed by HCG. Injection of HCG alone did not induce ovulation in 24-day old rats. Injection of PMS followed by HCG induced ovulation but not superovulation in 8–11 week old rabbits. Superovulation, however, was induced by such treatment in a few 12–15 week old rabbits. Thus, the reaction to hormonal treatment at a particular age in different species can be seen.

We are uncertain whether the lower rate of egg recovery and fertilization in the 10–15 week old rabbits (table III) but not for the young rats (tables VI and VII) can be attributed to a species difference or to a hormonal treatment difference.

Time of ovulation is an important factor in determining the fertilizable life of eggs following delayed insemination. In the mature rabbit ovulation occurs 9.5–13 h after injection of HCG [Harper, 1961] and the fertilizable life of rabbit eggs after ovulation lasts about 6–8 h [Chang, 1952; Hammond, 1934]. It has been reported that none of 68 eggs in 7 mature rabbits mated 14 h after injection of HCG was fertilized [Adams and Chang, 1962]. In the present study 6% of 67 eggs from six 16-week-old rabbits were fertilized under the same experimental condition (table V). It is possible that this difference is due to delayed ovulation in the immature rabbits rather than to a longer fertilizable life of eggs from immature rabbits. We have checked the time of ovulation very carefully and patiently in mature and immature rats treated with PMS and HCG. We are confident about the accuracy of the expected time of ovulation, yet we did not find a significant difference in the fertilizable life of eggs from mature and immature rats.

The fertilizing life of rat spermatozoa in the female has been determined as 14 h by counting the litter resulting from insemination before ovulation [Soderwall and Blandau, 1941]. We have found that the fertilizing life of rat spermatozoa lasted about 17-20 h by counting the proportion of fertilized eggs. Since one cannot expect all the fertilized eggs to develop into young, this discrepancy is, therefore, expected. It has been shown that the extreme limit of the fertilizable life of rat eggs is about 12 h after ovulation [Blandau and Jordan, 1941]. The effects of delayed fertilization on the development of the pronuclei in rat ova were further investigated by Blandau [1952]. It was found that the greatest decrease in fertilizability and increase in maldevelopment occurred in eggs aged 9-12 h before insemination. We have found that about 8–15% of eggs can be fertilized in the mature female rats inseminated 8-9 h after ovulation. Since we did not determine whether the rat eggs could be fertilized 10-12 h after ovulation, we cannot be sure whether the results of our study differ from those of Blandau [1952].

Summary

The presence of spermatozoa in the epididymis was observed in the New Zealand albino rabbits 13–15 weeks old and in the CD strain of Sprague-Dawley rats 64–68 days old. The fertilizing capacity of spermatozoa was not different from those obtained from immature or mature rabbits as long as there were enough spermatozoa in the male tract for insemination. The fertilizing life in the female tract of mature and immature rat spermatozoa lasted for 18–20 h. Whether sperm from old or immature rats were inseminated into mature or immature rats made no significant difference.

Ovulation was not induced by administration of HCG in the rabbits at the age of 4–8 weeks. A lower ovulation rate per rabbit was induced in the rabbits at the age of 10 to 13 weeks but very few eggs could be recovered, and not one of them was fertilized. At the age of 14–15 weeks, the recovery rate was high but the fertilization rate was low. Both the recovery and fertilization rates approached those of mature females at the age of 16–20 weeks. The fertilizing life of eggs was very much the same in the mature and immature rabbits between 14 and 18 weeks.

Superovulation by administration of PMS and HCG could be achieved regularly in the 22- to 26-day-old rats. The fertilizable life of eggs from the mature or immature rats lasted about 8–9 h after ovulation. No difference was found between the eggs from mature and immature rats. However, the fertilization rates were lower when sperm from the immature rats were inseminated into immature females. Abnormal fertilization, especially the presence of supplementary spermatozoa in the eggs, was more frequently observed in the rats inseminated after ovulation than before ovulation.

Acknowledgment

This work was supported by grants from the National Institute of Child Health and Development (HD 03472) and from the Ford Foundation. Thanks are due to Mrs. ROSE BARTKE and Mr. JOHN ZUCKER for the care of animals.

References

ADAMS, C.E. and CHANG, M.C.: The effect of delayed mating on fertilization in the rabbit. J. exp. Zool. *151:* 155 (1962).

ASDELL, S.A.: Patterns of mammalian reproduction; 2nd ed. (Cornell University Press, Ithaca 1964).

BLANDAU, R.J.: The female factor in fertility and infertility. I. Effects of delayed fertilization on the development of the pronuclei in rat ova. Fertil. Steril. *3:* 349 (1952).

BLANDAU, R.J. and JORDAN, E.S.: The effect of delayed fertilization on the development of the rat ovum. Amer. J. Anat. *68:* 275 (1941).

CHANG, M.C.: Fertilizability of rabbit ova and the effects of temperature *in vitro* on their subsequent fertilization and activation *in vivo*. J. exp. Zool. *121:* 351 (1952).

Hammond, J.: The fertilization of rabbit ova in relation to time. A method of controlling litter size, the duration of pregnancy and the weight of young at birth. J. exp. Biol. *11:* 140 (1934).

Harper, M.J.K.: The time of ovulation in the rabbit following the injection of luteinizing hormone. J. Endocrin. *22:* 147 (1961).

Soderwall, A.L. and Blandau, R.J.: The duration of the fertilizing capacity of spermatozoa in the female tract of the rat. J. exp. Zool. *88:* 55 (1941).

Toyoda, Y. and Chang, M.C.: Fertilization of rat eggs *in vitro* by epididymal spermatozoa and the development of such eggs following transfer. J. Reprod. Fertil. *36:* 9 (1974).

Author's address: Dr. M.C. Chang, Worcester Foundation for Experimental Biology, 222 Maple Avenue, *Shrewsbury, MA 01545* (USA)

Aging Gametes. Int. Symp., Seattle 1973, pp. 179–200 (Karger, Basel 1975)

The Gametogenic Function of the
Aging Ovary in the Mammal

R.H. Foote

Department of Animal Science, Cornell University, Ithaca, N.Y.

The intent of this chapter is to focus attention on the changing gameto-genic function of the aging ovary in the female. With most organs one might limit the examination of a particular aging organ to changes in the aged female. However, considering the fact that the gametogenic function in the female is initiated as soon as the definitive gonad is formed early in fetal life, aging of certain ovarian components truly begins prenatally. The gametogenic function is influenced by endocrine secretions, but it is only necessary to call attention here to a few of the more important interactions. Although the body of endocrine information is proliferating rapidly, the nature of the interactions still is imprecisely understood.

Throughout the chapter the terms 'gametogenic function' and 'oogenesis' will be used synonymously to include the formation, development, and maturation of the female gamete. In the definitive female gonad, the ovary, the diploid germinal cells that undergo repeated mitotic divisions are called 'oogonia'. The last mitotic division gives rise to 'primary oocytes' that enter prophase I of meiosis. The term 'egg' will be used somewhat loosely in reference to ovarian oocytes. At the time of ovulation the egg is usually shed as a secondary oocyte in the metaphase stage of the second meiotic division. The term 'ovum' will be little used since this correctly applies to the postovulatory haploid female gamete from which both polar bodies have been extruded. This condition seldom is realized because sperm penetration usually precedes extrusion of the second polar bodies.

I. Origin and Fate of the Germ Cells

More than 100 years ago WALDEYER [1870] suggested that during the neonatal period ovaries of mammals are stocked with a finite number of eggs.

The majority of evidence supports this concept for most species, although there have been many reports to the contrary [BAKER, 1972 a; BRAMBELL, 1956; FRANCHI et al., 1962; ZUCKERMAN, 1960]. Once the germ cells have moved to the genital ridge they lose their identifying morphological characteristics, making it difficult to interpret their fate by histological means.

KINGERY [1917] reported that oogenesis occurred from birth to sexual maturity in the mouse. He suggested that the primordial germ cells that proliferated before birth all degenerated, and that subsequent proliferations from the 'germinal epithelium' were responsible for the oocytes available at puberty. However, in order to conclude this the various authors [ZUCKERMAN, 1956] had to assume that typical meiosis did not occur in the adult. EVERETT [1943, 1945] presented convincing evidence that the primordial germ cells are the only source of oocytes in the adult. He transplanted genital ridges of mice before and after migration of the gonocytes or primordial germ cells. Gonads differentiated normally when transplanted after the migration, but were devoid of germ cells when transplanted before migration. From this and other work ZUCKERMAN [1956, 1960] concluded that the primordial germ cells were responsible for oocytes found in the adult ovary. Additional evidence to support this view is included in a subsequent section on neogenesis. Certain prosimians exhibit meiosis in oocytes found in sexually mature animals [GÉRARD and HERLANT, 1953], but these species are considered to be exceptions.

II. Oogenesis

The fetal gonads undergo sexual differentiation within a few weeks of conception (fig. 1). The primordial germ cells in the ovary are transformed into larger cells, oogonia, with a different arrangement of cytoplasmic components [BAKER, 1966; BRAMBELL, 1956]. Oogonia rapidly proliferate by mitoses. After a certain number of mitoses have occurred the oogonia are transformed into oocytes that enter prophase of the first meiotic division. As can be seen from figure 1, following sexual differentiation the succession of events of oogonial divisions, the stages of meiotic prophase I, and degeneration occur rapidly and they overlap. Prophase I proceeds through leptotene, zygotene, pachytene and diplotene before being arrested in the so-called dictyate or dictyotene stage. Chromosomes during this stage are diffuse. This is not a resting stage as RNA and protein are manufactured; growth of the oocyte occurs [BAKER, 1972 a].

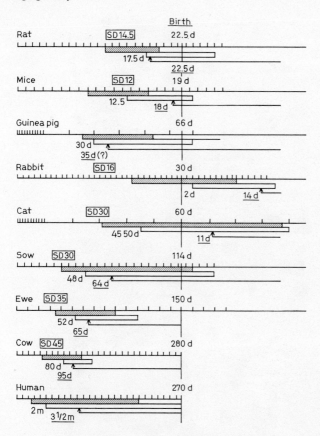

Fig. 1. Comparative aspects of oogenesis showing the age in days of the fetus at the time of sexual differentiation (SD), the duration of oogonial divisions (hatched bar) and the oocyte development until the dictyate stage (open bar). The number of days to the left of the bar represents the age at the beginning of meiosis and the second number gives the age when diplotene stages are first seen. The arrow points to the beginning of atresia. From MAULÉON [1969].

In rats, mice, guinea pigs, sheep, cattle, monkeys, and humans most oocytes have reached the dictyate condition considerably before or by the time of birth [BAKER, 1972a; MAULÉON 1969]. In the rabbit oocyte formation is initiated about the time of birth. This is also true of the golden hamster, ferret, mink, and vole.

The cytological appearance of the oocytes in different stages of prophase I in the rabbit is shown in figure 2 [KENNELLY *et al.*, 1970]. In leptotene fila-

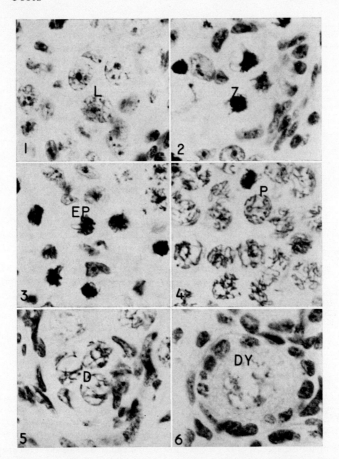

Fig. 2. Nuclear appearance of rabbit oocytes in the various stages of prophase I. *1,* Leptotene (L); *2,* zygotene (Z); *3,* early prophase (EP); *4,* prophase (P); *5,* diplotene (D); *6,* dictyotene (DY). × 850. From KENNELLY *et al.* [1970].

mentous threads visibly represent the chromatin network. In zygotene the thickened pairs of synapsed chromosomes are evident. By late zygotene the classical bouquet arrangement is reached, and the nuclear membrane is no longer visible. Pachytene is a relatively long stage in which the chromosomes are paired throughout their length. Chromosomes shorten and thicken owing to coiling. The chromosomes separate, except where still joined at specific points (chiasmata), in the diplotene stage. At this stage meiosis is interrupted and oocytes are stored in the dictyotene stage. This sequence was described in detail by DE WINIWARTER [1901].

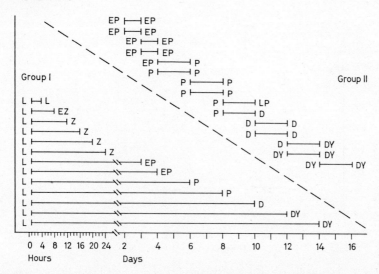

Fig. 3. The duration of the different stages of meiotic prophase I in the rabbit. To obtain the actual postnatal age of the animals studied add two days to group I and 3 days to group II. For key to abbreviations see figure 2. From KENNELLY *et al.* [1970].

The duration of the different stages and the time at which they occur in the rabbit are shown in figure 3 [KENNELLY *et al.*, 1970]. Rabbits in group I (fig. 3) received tritiated thymidine when 2 days old, at which time most oocytes were in the leptotene stage. In group II animals were 3 days old and the first ovaries were removed for study 2 days later. By identifying the stages of prophase I cytologically and by determining which were the most advanced cell types labeled through the use of autoradiography the duration of each stage was estimated. The oocytes were first seen in the dictyotene stage when the rabbits were 14 days old. The germ cells of the rabbit were fairly well synchronized in development, although not to the 90% extent reported for the rat [BEAUMONT and MANDL, 1962].

III. Follicular Growth

Soon after oocytes reach the dictyate stage they are surrounded by a single layer of flattened epithelial cells. This establishes the primary follicle. The follicular cells increase by mitosis. An oocyte surrounded by multiple layers of follicle cells, but with no evidence of any space (antrum 7), is referred to as

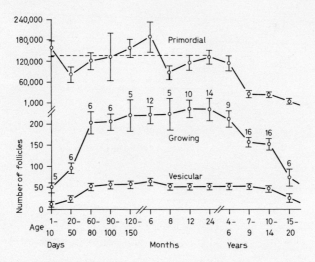

Fig. 4. Quantitative estimation of the number of primordial, growing and vesicular follicles in the postnatal bovine ovary. Vertical bars represent standard errors and numbers are the ovarian pairs examined. From ERICKSON [1966].

a secondary follicle. Finally antrum formation occurs, leading to an adult vesicular follicle capable of ovulation, the so-called Graafian follicle.

Before the primary follicle is established and through the early periods of follicular growth the oocyte itself enlarges. The zona pellucida is formed, and RNA and protein synthesis have been observed [BAKER, 1972 a]. A majority of the oocytes which do not undergo atresia continue to reside in primary follicles in the ovary. The number of follicles that develop into vesicular follicles is somewhat proportional to the total number of primary follicles present [ERICKSON, 1966; JONES and KROHN, 1961 a; PETERS and LEVY, 1966]. From the references cited [see also BAKER, 1972 b; TALBERT, 1968] it is clear that the reservoir of primary follicles in the ovaries of the aging female limits to some degree the number of follicles that mature and are potential sources of ovulatory eggs. It does not necessarily follow that such follicles will in fact rupture on a cyclical basis in aged females, since pituitary hormones and other factors must interact appropriately to induce ovulation [HANSEL and ECHTERNKAMP, 1972; JONES and KROHN, 1959].

The relationship in cattle among the number of primordial follicles (oocyte with a single layer of follicle cells), growing follicles (oocytes with more than one layer of follicle cells but an incomplete vesicle) and vesicular follicles is shown in figure 4 [ERICKSON, 1966]. Only follicles that were normal in appearance were counted. The number of growing follicles increases rapidly after birth. It is evident that the primordial cell population decreases rapidly in cattle after 4 years, and the number of growing follicles decreases appreciably at this time. There was considerable variation among animals. In humans the number of large follicles remains relatively uniform for many years. In contrast the number of large follicles in rats and some other species declines after puberty [JONES, 1970].

IV. Number of Oocytes and the Relationship to Fertility

In all species studied the mitotic activity of the primordial germ cells [HARDISTY, 1967] and oogonia (rat: BEAUMONT and MANDL [1962]; guinea pig: IOANNOU [1964]; pig: BLACK and ERICKSON [1968]; cow: ERICKSON [1966]; monkey: BAKER [1966]; GREEN and ZUCKERMAN [1951]; human: BAKER [1963]) lead to a rapid increase in the oocyte population of the ovary. Whereas only 700–1,300 cells are reported as migrating to the human ovary [WITSCHI, 1948], 7,000,000 germ cells have been tabulated at the fifth month of pregnancy. Thereafter, the number of germ cells decreases as oogonial mitoses cease, and degeneration of a high proportion of oocytes occurs even before birth. Actually degeneration starts before all mitoses cease but the net balance is an increase in the number of oocytes. The characteristic pattern of change in oocyte numbers with time for several species is shown in figure 5. The pattern is similar when an appropriate time scale is used.

As the female ages the ovarian population of oocytes continues to decrease through atresia, and after puberty, to a small extent through ovulation. Nevertheless some oocytes remain as long as reproductive life lasts or after it has ceased. Data reported by BLOCK [1952] for women is shown in table I. When these data are combined with reports by BAKER [1963, 1972 a] the pattern of germ cell numbers throughout human fetal and adult life is as shown in figure 6. The oocyte population in women approaches zero by 50 years of age. Thus, the human ovary is largely depleted of oocytes by the time of menopause. This change in ovarian oocyte content is illustrated dramatically by the ovarian sections (fig. 7) from women of different ages [VAN WAGENEN and SIMPSON, 1965]. At the oldest age (44 years) the section shown is nearly devoid of oocytes.

The oocyte population of a few species may not show this same dramatic increase followed by a continual decline as a result of oogenesis being limited

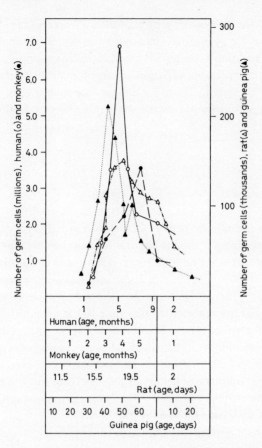

Fig. 5. Fluctuations in the total population of germ cells before birth. From Baker [1972a].

to the fetus or the neonate. These exceptions, reported to occur especially in prosimians, will be discussed under neogenesis of germ cells.

The characteristic reproductive life span (puberty to age at reproductive failure) is shown in table II. The average reproductive life for most species is less than is indicated in table II because most animals are not maintained after they become inefficient reproductively. It is of interest to compare the near maximum age at which reproduction still is known to occur sporadically with ovarian oocyte populations to determine to what extent depletion of oocytes might be fertility limiting. There is a paucity of quantitative information on oocyte numbers in aging females, particularly in primates. This is sur-

Table I. Maternal age and number of oocytes (human)

Age, years	Number of cases	Number of oocytes
Birth	7	733,000
4–10	5	499,200
11–17	5	389,300
18–24	7	161,800
25–31	11	62,500
32–38	8	80,200
39–45	7	10,900

Source: BLOCK [1952].

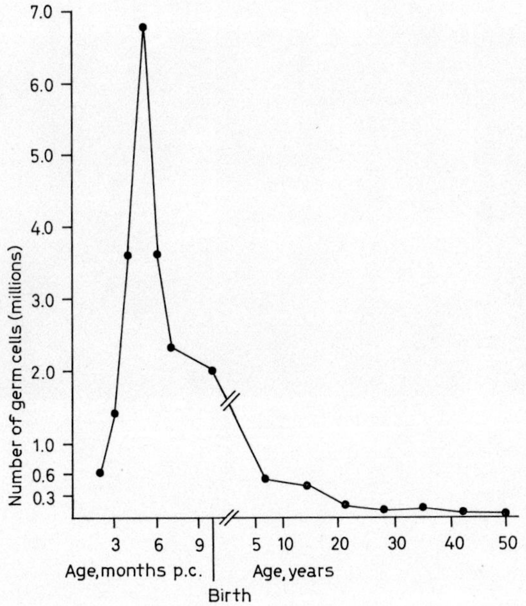

Fig. 6. Total germ cell population in the human ovary during reproductive life. From BAKER [1972a].

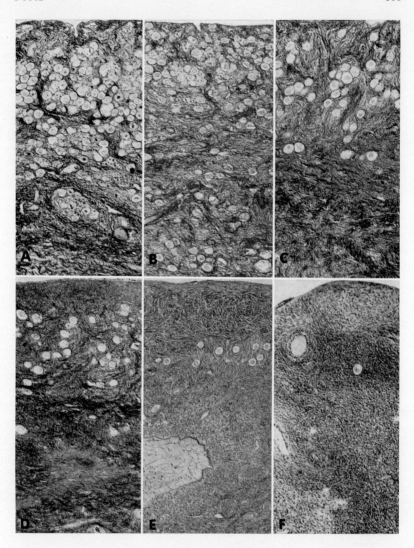

Fig. 7. Human ovary showing the changes in oocyte population with postnatal age. *A* 3 days; *B* 4 months; *C* 2.5 years; *D* 8 years; *E* 10 years; *F* 44 years. × 60. From VAN WAGENEN and SIMPSON [1965].

Table II. Approximate age at puberty and at reproductive failure in selected mammals

Species	Age at puberty, months	Near maximum age at reproductive failure, years
Human	140	45
Rhesus monkey	30	20
Horse	18	30
Cow	10	20
Ewe	7	15
Sow	6	10
Bitch	9	10
Guinea pig	4	4
Hamster	1	1.2
Mouse	1	1.3
Rat	1.5	1.3
Rabbit	5	6

Ages gathered from the literature. There is marked variation according to breed, nutrition, and environmental conditions.

prising considering all of the primates being used for experimental reproductive biology. However, proposals for such studies, although important to do and inexpensive to carry out, may be viewed as old fashioned by granting agencies. Well-conceived studies concerning the causes of cycle interruption and anovulation in senile ovaries still supplied with oocytes could provide invaluable information concerning infertility problems and fertility regulation.

It is difficult to define the average age at onset of menopause. However, from data collected [BLOCK, 1952; TALBERT, 1968] and the figures given in tables I and II it is apparent that in women the decline in fertility begins while the ovary still contains oocytes. By the time reproduction ceases the stock of oocytes may have largely disappeared.

MANDL and SHELTON [1959] found that when rats became sterile their ovaries still contained 1,200–1,500 oocytes. Mice still possess several hundred oocytes when the last litter is born, excepting in certain inbred strains. ERICKSON [1966] estimated that there were between 100 and 2,000 oocytes in the ovaries of two 2-year-old infertile cows. From these and other data [JONES, 1970; KROHN, 1964; TALBERT, 1968] it is clear that in several species reproductive failure does not result from a complete lack of oocytes. Defective oocytes or anovulatory conditions may lead to the inability of the aged female to produce young while still stocked with oocytes. Many studies show (see other

chapters in this book) that extra-ovarian factors associated with the aging hy-
pothalamic-pituitary-uterine axes may be the cause of reproductive failure in
old females [ADAMS, 1964; ASCHEIM, 1964–65; KROHN, 1964; MAURER and
FOOTE, 1971; TALBERT, 1968].

V. Neogenesis

It was pointed out earlier that several lines of evidence indicated that the
definitive ova are formed in most mammals in the prenatal or neonatal period and not in the adult [BRAMBELL, 1956; FRANCHI et al., 1962; ZUCKER-
MAN, 1956, 1960]. Both extirpation of the extra-embryonic germ cells before
their migrations and transplantation of the genital ridges before extra-embryonic germ cells migrated to the genital ridges led to sterile ovaries devoid
of oocytes. Other aspects, such as development of the mesonephric and genital ducts from the transplanted genital ridges, were normal. Irradiation of the
gonads, with the embryo shielded, results in destruction of the oocyte population, which is not replenished in the adults. However, X-ray studies have led
to equivocal results because of the great variability in oocytic sensitivity to
X-rays [KROHN, 1967]. MANDL [1964] and ROCHOWIAK [1967] using different
strains of rats reduced the oocyte population by 90 and 60%, respectively, by
a 200-r dose of X-rays. ROCHOWIAK [1967] concluded that oocytes are
formed to replace those destroyed by irradiation, but it is likely that the large
numbers of oocytes surviving irradiation were responsible for subsequent reproduction.

Unequivocal evidence that 'epithelial' cells are not transformed into
germ cells in the adult and that fetal oocytes persist in the adult female was
obtained in labeling studies [BORUM, 1967; CHIQUOINE, 1961; KENNELLY and
FOOTE, 1966; RUDKIN and GRIECH, 1962]. In the study by KENNELLY and
FOOTE [1966] the neonatal rabbits were injected with ^{3}H-methyl-thymidine.
The persistence of the label in both ovarian and ovulated oocytes was examined in the adult rabbit by autoradiography. The isotope persisted in the as
dult virtually undiminished. The proportion of ovarian and ovulated oocyte-
that were labeled was similar (table III). Injection of does at either 4 or 20
weeks of age resulted in extensive incorporation of tritiated thymidine into
follicle cells, but no labeled oocytes were ever found in animals injected at 4
weeks of age or more.

From an intensive analysis of the data KENNELLY and FOOTE [1966]
summarized their findings: 'From all the evidence obtained it is concluded

Table III. Proportion of labeled ovarian and ovulated oocytes or zygotes in rabbits injected with ³H-thymidine

Age at injection, weeks	Age when sampled, weeks	Cell type	Cells labeled, %
Birth	20	ovarian oocytes	83–90
		ovulated 'eggs'	90
	70	ovarian oocytes	74
		ovulated 'eggs'	78
4	4	ovarian oocytes	0
	12	ovarian oocytes	0
20	20	ovarian oocytes	0

From KENNELLY and FOOTE [1966].

that most, if not all oocytes in the adult rabbit originate during the neonatal period, and DNA is stored without appreciable turnover in the oocytes which survive the normal oocyte atresia characteristic of female mammals. A summation of the results obtained supporting these conclusions is as follows: (1) No cytological evidence was found of meiotic activity after the intense neonatal activity subsided; (2) the concentration of radioactive DNA incorporated at birth remained relatively constant in older animals and no appreciable decrease in the percentage of labeled oocyte nuclei was observed; (3) the changes noted in the population of oocytes were completely explainable by non-random degeneration of oocytes at the earlier ages; (4) the proportion of radioactive eggs obtained in the mature animal by superovulation was similar to the proportion of radioactive oocytes labeled neonatally and present in the ovaries of adults; (5) the radioactive ova are capable of fertilization and give rise to normal litters; (6) thy-H³ incorporated into oocyte nuclei was very slight at four weeks of age and it was not incorporated into oocyte nuclei at 20 weeks of age. Thus it is concluded that oocytogenesis ceases before reproductive life begins in rabbits, and from this evidence and other published work it is inferred that this is characteristic for most mammals.'

VI. Oogenesis in Prosimians

The pattern of oogenesis described for other mammals occurs in prosimians. However, the prediplotene stages of meiosis that are not seen in most other adult mammals are found in adult prosimians [ANAND KUMAR, 1966, 1968; BAKER, 1972 a; BUTLER, 1971; IOANNOU, 1967]. Oogonia and early prophase oocytes are found in the 'nests' of the ovarian cortex. They incorporate ³H-thymidine, indicating active DNA synthesis. Their origin and function are in doubt. BAKER [1972 b] suggests that the oogonia were formed from the primordial germ cells prenatally and escaped the waves of atresia that eliminate any remaining oogonia most in mammals. Oogonia also apparently persist occasionally in the hilar region of cat ovaries [BRAMBELL, 1956].

Do these germ cells migrate from the cortical 'nests' and become definitive germ cells in developing follicles? Oogonia in several species incorporate ³H-thymidine, and labeled oocytes have resulted. However, no labeled follicular oocytes have been detected [IOANNOU, 1967]. Thus, in view of no evidence to the contrary, the stock of oocytes potentially capable of participating in reproduction of the prosimians also appears to be fixed at birth.

The problem of postnatal oogenesis in prosimian primates is not entirely resolved, however. The number of germ cells in the cortical nests fluctuates during the sexual cycle, increasing from about 11,000 during anestrus to 164,000 at estrus in the slender loris [ANAND KUMAR, 1966]. A wave of atresia follows during diestrus, presumably under the influence of the gonadotropic hormones. To resolve the problem of postpubertal oogenesis in prosimians, isotopic labeling of the multiplying oogonia and oocytes in the adult should be combined with quantification of the follicular oocytes. Sufficient time should be allowed following injection of ³H-thymidine to permit follicular oocytes to develop from labeled precursor cells, if this potential in fact exists.

VII. Influence of Age on Oocytes Ovulated

Oocytes in women may be stored for more than 45 years before ovulation. Associated with this is a marked increase in the frequency of Down's syndrome or mongolism [EDWARDS, 1970 a]. It has been hypothesized that the cause of this genetic defect is either impairment with age of the placement of chromosomes on the spindle during the first meiotic division or impairment of the process of ovulation leading to oocytes that deteriorate just prior to fertilization.

A third hypothesis has been suggested: the time at which oocytes are formed affects the time of life they will be ovulated, and those formed last carry a greater risk of having chromosome abnormalities [EDWARDS, 1970 b;

HENDERSON and EDWARDS, 1968]. Based upon this line of reasoning, more of the oocytes ovulated in older animals would come from oocytes formed abnormally.

In the aging female, preovulatory and postovulatory oocyte aging and many other factors may reduce reproductive efficiency. These topics are treated in other chapters.

VIII. Oocyte Loss by Ovulation and Atresia

From table II, plus data on cycle length, average ovulation rate per estrus, and a correction for several pregnancies, the potential total number of oocytes ovulated per female can be calculated. The maximum that would be expelled from the ovary by ovulation is a few hundred. In the human, ovaries contain about 700,000 oocytes at birth. The maximum number of oocytes ovulated represents less than 0.1 % of the total present at birth. Adjusting the statistics for the fact that there may be a few oocytes remaining in the human when menstrual cycles cease (table II), over 98 % of the oocytes are still unaccounted for. These 98 % are lost by atresia.

The degenerative process of atresia by which most oocytes are removed is poorly understood. Changes that occur and factors affecting atresia have been described [INGRAM, 1962; RINGROSE, 1963]. Not all oogonia survive successive divisions leading to oocytes. By far the greatest loss of oocytes occurs before birth in most species (fig. 5). The rate of atresia appears to be partly dependent on the ovarian stock of oocytes at the time.

Many oocytes undergo atresia during meiotic prophase, especially during pachytene [BEAUMONT and MANDL, 1962]. Degenerating oocytes have an irregular nuclear outline with unevenly distributed chromatin. However, it is difficult to diagnose atresia with certainty in many primordial germ cells unless degeneration is severe. Repeated observations to study progressive changes are not feasible. Obviously histological processing to avoid artifacts is extremely important.

Small oocytes are also eliminated through the ovarian wall into the periovarian space [JONES and KROHN, 1961 a]. The oocyte normally becomes surrounded by a layer of follicle cells and grows. If it does not become enveloped in follicle cells it probably will not survive [BLANDAU, 1967] With the multiplication of follicle cells (granulosa cells) atresia, represented by pyknosis of the nuclei, nuclear fragmentation or breakdown of the nuclear membrane, becomes more obvious. Mitotic divisions of granulosa cells stop in the atretic follicle. It is not certain whether the oocyte or its layer of granulosa cells is affected first. In a multilayered follicle INGRAM [1962] suggests that atresia originates with the oocyte nucleus. EL-FOULY *et al.* [1970] showed that puncturing an oocyte can alter the granulosa cell layer. Thus the oocyte may contain a factor controlling the morphological fate of the granulosa cells. It follows that death of the oocyte also could induce follicular degeneration.

During nuclear fragmentation polar bodies may be extruded, but development is abortive. The follicle undergoes rapid degeneration, and its granulosa cells become pyknotic. These cells break down and are resorbed or may become phagocytized [INGRAM, 1962]. The zona pellucida may persist for some time and frequently is the last part of the follicle to disappear [HARRISON, 1948]. Cysts may also develop, enclosed in a single layer of cells [INGRAM, 1962]. The length of time required to eliminate an atretic follicle from the ovary is not known.

The reason for the mass production of oocytes and massive destruction before reproductive life in the female begins remains obscure. It is not known to what extent, if any, surviving oocytes represent a selected group, minimal in genetic defects and normal in metabolism. MINTZ and RUSSELL [1957] showed that mice with the W^j mutation had lost all of their oocytes by birth, but this does not mean that genetic selection is practiced under more usual conditions. If genetic defects were the principal cause of atresia an enormous load of gene and chromosomal aberrations would be implied. This seems unlikely. Human patients with XO karyotype (Turner's syndrome) usually have no oocytes, but this may also reflect a hormonal disturbance. Rabbit eggs collected following superovulation are as fertile and develop into normal young as readily as oocytes ovulated naturally [MAURER *et al.*, 1968]. Since some of the superovulated follicles yield oocytes that would ordinarily degenerate there seems to be no selection on a cyclical basis.

If the oocyte is removed from the follicle, meiosis is resumed. In the intact fully developed follicle the oocyte remains in the dictyate stage until ovulation is imminent. Resumption of meiosis and ovulation normally is somewhat synchronized [DONAHUE, 1972]. Resumption of meiosis without ovulation leads to atresia, and oocytes in many follicles undergoing atresia show evidence that meiosis was resumed. Clearly the oocyte and its follicle are in a delicate balance [NALBANDOV, 1972]. It would be most instructive and useful to know what the difference in this balance is in the aged ovary and in the ovary during the prime reproductive years. Study of the intrafollicular interactions along with pituitary influence should be helpful in understanding why most oocytes undergo atresia and only some ovulate. An understanding of the regulation of these events could lead to ingenious methods of exerting control over them.

IX. Factors Affecting Rate of Atresia

Rate of atresia is age related. The number of oocytes lost throughout life bears a relationship to the residual ovarian stock. Once oogonial divisions have ceased oocytes are lost at a decreased rate.

Genetic factors are involved, as indicated by the W^j strain of mice previously referred to [MINTZ and RUSSELL, 1957]. In the CBA strain of mice the oocyte population approaches zero at 450 days of age, whereas in the RIII strain about 1,000 oocytes are still present at this age [JONES and KROHN, 1961 a].

At sexual maturity a few oocytes leave the ovary by ovulation. If part of an ovary or a complete ovary has been removed the remaining ovarian tissue responds to hormone stimulation to maintain a fairly constant ovulation rate per animal [FRANCHI et al., 1962; McLAREN, 1966]. At the same time those follicles that grow with each cycle but are not selected for ovulation eventually decay.

Hypophysectomy retards the loss of oocytes [JONES and KROHN, 1961 b]. The proportion of oocytes judged to be normal is higher, but atresia continues after pituitary removal. Presumably this change is due to the interaction of the gonadotropins with the ovary and the production of ovarian steroids. WILLIAMS [1956] reported that estrogen promotes follicular growth following hypophysectomy of immature animals, and INGRAM [1962] found estrogen protection of follicles in the adult rat. The withdrawal of gonadotropins following hypophysectomy in rats causes atresia of the more developed follicles.

The hormonal studies done on aging animals clearly indicate a pituitary-ovarian relationship.

X. Consequences of Atresia

The development of several more large follicles than are destined to ovulate may provide additional estrogen to properly stimulate the reproductive tract, trigger LH release, and aid in maintaining the normal cyclical behavior characteristic of fertile females. Whether any genetic selection ordinarily is accomplished by cyclical atresia of the developed follicles, as well as by the degeneration of the many primordial follicles throughout life, seems doubtful.

The decrease in oocytes throughout life eventually decreases the probability of there being oocytes available for ovulation. Some oocytes ovulated may be atretic [DONAHUE, 1972], but evidence is lacking that the proportion of atretic oocytes ovulated increases with aging. With fewer large follicles, including atretic ones, there may be less estrogen feedback inhibition of the pituitary. This could account for the elevated gonadotropins seen in the blood and urine of postmenopausal women [TALBERT, 1968]. With inadequate circulating estrogen a normal LH surge may not occur, thus causing luteinization rather than rupture of Graafian follicles. Thus the problem of infertility with advancing age due to fewer oocytes and possible interference with ovulation is compounded. Detailed hormonal studies on the aged female similar to those published for younger cycling mammals [HANSEL and ECHTERNKAMP, 1972; KNOBIL, 1972] are needed and, it is hoped, will soon be forthcoming [BELLAMY, 1970].

XI. Conclusions

The gametogenic function of the aging ovary was considered in terms of formation, development, and maturation of female gametes.

1. The evidence is overwhelming that in most species of mammals oogenesis is limited to the prenatal or neonatal period of life in the female. Even in prosimians, where oogonia divide and oocyte formation continues in adults, there is as yet no evidence to show that the germ cells so produced undergo follicular development and utilization. Therefore, as a rule, a finite stock of gametes is formed in the female long before cyclical behavior and actual reproduction at the organism level begin.

2. The early fetal period characterized by the banking of a large stock of primary oocytes is followed by an incessant loss of the primordial oocytes and follicular populations until reproductive life ceases. Some oocytes are selected randomly undergo follicular development, and a few of these may ovulate and potentially contribute to the next generation. As a result of this constant atresia the entire stock of oocytes may be essentially depleted in some species (e.g., humans and certain inbred strains of mice) and be of primary importance in limiting reproductive life.

3. In other species a substantial number of oocytes persist in reproductively senescent females, and therefore a lack of oocytes *per se* is not limiting reproductive life. Rather oocytes may fail to develop or mature properly or may not be ovulated. They are probably subjected to unfavorable hypothalamic-pituitary-ovarian interactions, and may be further subjected to a hostile environment once ovulated in the aging female.

4. The process of atresia is poorly understood. Intrafollicular biochemical and hormonal studies offer exciting opportunities for uncovering mechanisms regulating normal development as well as causes of degeneration of most oocytes and associated follicles.

5. Further cytological and physiological evaluation of the oocytes 'selected' for ovulation, which therefore potentially contribute during reproductive life to the next generation, is needed.

References

ADAMS, C.E.: The influence of advanced maternal age on embryo survival in the rabbit. 5th Int. Congr. Animal Reprod., vol. 2, p. 305 (1964).

ANAND KUMAR, T.C.: Effects of sex-steroids on the reproductive organs of the female Loris; in MARTIN, FRANSCHINI and MOTTA Hormonal steroids. Proc. 2nd Int. Congr. Hormonal Steroids, ICS No. 132, p. 369 (Excerpta Medica, Amsterdam 1966).

ANAND KUMAR, T.C.: Oogenesis in lorises; *Loris tardingradus lydekkerianus* and *Nyceticebus coucang*. Proc. roy. Soc. B *169:* 167 (1968).

ASCHEIM, P.: Résultats fournis par la greffe hétérochrone des ovaires dans l'étude de la régulation hypophyso-ovarienne de la ratte sénile. Gerontologia, Basel *10:* 65 (1964–65).

BAKER, T.G.: A quantitative and cytological study of germ cells in human ovaries. Proc. roy. Soc. B *158:* 417 (1963).

BAKER, T.G.: A quantitative and cytological study of oogenesis in the rhesus monkey. J. Anat., Lond. *100:* 761 (1966).

BAKER, T.G.: Gametogenesis. Acta endocrin., Kbh. *71:* suppl. 166, p. 18 (1972a).

BAKER, T.G.: Oogenesis and ovarian development; in BALIN and GLASSER Reproductive biology, p. 398 (Excerpta Medica, Amsterdam 1972b).

BELLAMY, D.: Ageing and endocrine responses to environmental factors: with particular reference to mammals; in BENSON and PHILLIPS Hormones and the environment, p. 303 (Cambridge University Press, London 1970).

BEAUMONT, H.M. and MANDL, A.M.: A quantitative and cytological study of oogonia and oocytes in the foetal and neonatal rat. Proc. roy. Soc. B *155:* 557 (1962).

BLACK, J.L. and ERICKSON, B.H.: Oogenesis and ovarian development in the prenatal pig. Anat. Rec. *161:* 45 (1968).

BLANDAU, R.J.: Oogenesis – ovulation and egg transport; in BENIRSCHKE Comparative aspects of reproductive failure, p. 194 (Springer, Berlin 1967).

BLOCK, E.: Quantitative morphological investigations of the follicular system in newborn female infants. Acta anat. *17:* 201 (1952).

BORUM, K.: Oogenesis in the mouse: a study on the origin of the mature ova. Exp. Cell Res. *45:* 39 (1967).

BRAMBELL, F.W.R.: Ovarian changes; in PARKES Marshall's physiology of reproduction, vol. 1, part 1, p. 397 (Longmans, London 1956).

BUTLER, H.: Oogenesis and folliculogenesis (non-human primates); in HAFEZ Comparative reproduction of nonhuman primates, p. 243 (Thomas, Springfield 1971).

CHIQUOINE, A.D.: An electron microscope study of vitally stained ovaries from argyric mice. Anat. Rec. *139:* 29 (1961).

DONAHUE, R.P.: The relation of oocyte maturation to ovulation in mammals; in BIGGERS and SCHUETZ Oogenesis, p. 413 (University Park Press, Baltimore 1972).

EDWARDS, R.G.: Meiosis in oocytes and in origin of mongolism and infertility in older mothers; in HOLBRECHT Proc. 6th World Congr. Fertil. Steril., p. 64 (1970a).

EDWARDS, R.G.: Are oocytes formed and used sequentially in the mammalian ovary? Philos. Trans. roy. Soc. B *259:* 103 (1970b).

EL-FOULY, M.A.; COOK, B.; NEKOLA, M., and NALBANDOV, A.V.: Role of the ovum in follicular luteinization. Endocrinology *87:* 288 (1970).

ERICKSON, B.H.: Development and senescence of the postnatal bovine ovary. J. anim. Sci. *25:* 800 (1966).

EVERETT, N.B.: Observational and experimental evidence relating to the origin and differentiation of the definitive germ cells in mice. J. exp. Zool. *92:* 49 (1943).

EVERETT, N.B.: The present status of the germ-cell problem in vertebrates. Biol. Rev. *20:* 45 (1945).

FRANCHI, L.L.; MANDL, A.M., and ZUCKERMAN, S.: The development of the ovary and the process of oogenesis; in ZUCKERMAN, MANDL and ECKSTEIN The ovary, vol. 1, p. 1 (Academic Press, New York 1962).

GÉRARD, P. et HERLANT, M.: Sur la persistance de phénomènes d'oogenèse chez les lémuriens adultes. Arch. Biol. *64:* 97 (1953).

GREEN, S.H. and ZUCKERMAN, S.: The number of oocytes in the mature rhesus monkey *(Macaca mulatta)*. J. Endocrin. *7:* 194 (1951).

HANSEL, W. and ECHTERNKAMP, S.E.: Control of ovarian function in domestic animals. Amer. Zool. *12:* 225 (1972).

HARDISTY, M.W.: The numbers of vertebrate primordial germ cells. Biol. Rev. *42:* 265 (1967).

HARRISON, R.J.: The changes occurring in the ovary of the goat during the oestrus cycle and in early pregnancy. J. Anat., Lond. *82:* 21 (1948).

HENDERSON, S.A. and EDWARDS, R.G.: Chiasma frequency and maternal age in mammals. Nature, Lond. *218:* 22 (1968).

INGRAM, D.L.: Atresia; in ZUCKERMAN, MANDL and ECKSTEIN The ovary, vol. 1, p. 247 (Academic Press, New York 1962).

IOANNOU, J.M.: Oogenesis in the guinea-pig. J. Embryol. exp. Morph. *12:* 673 (1964).

IOANNOU, J.M.: Oogenesis in adult prosimians. J. Embryol. exp. Morph. *17:* 139 (1967).

JONES, E.C.: Ageing ovary and its influence on reproductive capacity. J. Reprod. Fertil. Suppl. *12:* 17 (1970).

JONES, E. C. and KROHN, P. L.: Influence of the anterior pituitary on the ageing process in the ovary. Nature, Lond. *185:* 1155 (1959).

JONES, E. C. and KROHN, P. L.: The relationship between age, numbers of oocytes and fertility in virgin and multiparous mice. J. Endocrin. *21:* 469 (1961a).

JONES, E. C. and KROHN, P. L.: The effect of hypophysectomy on age changes in the ovaries of mice. J. Endocrin. *21:* 497 (1961b).

KENNELLY, J. J. and FOOTE, R. H.: Oocytogenesis in rabbits. The role of neogenesis in the formation of the definitive ova and the stability of oocyte DNA measured with tritiated thymidine. Amer. J. Anat. *118:* 573 (1966).

KENNELLY, J. J.; FOOTE, R. H., and JONES, R. C.: Duration of premeiotic deoxyribonucleic acid synthesis and the stages of prophase I in rabbit oocytes. J. Cell Biol. *47:* 577 (1970).

KINGERY, H. M.: Oogenesis in the white mouse. J. Morph. *30:* 261 (1917).

KNOBIL, E.: Hormonal control of the menstrual cycle and ovulation in the rhesus monkey; in DICZFALUSY and STANLEY The use of non-human primates in research on human reproduction, Acta endocrin., Kbh. *71:* suppl. 166, p. 137 (1972).

KROHN, P. L.: The reproductive lifespan. 5th Int. Congr. Animal Reprod., vol. 3, p. 23 (1964).

KROHN, P. L.: Factors influencing the number of oocytes in the ovary. Arch. Anat. micr. Morph. exp. *56:* 151 (1967).

MANDL, A. M.: The radiosensitivity of germ cells. Biol. Rev. *39:* 288 (1964).

MANDL, A. M. and SHELTON, M.: A quantitative study of oocytes in young and old nulliparous laboratory rats. J. Endocrin. *18:* 444 (1959).

MAULÉON, P.: Oogenesis and folliculogenesis; in COLE and CUPPS Reproduction in domestic animals, p. 187 (Academic Press, New York 1969).

MAURER, R. R. and FOOTE, R. H.: Maternal aging and embryonic mortality in the rabbit. J. Reprod. Fertil. *25:* 329 (1971).

MAURER, R. R.; VAN VLECK, L. D., and FOOTE, R. H.: Developmental potential of superovulated ova. J. Reprod. Fertil. *15:* 171 (1968).

McLAREN, A.: Regulation of ovulation rate after removal of one ovary in mice. Proc. roy. Soc. B *166:* 316 (1966).

MINTZ, B. and RUSSELL, E. S.: Gene-induced embryological modifications of primordial germ cells in the mouse. J. exp. Zool. *134:* 207 (1957).

NALBANDOV, A. V.: Interaction between oocytes and follicular cells; in BIGGERS and SCHUETZ Oogenesis, p. 513 (University Park Press, Baltimore 1972).

PETERS, H. and LEVY, E.: Cell dynamics of the ovarian cycle. J. Reprod. Fertil. *11:* 227 (1966).

RINGROSE, C. A. D.: Controversial and dynamic ovary. Canad. med. Ass. J. *86:* 641 (1963).

ROCHOWIAK, M. W.: Postpubertal oogenesis following Co[60] irradiation in the albino rat. Obstet. Gynec. *29:* 173 (1967).

RUDKIN, G. T. and GRIECH, H. A.: On the persistence of oocyte nuclei from fetus to maturity in the laboratory mouse. J. Cell Biol. *12:* 169 (1962).

TALBERT, G. B.: Effect of maternal age on reproductive capacity. Amer. J. Obstet. Gynec. *102:* 451 (1968).

VAN WAGENEN, G. and SIMPSON, M. E.: Embryology of the ovary and testis in *Homo sapiens* and *Macaca mulatta* (Yale University Press, New Haven 1965).

WALDEYER, W.: Eierstock und Ei (Engelmann, Leipzig 1870); cited by FRANCHI *et al.* (1962).

WILLIAMS, P.C.: The history and fate of redundant follicles; in WOLSTENHOLME and MILLAR Ciba Found. Colloq. on Ageing, vol. 2, p. 59 (Churchill, London 1956).

WINIWARTER, H. DE: Recherches sur l'ovogenèse et l'organogenèse de l'ovaire des mammi-fères (lapin et homme). Arch. Biol. *17:* 33 (1901).

WITSCHI, E.: Migration of the germ cells of human embryos from the yolk sac to the primitive gonadal folds. Contrib. Embryol. Carneg. Inst. *32:* 67 (1948).

ZUCKERMAN, S.: The regenerative capacity of ovarian tissues; in WOLSTENHOLME and MILLAR Ciba Found. Colloq. on Ageing, vol. 2, p. 31 (Churchill, London 1956).

ZUCKERMAN, S.: Origin and development of oocytes in foetal and mature mammals; in AUSTIN Sex differentiation and development, Mem. Soc. Endocrin., vol. 7, p. 63 (1960).

Author's address: Dr. R.H. FOOTE, Department of Animal Science, Cornell University, *Ithaca, NY 14850* (USA)

Aging Gametes. Int. Symp., Seattle 1973, pp. 201–218 (Karger, Basel 1975)

The Role of Intrauterine Environment and Intrafollicular Aging of the Oocyte on Implantation Rates and Development

Roy L. Butcher

Departments of Obstetrics and Gynecology and of Anatomy, School of Medicine, West Virginia University, Morgantown, W.Va.

Causes of decreased fertility with advancing maternal age have been the subject of many investigations and numerous reviews. Reasons for infertility in aging females are undoubtedly related to a multitude of changes at all levels of the reproductive system. Alterations in intrauterine environment due to chronological aging of the uterus seem to have received the bulk of the blame for reduced fertility. The increase in congenital anomalies, which are associated with advanced maternal age, has been considered by many investigators to result from an accumulation of abnormal oocytes as a consequence of chronological aging.

Clinical observations and experimental findings now suggest that alterations in the pattern of secretion of hormones associated with reproduction occur with advancing age and that a delay in ovulation in the aging female is important both in the decline of fertility and the increase in birth defects. Major factors of infertility and abnormal embryonic development are probably associated with hormonal levels and the sequence of events during a few days immediately prior to ovulation and early in the postovulatory period rather than with an accumulation of nonreversible alterations in the uterus and oocytes with advancing age. Undoubtedly, permanent changes do occur late in the period of declining reproduction, the period that has been used for many studies. However, less attention has been given to the subtle changes leading to the decline of fertility and the increase in abnormal embryonic development.

Extensive reviews have been written on the factors associated with infertility and developmental defects concomitant with aging [Adams, 1970; Austin, 1970; Biggers, 1969; Butcher, 1972; Francis, 1970; Hertig, 1967; Jones, 1970; Krohn, 1964; Talbert, 1968]. It is not the purpose of this paper to make a comprehensive review of the decline in reproduction with advancing maternal age but rather to discuss various factors of intrauterine environment and intrafollicular aging of the oocyte as they affect implantation rate and embryonic development.

I. Effect of Intrauterine Environment on Implantation and Development

The effects of intrauterine environment on implantation and embryonic development are difficult to separate from those of defective oocytes, since certain factors that produce changes in the oocyte also alter intrauterine environment. Even more difficult is the separation of postimplantation effects of intrauterine environment from those effects on the conceptus during the preimplantation period. Changes in many oocytes are not severe enough to prevent implantation, although the affected embryo dies or develops abnormally after implantation. One of the most efficient techniques for separation of the effects of intrauterine environment is transfer of ova. Not only can the uterine factors be separated from intrinsic factors in the oocyte but, by timing the stage of development when ova or embryos are transferred, the pre- and postimplantation effects of the intrauterine environment can be studied. Transfer of oocytes immediately after ovulation should remove almost all the uterine effects and allow factors intrinsic to the oocyte to be evaluated.

A. Delayed Ovulation and Intrauterine Environment

Although deleterious changes are now known to occur in the oocyte during the period of delayed ovulation, a definitive study of alterations in intrauterine environment associated with intrafollicular aging has not been made. The only attempt in this area [BUTCHER et al., 1969 b] did not separate completely the changes in the oocyte from those of intrauterine environment during the preimplantation period with regard to embryonic development, but demonstrated changes in implantation rate as a result of altered environment within the uterus.

The ova-transfer technique was used in the above study with donor and recipient rats at day 4 of pregnancy and pseudopregnancy, respectively, at the time of transfer (estrus was day 0). An ovulatory delay of 48 h was produced with sodium pentobarbital by the method of EVERETT and SAWYER [1950]. Three types of transfers were made: control blastocysts to control uteri, control blastocysts of uteri of delayed ovulatory rats, and blastocysts from delayed ovulatory animals to control uteri. To prevent biasing data on intrauterine environment, degenerating, retarded and visibly abnormal embryos were not transferred. The 20 recipients in each group were killed at day 11 of gestation, and implantation rate, embryonic mortality, and embryonic development were assessed.

Blastocysts from delayed ovulation, when transferred to uteri of control animals, implanted as well as those from control rats (73.2 versus 72.8%). However, the implantation rate was significantly decreased when control blastocysts were placed in uteri of rats in which ovulation had been delayed for 48 h (49.7%). There was a trend toward an increase in embryonic death and defective embryonic development in uteri of delayed ovulatory rats. These data demonstrate alterations in intrauterine environment that markedly affect implantation and possibly later embryonic development. The highly significant increase in the incidence of abnormal and degenerating embryos after implantation of aged blastocysts into control uteri (33.0 versus 15.8% in control transfers) is in agreement with an alteration of the preovulatory oocyte. However, a detrimental effect of the environment within the reproductive tract during the 4-day period before transfer was not ruled out as a contributing cause of abnormal postimplantation development. Additional work in which ova are transferred immediately after ovulation is needed to clarify this point.

An altered intrauterine environment was expected, since there is a prolonged period of vaginal cornification and uterine ballooning when ovulation is delayed for 48 h in the rat. Also, the uterine ballooning subsides earlier in relation to the time of ovulation in animals with a delayed ovulation than it does in controls [BUTCHER, unpublished]. These observations indicate an altered level or pattern in secretion of ovarian steroid. Our recent analyses of gonadotropins and steroids [BUTCHER, unpublished] indicate a prolongation in the secretion of estrogen during the period of delayed ovulation. This prolonged secretion of estrogen is probably the main factor involved in the alteration of intrauterine environment during delayed ovulation.

B. Maternal Age and Intrauterine Environment

Extensive reviews of aging influences on the uterus have been made [ADAMS, 1970; BIGGERS, 1969; TALBERT, 1968]. Definite alterations take place in the uterus with increasing age, but the significance of these is not clear. Effects of altered concentrations of hormones and changes in the sequence of their release, as well as the general aging process, must be considered as factors in modified intrauterine environment of aging females. Endocrine changes with increasing age can affect the oocyte directly and should be considered when designing experiments dealing with the environment within the reproductive tract. When studying the uterine contribution to infertility in aging animals, we should give consideration to the stage of decline in reproduction, circulating levels of hormones, responsiveness of the uterus to these hormones, and timing of ovulation in relation to hormonal changes.

Whether changes in the uterus (e.g., increased collagen, decreased ability to form decidual tissue, and decreased sensitivity to ovarian steroids) are due to aging of that organ *per se* or to altered levels of circulating steroids has not been satisfactorily assessed. Nor has the role of delayed ovulation as it affects intrauterine environment in aged animals been evaluated.

An elevation in collagen content of the uterus with increasing age has been reported in the mouse [FINN *et. al.*, 1963], the rat [KOA *et al.*, 1962; KOA and McGAVACK, 1959], and the rabbit [MAURER and FOOTE, 1972]. In the human uterus, collagen content increased to 30 years of age, remained stable to age 50 and then decreased [WOESSNER, 1963]. However, the collagen became progressively more resistant to digestion by collagenase. Whether or not the increase in amount of collagen or change in its quality contributes significantly to infertility is not known. KOA and McGAVACK [1959] found that the increase in both insoluable and total collagen had occurred by 8 months of age in the rat, which is prior to a significant decrease in reproductive performance.

Amount of decidual tissue has been shown to decrease with increasing age in the mouse [FINN, 1966; SHAPIRO and TALBERT, 1969], and the hamster [BLAHA, 1966, 1967]. Unfortunately, most of the comparisons were made near the end of reproductive life rather than during the decline in fertility. At the end of reproductive life, nonreversible changes in the uterus probably have resulted from a number of influences (e.g., chronological aging, modified levels of ovarian steroids, number of pregnancies, and infections) that allow the consequences, but not the mechanism, of uterine aging to be studied. SHAPIRO and TALBERT [1969] studied decidual cell response in intact mice at 4–7, 9, 11, and 13 months of age. Studies also were made of mice of similar ages after ovariectomy and priming with estrogen and progesterone. In intact mice, fewer old mice (38%) responded with a decidual reaction than did young mice at 4–7 months of age (86%). No difference was found in response among 9-, 11-, and 13-month-old intact animals, but in ovariectomized mice 4–7 months old the positive decidual cell response was 63%, in those 9 months old 37%, and in those 11–13 months old 15%. This study suggests a decrease in sensitivity of the uterus either to trauma or to steroid stimulation with increasing age.

BLAHA [1966, 1967] found a greater decidual cell reaction in aged hamsters treated in the previous cycle with pregnant mares serum gonadotropin than in aged controls, which suggests insufficient endogenous hormonal stimulation for a maximum response in old hamsters. Progesterone treatment after uterine trauma was ineffective in increasing decidual response. WOESSNER [1969] found a difference in collagen depletion as a result of estradiol treatment following parturition in the rat. Rate of steroid secretion, timing of secretion in relation to time of trauma or implantation, sensitivity of the uterus to steroids, as well as permanent changes in the uterus, should be considered simultaneously in future studies.

Prepuberal unilateral ovariectomy has been used to study the effect of life-time reproduction in the mouse [BIGGERS et al., 1962 a; JONES and KROHN, 1960], the hamster [BLAHA, 1964 a], the rat [ADAMS, 1970; PEPPLER, 1971] and the rabbit [ADAMS, 1970]. In all studies, about half as many total offspring were produced during a life time as in intact animals. Litter size and number of litters were decreased and the mothers were younger at the time of birth of their last litter. In comparing a single ovary from intact mice and a single ovary from mice that had had unilateral ovariectomy, JONES and KROHN [1960] found that they had about the same number of large follicles and the same number of oocytes. They concluded that the reduction in litter size was due to overcrowding in the uterus as there was no indication that oocytes were being depleted. However, this does not account for termination of reproduction at an earlier age following unilateral ovariectomy. BIGGERS et al. [1962 a] found no difference between the weight of the single ovary of unilaterally ovariectomized mice and the combined weight of both ovaries in intact animals 16 weeks after production of their last litter. BIGGERS et al. [1962 b] concluded that overcrowding caused a reduction in litter size and a premature aging of the uterus in unilaterally ovariectomized mice. The premature aging of the uterus was considered to be the cause of the earlier onset in the decline in reproduction. Tying off one oviduct in the mouse reduced litter size and the total number of offspring by about one half [FINN, 1963] but did not reduce the number of litters produced. FINN also concluded that decreased fertility with increasing age is due to chronological aging and that overloading the uterus of unilaterally ovariectomized animals results in earlier aging than usual. In contrast to this work in the mouse, ADAMS [1970] found no decrease in the age at last litter following unilateral ovariectomy in either the rat or the rabbit, although litter size was reduced. This decrease in litter size was due to embryonic mortality and not ovulation rate. It seems probable that removal of one ovary would alter hormonal levels, which could accelerate the aging process of the hormonal control of the ovary. With the sensitive techniques for hormone assays now available the effect of hemiovariectomy on intrauterine environment should be investigated in relation to plasma levels of ovarian steroids.

The effect of aging on reproduction also has been studied by using the technique of ova transfer between young and old mice [TALBERT and KROHN, 1965, 1966], hamsters [BLAHA, 1964 a, b] and rabbits [ADAMS, 1970]. Both the intrauterine environment and oocytes of aged animals appear to exert a detrimental effect although not uniformly as the reaction varies in different species. This subject is covered in detail by BLAHA elsewhere in this volume and will not be reviewed here. However, it should be pointed out that studies to date have considered only the chronological ages of donor and recipient. In none of these investigations has the preovulatory development of the oocyte been considered, nor has the hormonal secretion during the preovulatory interval been evaluated.

FUGO and BUTCHER [1971] have reported that a spontaneous 6-day estrous cycle in the aged rat results in a greater incidence of abnormal embryonic development and of embryonic death than occurs if the cycle is 4 days in length. Since both the rat and the mouse have a high incidence of irregular cycle lengths with advancing age, studies of uterine environment in aged animals should include the length of the estrous cycle. The decline in fertility in the aged rabbit (an induced ovulator) and the hamster (which has a 4-day estrous cycle throughout life) does not appear to be related to delayed ovulation. However, this does not preclude the possibility of ovulation of oocytes that are past their peak of maturation and a change in secretion of ovarian steroids associated with postmaturity of the follicle. A prolonged elevation of estrogen could occur in aged animals as it does during sodium pentobarbital delay of ovulation in the rat. Levels of hormones in plasma of the aged rat need to be investigated, both in relation to preovulatory changes and to progressive changes with advancing age.

II. Intrafollicular Aging of the Oocyte on Development and Implantation

Clinical observations and experimental evidence suggest that the time of ovulation in relation to preovulatory events is an important factor in infertility and the production of congenital anomalies. The decrease of fertility following alterations in the time of ovulation is often attributed to a hostile intrauterine environment or time of insemination without considering modifications that have occurred in the oocyte. Likewise, the decreased fertility and abnormal embryonic development with advanced maternal age have generally been thought to be due to age-related changes in the uterus and to an accumulation of changes in the oocyte brought about by chronological aging without considering the timing of events that occur in the immediate reproductive cycle.

The process of meiosis has been studied in many species [DONAHUE, 1968; EDWARDS, 1965, 1966; MANDL, 1963; SCHUETZ, 1969; TSAFRIRI et al., 1972], but the factors that are responsible for the preovulatory resumption of maturation are not fully understood. Most studies in mammals have concluded that the resumption of meiosis is due to the preovulatory surge of LH. However, maturation of the oocyte occurs in vitro in the absence of hormones following mechanical rupture of the follicle [EDWARDS, 1966; PINCUS and ENZMANN, 1935], but not if the intact follicle is cultured [TSAFRIRI et al., 1972]. Histochemical and ultrastructural changes occur within the oocyte and the surrounding cumulus cells during follicular growth and oocyte maturation [ADAMS et al., 1966; HERTIG and ADAMS, 1967; LOBEL and LEVY, 1968]. Control of these biochemical and ultrastructural processes is not understood. Alterations in the timing of the biochemical events within the oocyte in relation to the resumption of meiosis and the time of ovulation could lead to a defective zygote.

A. Delayed Ovulation in the Human Female

For many years it has been known that the incidence of abortions, stillbirths, and congenital anomalies increases as maternal age advances [HENDRICKS, 1955; HERTIG, 1967; IFFY and WINGATE, 1970; LANMAN, 1968; MILHAM and GITTELSOHN, 1965; PENROSE, 1954; TALBERT, 1968]. Congenital malformations also occur with a relatively high frequency when mothers are under 15 years of age [HENDRICKS, 1955]. Only maternal age as it relates to delayed ovulation will be presented, since a detailed discussion of the effects of maternal age is presented elsewhere in this volume by ADAMS.

At puberty and during the climacteric period changes occur in the secretion of gonadotropic hormones with the consequence that the menstrual cycles are irregular and often prolonged. It has been proposed [FUGO and BUTCHER, 1970] that during these periods of adjustments a delay in ovulation can occur that could result in congenital anomalies. Intrafollicular aging of the oocyte as a result of prolonged menstrual cycles could result in birth defects at any time during reproductive life when a delay in ovulation occurs. HERTIG [1967] states: 'If an oocyte lingers longer than day 14 in the follicle, it has an increasing chance of becoming a "bad egg" when fertilized.' He examined a group of 34 fertilized human ova from patients with dated coitus. Only 1 of 13 ova ovulated on or before day 14 of the menstrual cycle was abnormal; 12 of 21 of those ovulated after day 14 exhibited abnormal development. HERTIG and SHELDON [1943] examined 1,000 abortuses from women with known reproductive histories and classified 617 abortions as related to defects in the oocytes and 383 as due to other causes. These studies suggest that defective oocytes are more the cause of abortion and developmental anomalies than is hostile intrauterine environment.

The conceptus in a large proportion of spontaneous abortions has an abnormal number of chromosomes. CARR [1969] reported that 21% of 811 abortuses had chromosomal anomalies. This subject is discussed elsewhere in this volume by BOUÉ. Degenerative changes in occytes during a preovulatory overripeness have been suggested as a cause of chromosomal abnormalities [MIKAMO, this volume]. Others [KNÖRR and UEBELE-KALLHARDT, 1967] have concluded that abortion and abnormal development are increased by ovulation of eggs that are not at the peak of maturation.

Delayed ovulation in the human female has been reviewed by IFFY and WINGATE [1970] and by JONGBLOET [this volume] as it relates to congenital anomalies and abortion. Although some data are open to criticism owing to uncertainty of conception date, the data suggest that delayed ovulation is an important factor in human abortion and congenital anomalies. Midcycle abstinence as a method of contraception has been reported to result in an increase in birth defects [CROSS, 1968; NAGGAN and MACMAHON, 1967]. These defects could result from either delayed ovulation or delayed fertilization. CARR [1969] found an increase in the incidence of polyploidy in abortuses from conception within 6 months after discontinuing oral contraceptives. Irregular and prolonged menstrual cycles often occur for a time after discontinuing oral contraceptives. Such alteration in length of the menstrual cycle could result in an intrafollicular aging of the oocyte. If an intrafollicular aging of the occyte produces abnormal development of the conceptus in the human female as it does in the rat, then any condition that produces a delay in ovulation holds the potential for the production of congenital anomalies.

B. Delayed Ovulation in the Rat

Many studies have been made on the effect of advancing maternal age and of delayed fertilization on infertility and abnormal embryonic development. However, relatively little has been done on the relationship of delayed ovulation to decreased fertility and to increased abnormalities of embryonic development.

A series of experiments has been carried out in my laboratory by delaying ovulation in young rats with sodium pentobarbital and with spontaneous delay of ovulation in the aged rat. These experiments were undertaken to determine in an animal model whether intrafollicular overripeness of oocytes might account for the increased incidence of abortions and birth defects observed with advancing maternal age in the woman. Ovulation was delayed with sodium pentobarbital [EVERETT and SAWYER, 1950] for 48 h in rats with 4-day estrous cycles and for 24 h in animals with 4- or 5-day cycles. Effects of the ovulatory delay were determined for the preovulatory oocyte, preimplantation stages, midgestation, and near term.

A 48-hour delay of ovulation resulted in a 2-day postponement in the resumption of meiosis in oocytes [FREEMAN et al., 1970] although the follicles continued to grow and reached a greater preovulatory diameter than those in control animals. Resumption of meiosis, ovulation, mating, fertilization, and implantation all occurred at the usual time of day, but 48 h later than would have occurred had ovulation not been delayed [BUTCHER, unpublished; FREEMAN, 1970]. Studies during the preimplantation stages of development [FUGO and BUTCHER, 1966] demonstrated that a 48-hour delay of ovulation resulted in a decrease in fertilization rate (78 versus 93%) and an increase in the incidence of fertilized ova that were abnormal at the pronuclear, 2-cell, and blastocyst stages (29.0 versus 3.6%, 14.1 versus 4.3% and 53.6 versus 20.3%, respectively). Some of the anomalies found included an increase in polyspermy, degeneration of fertilized ova, irregular cell membranes, unequal cleavage, large polar bodies, retarded development, and accessory spermatozoa.

At midgestation following a 48-hour delay of ovulation, BUTCHER et al. [1969 a] reported a signifiicant decrease in implantation (62 versus 89%), an increase in the incidence of abnormal or retarded fetuses (17 versus 7.4%), and an increase in degenerating embryos (10.2 versus 4.4%). Embryonic development following either pentobarbital at 8.30 a.m. on the day of proestrus or a 24-hour delay of ovulation during 4-day cycles did not differ from that of the uninjected controls. However, a 24-hour delay during a 5-day cycle was as detrimental as a 48-hour delay in a 4-day cycle in rats. This suggests that the lapse of time from the previous ovulation (6 days) rather than the length of delay by pentobarbital is the important factor. When ovulation does not take place by day 5, some process must be occurring in the follicular occyte that is detrimental to its future development. The incidence of anomalies found at day 20 of gestation had decreased owing to embryonic death and resorption but was still significantly elevated in the treated group (3.6 versus 0.4%).

Reciprocal transfers of blastocysts between control and delayed ovulatory rats and between controls were made on the morning of day 4 of gestation, and fetuses were examined at midgestation [BUTCHER et al., 1969 b]. This investigation demonstrated that the decrease in implantation rate is due to altered intrauterine environment but indicates that embryonic death and abnormal development are the result of preovulatory overripeness of the oocyte. However, the possibility of an environmental effect within the reproductive tract during the 4 days prior to transfer cannot be discounted. In another study at midgestation [BUTCHER and FUGO, 1967], the incidence of chromosomal anomalies was 3 times as great in fetuses after delayed ovulation as in control fetuses (18 of 390 versus 6 of 410).

After one year of age, estrous cycles of the rat become irregular with periods of constant vaginal estrus and diestrus. This phenomenon was used to investigate the effect of spontaneously delayed ovulation on developmental anomalies resulting from conception at the estrus ending a 6-day estrous cycle as compared to conception at the end of a 4-day cycle in the aging rat. The incidence of abnormal development at the one-cell, blastula, and 11- and 20-day stages of gestation was significantly greater when conception occurred during a 6-day cycle than when the cycle was 4 days in length. The type and incidence of anomalies were similar to those found in the young adult rat after pentobarbital delay of ovulation. This demonstrates that a spontaneous as well as an induced delay of ovulation is detrimental to embryonic development.

Additional studies have been made to determine what alterations occur in the oocyte and in circulating levels of hormones as a result of delayed ovulation. The plasma concentrations of LH, FSH, prolactin, progesterone, and estradiol were measured at 3-hour intervals from the initiation of delay of ovulation by pentobarbital until midnight of the fourth day of gestation [BUTCHER, unpublished]. Measurements also were made at 30-min intervals on the afternoon of the ovulatory peak of gonadotropins. Control rats received injections of vehicle only. Blood was collected in 8 replicates from one treated and one control rat simultaneously at each time period. The paired samples were analyzed in adjacent tubes of an assay that included a complete replicate for the gonadotropins or one fourth replicate for the steroids. The proestrous peaks of LH, FSH, and progesterone were suppressed on both days of treatment but occurred at the expected time on the afternoon prior to ovulation. Peaks of prolactin occurred on both treatment days and along with the LH and FSH peaks on the following day. Plasma levels of estradiol were elevated on all 3 days but dropped back to base level at the usual time in relation to ovulation. The prolonged secretion of estrogen was reflected in a 2-day increase in vaginal cornification and in uterine ballooning. Concentrations of all 5 hormones during estrus and the first 4 days of gestation did not differ from those in the controls. Since estradiol is elevated throughout the period of delayed ovulation, this hormone needs to be studied for a possible role in the alteration in the oocyte during intrafollicular aging.

Studies of oocytes obtained at 8 a.m. on the day of estrus from control rats and from rats after a 48-hour delay of ovulation were examined by electron microscopy [PELUSO and BUTCHER, unpublished]. Following intrafollicular overripeness, oocytes showed a number of cytoplasmic alterations. These changes in ultrastructure varied in degree among oocytes, which could account for variations from normal to grossly abnormal development within the same litter in our previous studies. Numbers of cortical granules were reduced by 50%, which could account both for failure to fertilize and for polyspermy, depending on whether the reduction in number of cortical granules was due to early expulsion of their contents into the perivitelline space, to degeneration or to production of insufficient numbers to block polyspermy. Mitochondria in the intrafollicularly aged oocyte were elongated with shelf-like cristae, whereas those of the controls were spherical with peripheral cristae. The elongated mitochondria with shelf-like cristae are suggestive of increased metabolism since this type of mitochondria usually is not present until about the 8-cell stage [STERN et al., 1971]. Additional work needs to be done in this area, particularly in relation to metabolic changes, RNA synthesis, and hormonal action.

Present data on delayed ovulation suggest that most of the deleterious effects on embryonic development are due to alterations in the preovulatory oocyte, whereas failure of implantation arises from changes in intrauterine environment. Upon delay of ovulation by sodium pentobarbital, a prolonged secretion of estrogen occurs that is probably responsible for a hostile intrauterine environment. Further studies are needed to investigate the effect of this prolonged secretion of estrogen and to determine whether a similar pattern occurs during lengthened estrous cycles in aged animals. Intrauterine environment has been shown to affect implantation, but additional work is needed to determine whether intrauterine environment contributes to the production of defective embryonic development.

The available evidence indicates that defective oocytes produced by intrafollicular aging are the result of some event initiated before 2 p.m. of the third day of the estrous cycle in the rat. If ovulation does not take place by the fifth day following the previous estrus, the chance of defective embryonic development is markedly increased. The exact point at which these time-dependent events occur in the oocyte is not known. There is undoubtedly a series of biochemical reactions occurring continuously, starting at the time of initiation of growth of the primary oocyte. Whether these processes can be interrupted during growth of the oocyte without harmful effects or whether development from time of activation until ovulation is regulated rigidly is not known. Likewise, we do not understand the role or the timing of hormones in initiating various biochemical events in the growing oocyte and follicle. Does the follicle suppress some processes in the oocyte until a hormonal dependent mechanism, such as the preovulatory peak of estrogen or LH, releases the oocyte from this suppression? What is the mechanism that activates growth of certain primary oocytes and not others? This activation takes place to some degree in hypophysectomized animals. Might the growing follicles play a role in initiation of oocyte growth and development?

Knowledge of activation and early growth of the follicle, as well as knowledge of biochemical events in the growing oocyte, is almost completely lacking. This is a fruitful area for research that would contribute much to our understanding of the mechanism of aging of gametes.

III. Approaches to Investigation of Intrafollicular Aging of Oocytes

Intrafollicular aging of oocytes resulting from prolonged reproductive cycles has similar effects whether it occurs as a consequence of increased maternal age or from pentobarbital blockage of ovulation. However, other factors related to somatic aging probably contribute in various ways to defective development with increasing maternal age. Studies of reproduction in aging animals present many difficult technical and scientific problems in carrying out experiments and in interpreting results. Although several studies can be made on this problem in aged animals, certain investigations in which induced delayed ovulation is used would be more realistic. Many areas of importance to the complete understanding of gamete aging, such as the control of early growth of the follicle and oocyte, should first be elucidated during the normal reproductive cycle.

Some of the questions that need to be answered in relation to the normal reproductive cycle are: What initiates growth of the follicle and oocyte? What are the growth rates of the follicle and oocyte at all stages of development? What determines which oocyte will develop to an ovulatory size? What controls follicular atresia? What are the biochemical and ultrastructural changes in the follicle and oocyte during growth? What is the relationship of the cyclic nature of the secretion of gonadotropic and gonadal hormones in all the above questions? Considerable information is available for limited time periods in some of these areas, whereas little or nothing is known about many of the mechanisms. A knowledge of the normal oocyte during preovulatory development must be achieved before aging of the oocyte can be completely understood.

A. Studies on Normal Mechanisms

Pulse labeling has been used for evaluating follicular growth [PEDERSEN, 1970]; and it seems that a great deal of progress could be made on initiation and rate of follicular growth with this technique. With the correct dose and timing of isotope-labeled precursors, the pattern of initiation of growth of follicles and number of follicles involved could be obtained. Synthesis within the follicular cells and oocytes could be studied by the use of radioactive precursors and autoradiography. Autoradiography in conjunction with electron microscopy, histochemistry, and micro-biochemical techniques could be used in the investigation of biochemical events during growth and development. For greatest progress into the mechanisms involved in all the above studies, the hormonal patterns should be known in relation to the timing of the events under investigation.

B. Studies with Induced Delay of Ovulation

From previous work with pentobarbital delay of ovulation, a number of areas are suggested for additional study. One of these areas is the effect of preimplantation environment on developmental defects. Following delayed ovulation, embryos exposed for the first 4 days of gestation to the environment within the reproductive tract implant as well as control blastocysts that have been transferred to control uteri [BUTCHER *et al.*, 1969 b]. However, it has not been determined whether this 4-day exposure in the reproductive tract following delayed ovulation affects future development of the embryos after implantation. This can be accomplished by reciprocal transfer of ova immediately after ovulation.

The effect of prolonged secretion of estrogen during delayed ovulation in the production of a hostile intrauterine environment could be studied by using an anti-serum to estrogens. Estrogen antiserum alone will block ovulation or it can be used in combination with sodium pentobarbital. This use of estrogen antiserum in combination with ova transfer would be useful in studying the effects of estrogen on both the oocyte and the intrauterine environment.

As suggested earlier, a difference was found between the ultrastructure of oocytes following delayed ovulation and that of control oocytes. Ultrastructural studies of oocytes need to be made during the period of delayed ovulation to determine when changes occur. Autoradiography could be combined with electron microscopy to discover what metabolic alterations produce, or are regulated by, ultrastructural changes. This investigation also should be correlated with plasma patterns of gonadotropins and ovarian steroids. Treatments with hormones and antisera to hormones would be valuable in these investigations.

C. Studies of Intrafollicular Overripeness in Aging Animals

Investigations of intrafollicular overripeness of oocytes in aged animals face a number of problems. Many physiological alterations related to age occur that probably affect the hypothalamus, pituitary gland, ovaries, and uterus to varying degrees in different animals. Although some changes are probably of a permanent nature, others are dependent on the hormonal levels in the immediate or recent reproductive stage. With advanced age, neither an estrous cycle of normal length nor an induced ovulation assures that oocytes are not postmature. With increasing age, changes have been shown to occur in circulating levels of hormones. Such changes in hormonal levels could be expected to alter the rate of biochemical development of the oocyte.

Again, the technique of ova transfer immediately after ovulation should be productive in determining the extent to which intrafollicular aging of the oocyte and intrauterine environment are involved in reduced fertility of aging animals. Ova transfers would be between young and aging animals, and the length of estrous cycles, previous reproductive history, and circulating levels of gonadotropins and ovarian steroids should be taken into consideration.

The number of developing follicles may be important in the development of oocytes and of follicles destined to ovulate. If all but one or two follicles are destroyed during the follicular phase, the remaining follicles do not reach ovulatory size or ovulate [NALBANDOV, 1964]; but with exogenous estrogen injections, these remaining follicles grow and ovulate. DUFOUR et al. [1972] reported continual growth and atresia of follicles in the heifer, but the follicle destined to ovulate was not the largest follicle until about 3 days before ovulation. A steady decline in the number of large follicles with increasing age has been reported in rats [MANDL and SHELTON, 1959] and mice [JONES and KROHN, 1961] without a decrease in ovulation rate. Changes in the number of nonovulatory-sized follicles in aging females could be of great importance to intrafollicular aging of oocytes and should be examined.

Most of the above studies suggested for normal animals or for animals in which ovulation has been delayed also are applicable to aged animals. However, a greater understanding of the normal function should be achieved in many areas before studies are made during advanced maternal age.

Summary

Either an induced delay of ovulation with sodium pentobarbital or a spontaneous delay of ovulation in the aged rat produces decreased fertility and an increased incidence of developmental anomalies. Alterations in the oocyte during intrafollicular aging are primarily responsible for developmental defects and postimplantation deaths and contribute to preimplantation losses. Changes in intrauterine environment accompany intrafollicular aging of oocytes and appear to result mainly in a marked decrease in implantation rate. Intrauterine environment has received much blame for embryonic death and developmental abnormalities related to aging without consideration of the effects of alterations within the oocytes.

Some possible experimental approaches for further separation of alterations in the oocytes and in the intrauterine environment have been suggested. Additional studies of the aged oocyte have been proposed. Suggestions for needed investigations of the growth and maturation of normal follicles and oocytes have been discussed. Much still remains to be learned about the role of oocyte aging and related changes in intrauterine environment. Knowledge of many phases of normal growth and development of oocytes and follicles is completely lacking. These areas need to be understood before the mechanisms involved in oocyte aging can be fully comprehended.

References

ADAMS, C.E.: Ageing and reproduction in the female mammal with particular reference to the rabbit. J. Reprod. Fertil. Suppl. *12:* 1 (1970).

ADAMS, E.C.; HERTIG, A.T., and FOSTER, S.: Studies on guinea pig oocytes. II. Histochemical observations on some phosphatases and lipids in developing and in atretic oocytes and follicles. Amer. J. Anat. *119:* 303 (1966).

AUSTIN, C.R.: Ageing and reproduction. Post-ovulatory deterioration of the egg. J. Reprod. Fertil. Suppl. *12:* 39 (1970).

BIGGERS, J.D.: Problems concerning the uterine causes of embryonic death, with special reference to the effects of ageing of the uterus. J. Reprod. Fertil. Suppl. *8:* 27 (1969).

BIGGERS, J.D.; FINN, C.A., and MCLAREN, A.: Long-term reproductive performance of female mice. I. Effect of removing one ovary. J. Reprod. Fertil. *3:* 303 (1962a).

BIGGERS, J.D.; FINN, C.A., and MCLAREN, A.: Long-term reproductive performance of female mice. II. Variation of litter size with parity. J. Reprod. Fertil. *3:* 313 (1962b).

BLAHA, G.C.: Reproductive senescence in the female golden hamster. Anat. Rec. *150:* 405 (1964a).

BLAHA, G.C.: Effect of age of the donor and recipient on the development of transferred golden hamster ova. Anat. Rec. *150:* 413 (1964b).

BLAHA, G.C.: Deciduoma formation in aged golden hamsters. Anat. Rec. *154:* 318 (1966).

BLAHA, G.C.: Effect of age, treatment, and method of induction of deciduomata in the golden hamster. Fertil. Steril. *18:* 477 (1967).

BUTCHER, R.L.: Aberrant ovulation-consequences on fertility and embryonic development. J. anim. Sci. *34:* suppl. 1, p. 39 (1972).

BUTCHER, R.L.; BLUE, J.D., and FUGO, N.W.: Overripeness and the mammalian ova. III. Fetal development at midgestation and at term. Fertil. Steril. *20:* 223 (1969a).

BUTCHER, R.L.; BLUE, J.D., and FUGO, N.W.: Role of intrauterine environment on ova after normal and delayed ovulation. Biol. Reprod. *1:* 149 (1969b).

BUTCHER, R.L. and FUGO, N.W.: Overripeness and the mammalian ova. II. Delayed ovulation and chromosome anomalies. Fertil. Steril. *18:* 297 (1967).

CARR, D.H.: Chromosomal errors and development. Amer. J. Obstet. Gynec. *104:* 327 (1969).

CROSS, R.G.: Anencephalus and spina bifida. Brit. med. J. *iii:* 253 (1968).

DONAHUE, R.P.: Maturation of the mouse oocyte *in vitro*. I. Sequence and timing of nuclear progression. J. exp. Zool. *169:* 237 (1968).

DUFOUR, J.; WHITMORE, H.L.; GINTHER, O.J., and CASIDA, L.E.: Identification of the ovulating follicle by its size on different days of the estrous cycle in heifers. J. anim. Sci. *34:* 85 (1972).

EDWARDS, R.G.: Maturation *in vitro* of mouse, sheep, cow, pig, rhesus monkey and human ovarian oocytes. Nature, Lond. *208:* 349 (1965).

EDWARDS, R.G.: Mammalian eggs in the laboratory. Sci. Amer. *215:* 72 (1966).

EVERETT, J.W. and SAWYER, C.H.: A 24-hour periodicity in the 'LH-release apparatus' of female rats, disclosed by barbiturate sedation. Endocrinology *47:* 198 (1950).

FINN, C.A.: Reproductive capacity and litter size in mice. J. Reprod. Fertil. *6:* 205 (1963).

FINN, C.A.: The initiation of the decidual cell reaction in the uterus of the aged mouse. J. Reprod. Fertil. *11:* 423 (1966).

FINN, C.A.; FITCH, S.M., and HARKNESS, R.D.: Collagen content of barren and previously pregnant uterine horns in old mice. J. Reprod. Fertil. *6:* 405 (1963).

FRANCIS, W.J.A.: Reproduction at menarche and menopause in women. J. Reprod.
Fertil. Suppl. *12:* 89 (1970).

FREEMAN, M.E.: Functional changes associated with delayed ovulation; Ph.D. diss.,
Morgantown (1970).

FREEMAN, M.E.; BUTCHER, R.L., and FUGO, N.W.: Alteration of oocytes and follicles
by delayed ovulation. Biol. Reprod. *2:* 209 (1970).

FUGO, N.W. and BUTCHER, R.L.: Overripeness and the mammalian ova. I. Overripeness
and early embryonic development. Fertil. Steril. *17:* 804 (1966).

FUGO, N.W. and BUTCHER, R.L.: Irregular menses. Overripeness and fetal anomalies.
J. Reprod. Med. *4:* 75 (1970).

FUGO, N.W. and BUTCHER, R.L.: Effects of prolonged estrous cycles on reproduction in
aged rats. Fertil. Steril. *22:* 98 (1971).

HENDRICKS, C.H.: Congenital malformations, analysis of the 1953 Ohio records. Obstet.
Gynec. *6:* 592 (1955).

HERTIG, A.T.: The overall problem in man; in BENIRSCHKE Comparative aspects of reproductive failure (Springer, Berlin 1967).

HERTIG, A.T. and ADAMS, E.C.: Studies on the human oocyte and its follicle. I. Ultrastructural and histochemical observations on the primordial follicle stage. J. Cell
Biol. *34:* 647 (1967).

HERTIG, A.T. and SHELDON, W.H.: Minimal criteria required to prove prima facie case
of traumatic abortion or miscarriage. Ann. Surg. *117:* 596 (1943).

IFFY, L. and WINGATE, M.B.: Risks of rhythm method of birth control. J. Reprod. Med. *5:*
96 (1970).

JONES, E.C.: The aging ovary and its influence on reproductive capacity. J. Reprod. Fertil.
Suppl. *12:* 17 (1970).

JONES, E.C. and KROHN, P.L.: The effect of unilateral ovariectomy on the reproductive
lifespan of mice. J. Endocrin. *20:* 129 (1960).

JONES, E.C. and KROHN, P.L.: The relationship between age, number of oocytes and
fertility in virgin and multiparous mice. J. Endocrin. *21:* 469 (1961).

KNÖRR, K. und UEBELE-KALLHARDT, B.: Zytogenetische Untersuchungen an einem Spon-
tanabort nach induzierter Ovulation. Med. Welt, Stg. *18:* 1812 (1967).

KOA, K.-Y.T. and MCGAVACK, T.H.: Connective tissue. I. Age and sex influence on
protein composition of rat tissues. Proc. Soc. exp. Biol. Med. *101:* 153 (1959).

KOA, K.-Y.T.; LU, S.-D.C.; HITT, W., and MCGAVACK, T.H.: Connective tissue. VI.
Synthesis of collagen by rat uterine slices. Proc. Soc. exp. Biol. Med. *109:* 4 (1962).

KROHN, P.L.: The reproductive lifespan. Proc. 5th Int. Congr. Anim. Reprod. A.I.,
Trento 1964, vol. 3, p. 23 (1964).

LANMAN, J.T.: Delays during reproduction and their effects on the embryo and fetus.
New Engl. J. Med. *278:* 993, 1047, 1092 (1968).

LOBEL, B.L. and LEVY, E.: Enzymic correlates of development, secretory function and
regression of follicles and corpora lutea in the bovine ovary. Acta endocrin., Kbh. *59:*
suppl. 132, p. 7 (1968).

MANDL, A.M.: Pre-ovulatory changes in the oocyte of the adult rat. Proc. roy. Soc. B *158:*
105 (1963).

MANDL, A.M. and SHELTON, M.: A quantitative study of oocytes in young and old nulliparous laboratory rats. J. Endocrin. *18:* 444 (1959).

MAURER, R.R. and FOOTE, R.H.: Uterine collagenase and collagen in young and ageing rabbits. J. Reprod. Fertil. *30:* 301 (1972).

MILHAM, S., jr. and GITTELSOHN, A.M.: Parental age and malformations. Human Biol. *37:* 13 (1965).

NAGGAN, L. and MACMAHON, B.: Ethnic differences in the prevalence of anencephaly and spina bifida in Boston, Massachusetts. New Engl. J. Med. *277:* 1119 (1967).

NALBANDOV, A.V.: Reproductive physiology; 2nd ed. (W.H. Freeman, London 1964).

PEDERSEN, T.: in BIGGERS and SCHUETZ Oogenesis (University Park Press, Baltimore, and Butterworth, London 1970).

PENROSE, L.S.: Mongolian idiocy (Mongolism) and maternal age. Ann. N.Y. Acad. Sci. *57:* 494 (1954).

PEPPLER, R.D.: Effects of unilateral ovariectomy on follicular development and ovulation in cycling, aged rats. Amer. J. Anat. *132:* 423 (1971).

PINCUS, G. and ENZMANN, E.V.: The comparative behavior of mammalian eggs *in vivo* and *in vitro*. I. The activation of ovarian eggs. J. exp. Med. *62:* 665 (1935).

SCHUETZ, A.W.: in MCLAREN Advances in reproductive physiology, vol. 4, p. 99 (Academic Press, New York 1969).

SHAPIRO, M. and TALBERT, G.B.: Effect of maternal age upon decidualization. Anat. Rec. *163:* 261 (1969).

STERN, S.; BIGGERS, J.D., and ANDERSON, E.: Mitochondria and early development of the mouse. J. exp. Zool. *176:* 179 (1971).

TALBERT, G.B.: Effect of maternal age on reproductive capacity. Amer. J. Obstet. Gynec. *102:* 451 (1968).

TALBERT, G.B. and KROHN, P.L.: Effect of maternal age on the viability of ova and on the ability of the uterus to support pregnancy. Anat. Rec. *151:* 424 (1965).

TALBERT, G.B. and KROHN, P.L.: Effect of maternal age on viability of ova and uterine support of pregnancy in mice. J. Reprod. Fertil. *11:* 399 (1966).

TSAFRIRI, A.; LINDNER, H.R.; ZOR, U., and LAMPRECHT, S.A.: *In vitro* induction of meiotic division in follicle-enclosed rat oocytes by LH, cyclic AMP and prostaglandin E_2. J. Reprod. Fertil. *31:* 39 (1972).

WOESSNER, J.F., jr.: Age-related changes of the human uterus and its connective tissue framework. J. Geront. *18:* 220 (1963).

WOESSNER, J.F., jr.: Inhibition by oestrogen of collagen breakdown in the involuting rat uterus. Biochem. J. *112:* 637 (1969).

Author's address: Dr. ROY L. BUTCHER, Departments of Obstetrics and Gynecology and of Anatomy, School of Medicine, West Virginia University, *Morgantown, WV 26506* (USA)

Aging Gametes. Int. Symp., Seattle 1973, pp. 219–230 (Karger, Basel 1975)

Egg Transfer between Old and Young Mammals

GORDON C. BLAHA

Department of Anatomy, College of Medicine, University of Cincinnati, Cincinnati, Ohio

The decline of reproductive capacity with increasing maternal age is well documented in many species [TALBERT, 1968]. The increased incidence of abnormal offspring born to older women has also been repeatedly shown [BÖÖK et al., 1958; HAY and BARBANO, 1972]. Aging of biological systems seems to lead to an escape from homeostatic mechanisms, and there are likely to be multiple factors involved in the decline of aging biological processes [COMFORT, 1970; STREHLER, 1962]. Various approaches to the study of aging systems are needed to sort out all of the factors involved.

Transfer of eggs between old and young animals is one experimental approach to separating the effects of aging of the maternal reproductive system from intrinsic defects of the eggs themselves. That is not to say that these factors are independent of each other. Oocytes could be adversely influenced by maternal conditions while still in the follicles. Conversely, as we see in the human and some experimental animals, the loss of most or all oocytes leads to considerably different functioning of the ovary [JONES, 1970]. Even when ovaries of older females still have a supply of oocytes they will show declining fertility, and there is reason to believe that defective function of both the maternal system and the ova contribute to this decline [ADAMS, 1970; BLAHA, 1964 a, b; BOOT and MÜHLBOCK, 1954].

I. Past Studies on Egg Transfer between Old and Young

My own studies involving transfer of ova between old and young animals were done on golden hamsters *(Mesocricetus auratus)*. These animals were chosen because they were good breeders and had regular reproductive

Table I. Ova recovered from uteri of mated hamsters 63–68 h after estimated ovulation

Age, months	Total females	Total ova	Ova of four cells or less	Ova/hamster (mean ± SE)
2–1/2–6	21	209	2	9.95 ± 0.89
14–18	24	122	22	5.08 ± 0.71

cycles and a short life span. They were said to have a significant decline in the number of young per litter after 14 months of age [SODERWALL et al., 1960], an observation that resembled that in our own colony. The method used in my first study [BLAHA, 1964 b] consisted of flushing the eggs from the lumina of uterine horns with Hanks solution. This was done on the third day after mating (63–68 h after ovulation). The fluid was collected in a depression slide and the ova were observed at low magnification under a dissecting microscope. A glass micropipet was used to recover the ova and transfer them to the uterus of a recipient that had been mated 3 days before with a vasectomized male. The 3 groups in the study were: (1) young donors (2.5–6 months) whose ova were transferred to old recipients (14–18 months); (2) old donors to young recipients and (3) young donors to young recipients. The number of eggs recovered from all animals were counted (table I), and as much abnormality as could be seen at the low magnification was recorded. It is likely that in both young and old groups some abnormal eggs were not recorded as such. Even so there was an obvious difference between old and young donors both in the number of ova recovered and in the number regarded as abnormal. Abnormal ova were mostly those of four cells or fewer, including degenerated specimens.

The number of term fetuses that developed from the transfers are seen in table II. Neither old-to-young nor young-to-old transfers were as successful as the young-to-young controls. Some young recipients of ova from old donors were seen with small decidual swellings at midterm that were found to contain abnormal embryonic material or trophoblastic remnants. Failure of ova from young donors transferred to old uteri often seemed to be from a lack of decidualization.

TALBERT and KROHN [1966] performed a similar series of experiments in old and young mice. Their methods differed from mine in several respects. They used ova from donors 1 day more advanced in pregnancy than the stage of pseudopregnancy in recipients (day 4 donors to day 3 recipients). They also carefully selected out abnormal ova and did not transfer them, whereas I

Table II. Results of ova transfers between mated donor and sterile-mated recipient golden hamsters, 63–68 h after ovulation

Group[1]	Number of operations	Total ova transferred	Recipients with term fetuses	Total term fetuses	Percent success
Young to old	8	72	3	6	8.3
Old to young	11	88	1	4	4.5
Young to young	8	63	8	31	49.2

1 Young = 2.5–6 months; old = 14–18 months.
From BLAHA [1964b], reprinted with permission of the Wistar Press.

had transferred such ova along with the others. They found more abnormal ova in old mice than in young ones (13 versus 5%). Their results differed from those I obtained with hamsters. The ova from their old donors (400–750 days) transferred to young hosts did as well as their control young-to-young transfers. They also found that ova from young mice did not survive well in old hosts, suggesting again the lessened capability of the aging female reproductive tract.

In another species, the rabbit, ADAMS [1970] has done some egg transfers between old and young does. His results resemble mine in hamsters in that both old-young and young-old transfers demonstrated a low percentage of development compared to controls. More recently, MAURER and FOOTE [1971], using superovulated rabbit does, found that recipients showed less capacity to maintain pregnancy when they were 3 years old but that the embryos derived from donors of that age were just as viable. Donors of 4.5 years, however, showed significantly less capability both for superovulation and for the viability of their embryos that were transferred to younger recipients. Thus, it appeared that the ability of aging does to maintain pregnancy failed before they reached an age when their conceptuses showed impaired viability.

In most mammals the timing of implantation is a critical event; there is a need for blastocyst and endometrium to reach the proper condition at the same time. The blastocysts of some species can wait for a time until the uterus is brought to the proper state by hormonal action [KIRKHAM, 1918; KREHBIEL, 1941; MEYER and COCHRANE, 1962]. Experiments on egg transfers in these species show better results if the blastocysts are a day more advanced in development than the uterus of the recipients [McLAREN and MICHIE,

1956; NOYES and DICKMAN, 1960]. An additional factor here is that the procedure of transferring ova causes some delay in their development [TARKOWSKI, 1959].

Some species, such as hamsters, do not naturally have delayed implantation [ORSINI, 1963] and the blastocysts apparently cannot wait very long until proper conditions are brought about by hormonal action. Egg transfer in these animals should work best when the donor and recipient are synchronized in their preparation. Since even in the controls of my early experiments on hamsters only about 50% of transfers resulted in term fetuses, I attribute at least part of the loss to delay of blastocyst development caused by the transfer procedure.

Old hamsters appear to have a diminished capacity to develop decidual reactions [BLAHA, 1967] and a retarded development of implantation decidual swellings [CONNORS et al., 1972]. CONNORS [1969] has found a 12-hour delay in the formation of decidual cells during pregnancy in senescent hamsters. STOCKTON et al. [1973] have reported that 3-day-old ova from young hamsters survive best in senescent hamsters (14–15 months) when the old hosts are at 4 days of pseudopregnancy. This contrasts with a better survival in synchronous (3-day pseudopregnant) young hosts. This suggests that there is a delay in uterine receptivity in senescent hamsters.

II. Recent Observations on Ova from Old and Young Hamsters

We have recently begun some studies with old and young hamsters that are on different light schedules for purposes of asynchronous ovum transfer. It is too soon to give data here on the survival of transferred ova in these studies. There are some data and observations, however, on the recovery of ova from old and young animals in this study.

One factor that has delayed the accumulation of results in the present series is the low percentage of usable eggs recovered from the old hamsters. The kinds of ova recovered from young and old hamsters at various times after ovulation are shown in table III. There was no irregularity in the cycles of any of these hamsters and the time of ovulation in senescent hamsters of 15–22 months was within a range of 2 h, not notably different from the time in young ones. All hamsters were mated 3–6 h before the expected time of ovulation. Data shown are for ova collected on days 1, 3, and 4 after mating (table III). At the most advanced time, 3 days and 15 h after ovulation, ova were flushed from the uterus. This has recently been reported by SATO and

Table III. Observations on ova recovered from mated golden hamsters. Comparison between old (15–22 months) and young (3–6 months) donors

Time	Donors	Ova		
		fertile	unfertilized	empty zonae
15 h	6 old	32	14 normal	20
			14 degenerate	
	3 young	35	0	0
Two days 16–20 h	13 old	14	65	80 (estimate)
	8 young	78	5	0
Three days 14–16 h	7 old	29	36	3
	5 young	35	5	2

YANAGIMACHI [1972] to be the best time for successful ovum transfer in hamsters. Recovery at this time is difficult, however, because adherence of blastocyst and uterus may already be occurring. The uterine lumen in normal animals may close [FINN, 1970] making flushing a problem. Results could be biased in favor of less normal ova, which would be more easily flushed out. Most of the blastocysts from old animals were still in zonae pellucidae at this time, whereas blastocysts in young animals were out of their zonae. Many undeveloped ova were found in the old animals, some presumably because of lack of fertilization. At 2 days and 15–20 h after ovulation, ova were usually recovered from the uterus, but in many of the old animals cutting of the oviducts was also necessary. A large percentage of the ova in old hamsters appeared unfertilized at this time, particularly those found in oviducts. That some oviducts were blocked was indicated by a great number of empty zonae pellucidae that had accumulated in the tubes of at least two animals.

At 14–16 h after ovulation ova were recovered from the oviducts. Again, a larger number of abnormal or unfertilized ova were recovered from the old animals, including some shrunken oocytes or nearly empty zonae. Some ova recovered at the several stages are shown in figures 1–9.

At 13–18 h, normal ova in old or young had two polar bodies and two pronuclei (fig. 1). There was a large perivitelline space, and the granulosa cells had been shed. Unfertilized ova (fig. 2) had clinging granulosa cells, one polar body, and incomplete development of the second. Some interesting abnormalities include: a fertilized egg with many peculiar globules in the perivitelline space, collected from a young hamster (fig. 3); very shrunken ova found along with normal ova in an old female, probably atretic before ovula-

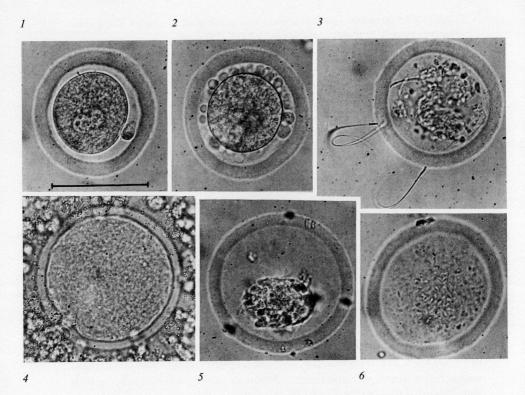

Fig. 1–6. Ova collected from mated hamsters 14–16 h after ovulation. Figure 1: Normal ovum with 2 pronuclei and 2 polar bodies. Figure 2: Unfertilized ovum from old female. Figure 3: Ovum with 2 pronuclei but with many globules in the perivitelline space. Figure 4: Ovum with degenerate vitellus. Figure 5: Disintegrated vitellus with 1 live spermatozoon swimming inside the zona pellucida and 3 more trying to enter. Figure 6: Zona pellucida with no vitellus. Figures 4–6 were from senescent females. Scale marker indicates approximately 100 μm.

tion (fig. 4); a disintegrated oocyte with a spermatozoon swimming inside the zona and three more trying to penetrate (fig. 5); and nearly empty zonae pellucidae (fig. 6). Only one ovum with three pronuclei was found. It contained two spermatozoan tails, suggestive of late fertilization [YANAGIMACHI and CHANG, 1961]. Other than this, delay in fertilization or ovulation has not been apparent in the old hamsters.

Ova recovered at later stages are shown in figures 7 and 8. At 2 days and 16–20 h, normal ova of 6–8 cells were recovered from the uterus of young hams-

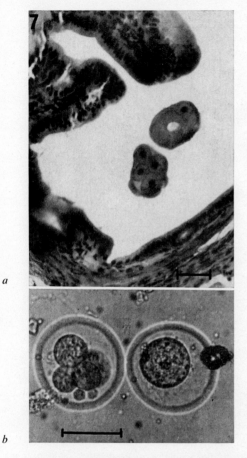

Fig. 7. Ova seen at 2 days, 16–18 h after ovulation in senescent hamsters. *a* Ova still in the oviduct, seen in section. One appears normal, the other has a large vacuolated cell. *b* Ova in fluid collected from the uterus. One has four cells, the other has only one. Scale markers indicate approximately 100 μm.

ters. Some ova in old hamsters were still in the oviduct (fig. 7a). Ova of four cells or fewer at this stage would probably be nonviable (fig. 7b). At 3 days and 14–16 h, blastocysts should have been in the uterus for about 1 day, but in at least one old hamster, they were still in the oviduct (fig. 8a). Most did reach the uterus in old hamsters, however, but were still in zonae pellucidae (fig.8b) at a time when blastocysts in young hamsters had shed their zonae (fig. 8c). These defects in transport of ova and shedding of zonae are suggestive of hormonal imbalance [BURDICK *et al.*, 1942; ORSINI, 1963].

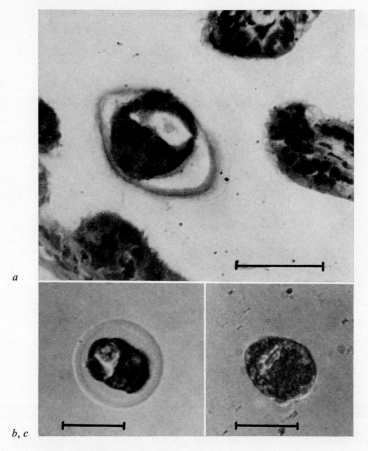

Fig. 8. Ova seen at 3 days, 14–16 h after ovulation. *a* Blastocyst in section of the oviduct from a senescent hamster. *b* Blastocyst still in its zona pellucida, collected from the uterus of a senescent hamster. *c* Blastocyst without its zona, collected from the uterus of a young hamster. Scale markers indicate approximately 100 μm.

Figure 9 shows some unfertilized ova and empty zonae pellucidae recovered from a blocked oviduct at 2 days and 18 h.

III. Studies of Chromosomes

The finding of a greater incidence of abnormal conceptuses from older females has given investigators reason to look for chromosomal defects as

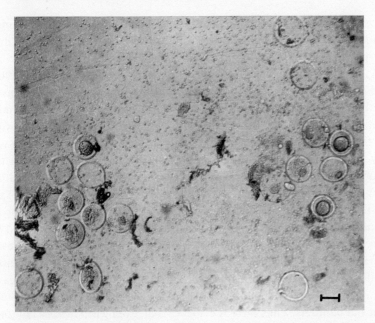

Fig. 9. Fluid with ova from the oviducts of a senescent hamster at 2 days, 18 h after ovulation. Note unfertilized ova, degenerate ova and empty zonae pellucidae. Scale marker indicates approximately 100 μm.

one possible cause of this increased abnormality. Even before cytogenetic studies had been done, it was found that delay in fertilization could cause abnormal development of ova [BLANDAU, 1952; BLANDAU and YOUNG, 1939]. Later studies have shown that such delayed fertilization may alter chromosomal distribution in the second meiotic division [RODMAN, 1971; YAMAMOTO and INGALLS, 1972], or else lead to digyny or polyspermy [AUSTIN, 1970]. Delaying ovulation for 2 days may also lead to chromosomal abnormalities in the conceptuses [BUTCHER and FUGO, 1967]. Neither of these kinds of delay may be needed as an explanation for chromosomal abnormalities in offspring of older females, however. HENDERSON and EDWARDS [1968] have found that the frequency of chiasmata between bivalent chromosomes in primary oocytes decreases with increasing age of the females (in mice). This was more notable in CBA mice, which are known to deplete their store of oocytes at a more rapid rate. They presented evidence that this decreased crossing over between bivalents led to premature separation of univalents. A resulting maldistribution of chromosomes during meiosis could lead to trisomy or monosomy. Studies on human abortuses show trisomy of many different chromosomes in early stages [CARR, 1967] but only a few varieties of trisomy survive until term. Perhaps in some species, such as mice, aneuploidies do not normally survive pregnancy, which would explain why GOODLIN [1965] failed to find any in the offspring of older mice. More likely, however, as in the rabbit does of MAURER and FOOTE [1971], the reproductive tracts of mice become incapable of maintaining any pregnancy long before the ovaries release the more abnormal oocytes. To detect the true incidence of chromosomally abnormal oocytes in these species, oocytes must be examined at the first or second meiotic division. Making suitable karyotypes from granulosa surrounded, yolk-filled oocytes is not an easy matter. The procedure of TARKOWSKI [1966] is useful in such studies but more data are needed to improve our understanding of this early period of development of oocytes in old females. As I pointed out earlier, some of the oocytes in old females may even degenerate before ovulation, judging by the examples I found at 14–16 h after ovulation. There is also an increased incidence of corpora lutea atretica in some old animals [JONES and KROHN, 1961], which I have observed in some of our old hamsters. Thus there is evidence that, even when ovaries continue to produce follicles, there can be multiple causes of reproductive failure ranging from failure to ovulate and production of nonviable or defective ova to defects in the physical or hormonal conditions of the reproductive tract. Egg transfer between old and young animals has given added evidence that both defective conceptuses and declining maternal capacity to maintain pregnancy contribute to senescent reproductive decline. Some treatments may improve the capacity of the aging maternal system to maintain pregnancy. This is suggested by experiments in which we were able to get improved development of transferred eggs in old hamsters after they had established pararenal ovarian grafts from young hamsters [BLAHA, 1970]. Measures to maintain pregnancy in older females will not be helpful, however, if the conceptuses themselves are defective.

Acknowledgments

Tables I and II are reprinted by permission of the Wistar Press. Recent work of the author has been supported by research grants from the Population Council.

References

ADAMS, C.E.: Ageing and reproduction in the female mammal with particular reference to the rabbit. J. Reprod. Fertil. Suppl. *12:* 1 (1970).

AUSTIN, C.R.: Ageing and reproduction. Post-ovulatory deterioration of the egg. J. Reprod. Fertil. Suppl. *12:* 39 (1970).

BLAHA, G.C.: Reproductive senescence in the female golden hamster. Anat. Rec. *150:* 405 (1964a).

BLAHA, G.C.: Effect of age of the donor and recipient on the development of transferred golden hamster ova. Anat. Rec. *150:* 413 (1964b).

BLAHA, G.C.: Effects of age, treatment, and method of induction on deciduomata in the golden hamster. Fertil. Steril. *18:* 477 (1967).

BLAHA, G.C.: The influence of ovarian grafts from young donors on the development of transferred ova in aged golden hamsters. Fertil. Steril. *21:* 268 (1970).

BLANDAU, R.J.: The female factor in fertility and infertility. I. The effects of delayed fertilization on the development of the pronuclei in rat ova. Fertil. Steril. *3:* 349 (1952).

BLANDAU, R.J. and YOUNG, W.C.: The effects of delayed fertilization on the development of the guinea pig ovum. Amer. J. Anat. *64:* 303 (1939).

BÖÖK, J.A.; FRACCARO, M.; HAGERT, C.G., and LINDSTEN, J.: Congenital malformations in children of mothers aged 42 and over. Nature, Lond. *181:* 1545 (1958).

BOOT, L.M. and MÜHLBOCK,:O. The ovarian function in old mice. Acta physiol. pharmacol. neerl. *3:* 463 (1954).

BURDICK, H.O.; WHITNEY, R., and EMERSON, B.: Observations on the transport of tubal ova. Endocrinology *31:* 100 (1942).

BUTCHER, R.L. and FUGO, N.W.: Overripeness and the mammalian ova. II. Delayed ovulation and chromosome anomalies. Fertil. Steril. *18:* 297 (1967).

CARR, D.H.: Cytogenetics of abortions; in BENIRSCHKE Comparative aspects of reproductive failure, p. 96 (Springer, Berlin 1967).

COMFORT, A.: Basic research in gerontology. Gerontologia, Basel *16:* 48 (1970).

CONNORS, T.J.: Reproductive senescence in the golden hamster: early development and implantation of the blastocyst; Ph. D. diss., Eugene (1969).

CONNORS, T.J.; THORPE, L.W., and SODERWALL, A.L.: An analysis of preimplantation embryonic death in senescent golden hamsters. Biol. Reprod. *6:* 131 (1972).

FINN, C.A.: The ageing uterus and its influence on reproductive capacity. J. Reprod. Fertil. Suppl. *12:* 31 (1970).

GOODLIN, R.C.: Non-disjunction and maternal age in the mouse. J. Reprod. Fertil. *9:* 355 (1965).

HAY, S. and BARBANO, H.: Independent effects of maternal age and birth order on the incidence of selected congenital malformations. Teratology *6:* 271 (1972).

HENDERSON, S.A. and EDWARDS, R.G.: Chiasma frequency and maternal age in mammals. Nature, Lond. *218:* 22 (1968).

JONES, E.C.: The ageing ovary and its influence on reproductive capacity. J. Reprod. Fertil. Suppl. *12:* 17 (1970).

JONES, E.C. and KROHN, P.L.: The relationships between age, numbers of oocytes and fertility in virgin and multiparous mice. J. Endocrin. *21:* 469 (1961).

KIRKHAM, W. B.: Observation on the relation between suckling and the rate of embryonic development in mice. J. exp. Zool. *27:* 49 (1918).

KREHBIEL, R. H.: The effects of theelin on delayed implantation in the pregnant lactating rat. Anat. Rec. *81:* 381 (1941).

MAURER, R. R. and FOOTE, R. H.: Maternal ageing and embryonic mortality in the rabbit. I. Repeated superovulation, embryo culture and transfer. J. Reprod. Fertil. *25:* 329 (1971).

MCLAREN, A. and MICHIE, D.: Studies on the transfer of fertilized mouse eggs to uterine foster mothers. J. exp. Biol. *33:* 394 (1956).

MEYER, R. K. and COCHRANE, R. L.: Induction of implantation in the ovariectomized progesterone-treated rat after adrenalectomy. J. Endocrin. *24:* 77 (1962).

NOYES, R. W. and DICKMAN, Z.: Relationship of ovular age to endometrial development. J. Reprod. Fertil. *1:* 186 (1960).

ORSINI, M. W.: Morphological evidence on the intrauterine career of the ovum; in ENDERS Delayed implantation, p. 155 (University of Chicago Press, Chicago 1963).

RODMAN, T. C.: Chromatid disjunction in unfertilized ageing oocytes. Nature, Lond. *233:* 191 (1971).

SATO, A. and YANAGIMACHI, R.: Transplantation of preimplantation hamster embryos. J. Reprod. Fertil. *30:* 329 (1972).

SODERWALL, A. L.; KENT, H. A.; TURBYFILL, C. L., and BRITENBAKER, A. L.: Variation in gestation length and litter of the golden hamster, *Mesocricetus auratus.* J. Geront. *15:* 246 (1960).

STOCKTON, B. A.; PARKENING, T. A., and SODERWALL, A. L.: Blastocyst transfer study in the senescent golden hamster. J. Reprod. Fertil. *32:* 145 (1973).

STREHLER, B. L.: Time, cells, and aging (Academic Press, New York 1962).

TALBERT, G. B.: Effect of maternal age on reproductive capacity. Amer. J. Obstet. Gynec. *102:* 451 (1968).

TALBERT, G. B. and KROHN, P. L.: Effect of maternal age on viability of ova and uterine support of pregnancy in mice. J. Reprod. Fertil. *11:* 399 (1966).

TARKOWSKI, A. K.: Experiments on the transplantation of ova in mice. Acta theriol. *2:* 251 (1959).

TARKOWSKI, A. K.: An air drying method for chromosome preparations from mouse eggs. Cytogenetics *5:* 394 (1966).

YAMAMOTO, M. and INGALLS, T. H.: Delayed fertilization and chromosome anomalies in the hamster embryo. Science *176:* 518 (1972).

YANAGIMACHI, R. and CHANG, M. C.: Fertilizable life of golden hamster ova and their morphological changes at the time of losing fertilizability. J. exp. Zool. *148:* 185 (1961).

Author's address: Dr. GORDON C. BLAHA, Department of Anatomy, College of Medicine, University of Cincinnati, *Cincinnati, OH 45219* (USA)

Aging Gametes. Int. Symp., Seattle 1973, pp. 231–248 (Karger, Basel 1975)

Effects of Maternal Age on
Ovulation, Fertilization and Embryonic Development

C.E. ADAMS

ARC Unit of Reproductive Physiology and Biochemistry, Cambridge

In the female mammal reproduction declines with advancing age and ceases well within the normal life span (see reviews by KROHN, 1964; TALBERT, 1968). For various reasons the terminal stages of the reproductive life-span are poorly documented except for man and a few short-lived laboratory animals. In the case of many species the only available records concern exceptional individuals that achieve recognition by virtue of reproducing in extreme old age.

Against this background it is not surprising that the experimental investigation of the causes of age-dependent changes in reproductive functions has comparatively recent origins. Nevertheless, significant advances have been made already that permit a more critical appraisal of the factors involved than was possible only 2 or 3 decades ago. Much of this work has been the subject of comprehensive reviews [ADAMS, 1970; BIGGERS, 1969; JONES, 1970].

Certain aspects of aging and reproduction are particularly important in relation to the human species, whose reproductive life span is so prolonged, now frequently exceeding 35 years, as noted by FRANCIS [1970] in her review of reproduction at menarche and menopause. It is perhaps fortunate that the trend towards earlier menarche seems to be halting [TANNER, 1973]. However, the menopause apparently still shows a tendency to occur later in life [FRANCIS, 1970].

In relation to the rise and fall in reproductive function, aging can be seen as a continuous process. This aspect is well illustrated by the degeneration of female germ cells, the loss of which is greatest before birth and then continues with advancing age [PETERS, 1970].

The scope of the present review will be restricted largely to the terminal stages of the reproductive life span and, in particular, to the preimplantation stages of pregnancy.

I. Ovulation

A. Monotocous Species

With the exception of man, little is known about any aspect of ovulation in aged monotocous species. Moreover, most of the data that are available have resulted from indirect observation. The lack of, and the consequent need for, direct observation of certain processes, has been noted earlier [JONES, 1970] in connection with the timing of ovulation. This applies equally to polytocous species.

The relationship between a declining oocyte population and fertility has been discussed by JONES [1970] and need not be considered further here, except to note that in women, where the oocyte population becomes totally exhausted, the position is rather exceptional. In other species, the ovaries usually contain a considerable number of oocytes long after reproduction has ceased.

The incidence of ovulation failure relative to age in women has been investigated both on the basis of endometrial biopsy material [SHARMAN, 1962] and by means of basal body temperature records [DÖRING, 1969]. SHARMAN [1962] found evidence of a high incidence of anovular menstruation (an anovular cycle was defined as one where periodical bleeding occurs without previous ovulation and without the formation of a corpus luteum), increasing with age, in women over 40. Of the premenstrual specimens taken within 10 days of a supervening menstruation, 75% were ovular in the age group 40–45, falling to 60% in the age group 46 and over. After the age of 52 there was no evidence of ovulation.

DÖRING's [1969] study included women of all ages; his results concerning the incidence of anovular and normal cycles as well as cycles with a shortened hyperthermic phase (= luteal insufficiency) are shown in figure 1. DÖRING [1969] concluded that his most striking finding was the high proportion of insufficient cycles in the early years after the onset of menstruation. In fact, the incidence of normal cycles was not maximal until 26–30 years of age, which is remarkable in view of the fact that menarche occurs at about 13 years [FRANCIS, 1970; TANNER, 1973]. Insufficient cycles were also common before

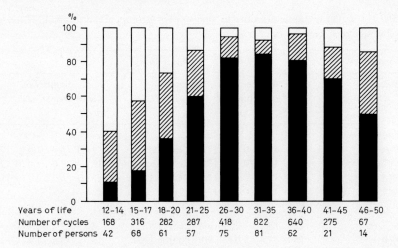

Years of life	12–14	15–17	18–20	21–25	26–30	31–35	36–40	41–45	46–50
Number of cycles	168	316	282	287	418	822	640	275	67
Number of persons	42	68	61	57	75	81	62	21	14

Fig. 1. Each column includes an age-group of 3 (later 5) consecutive years. The white areas represent the proportion of anovular cycles, the shaded areas the proportion of cycles with shortened hyperthermic phase, and the black areas the proportion of normal cycles.

the menopause, as previously suggested by the findings of COLLETT *et al.* [1954], who also noted a premature fall in the basal body temperature.

B. Polytocous Species

In polytocous species aging may lead to an increasing incidence of ovulation failure, which expresses itself in irregular cycles, and ultimately to a decreasing ovulation rate. For example, in the rabbit, ADAMS [1970] reported that the ovulation rate after 4 years of age declined to about 60% of that observed in young does (table I), whereas the incidence of ovulation failure in old does was double that recorded in young females; namely 11.5% compared with 5%. Confirmatory findings have been reported recently [LARSON *et al.*, 1973].

The position seems to be quite similar in the Mongolian gerbil, *Meriones unguiculatus*, a small cricetid rodent. In an experiment concerned primarily with the effect of semi-spaying on lifetime reproductive performance, the ovaries were examined histologically following autopsy, which was per-

Table I. Ovarian response, expressed as number of ovulations, in control and FSH-treated young and aged does

Young does			Aged does		
series	num-ber of does	number of ovulations[1]	series	num-ber of does[2]	number of ovulations[1]
Control					
1960	16	11.4 ±0.6 (8–17)	Nov. 1962	9 (1)	6.8 ±1.0 (0–10)
1962	160	10.4 ±0.2 (5–18)	July–Aug. 1963	12 (1)	7.9 ±1.0 (0–12)
1965	24	11.4 ±0.5 (8–17)	March 1964	5 (1)	6.2 ±2.2 (0–11)
1968	56	11.0 ±0.3 (4–17)			
FSH-treated					
1958–60	122	32.1 ±1.2 (8–69)	Nov. 1962	6	23.2 ±2.1 (16–31)
1960	15	57.6 ±5.0 (27–90)	March 1964	10	13.9 ±1.4 (7–22)
1964–65	25	39.8 ±2.3 (15–59)	Aug. 1966	10 (1)	11.0 ±2.6 (0–26)
Sept. 1965	11	47.3 ±4.1 (20–63)	Nov. 1968	6	11.8 ±0.9 (9–15)
March–June 1969	19	34.8 ±2.4 (19–58)	June 1969	3	25.0 ±4.6 (19–34)

1 Mean ± standard error, range in parentheses.
2 Number of does failing to ovulate in parentheses.

Table II. Effect of maternal age on ovulation in the Mongolian gerbil, *Meriones unguiculatus*

Age, days	One ovary				Two ovary			
	number of females	females without c.l.		corpora lutea, mean ±SE	number of females	females without c.l.		corpora lutea, mean ±SE
		num-ber	%			num-ber	%	
300–700	17	3	17.6	7.8 ±0.3	13	1	7.7	7.6 ±0.4
700–799	12	0	0	7.7 ±0.5	5	1	20.0	7.7 ±0.5
800–900	3	1	33.3	8.0 ±0.0	9	4	44.4	5.6 ±0.5

formed 3 months after production of the final litter, at ages ranging from 300 to 900 days [NORRIS and ADAMS, unpublished]. Some of the results are shown in table II. In the intact females an increasing proportion failed to ovulate but in those that did ovulate there was no decline in ovulation rate up to 800 days of age. Thereafter, however, a decline was apparent. The ovulation rate was exceptionally well maintained in the 1-ovary females although their apparent superiority after 800 days can be explained by differences in the age composition of the 2 groups. The 2 oldest 1-ovary females were aged 805 and 814 days whereas the 2 oldest intact females were nearly 100 days older. In this particular species the occurrence of cystic ovaries, which is strongly age-dependent [NORRIS and ADAMS, 1972], does create a somewhat abnormal situation.

In the mouse neither BIGGERS et al. [1962] nor HARMAN and TALBERT [1970] found any significant decline in ovulation rate in females aged 10–13 months compared with those aged 4–7 months. However, TALBERT and KROHN [1966], working with older mice (13–24 months), observed a reduction in the numbers of corpora lutea on day 4 of pregnancy.

In the hamster, too, different workers have reported varying results. Thus, in senescent, pregnant females aged 13–16 months, the mean number of corpora lutea was not significantly reduced in comparison with that in young females aged 3–6 months [CONNORS et al., 1972]. This finding accords with an earlier report, based on slightly older animals aged 14–19 months from the same colony [THORNEYCROFT and SODERWALL, 1969 a]. At variance is the report of BLAHA [1967], based on counts of corpora lutea on day 8 of pseudopregnancy; he found significantly fewer corpora lutea in females aged 15–18 months compared with those aged 4–7 months (12.2 versus 14.8; $p < 0.02$). However, even in this case, it is apparent that the ovulation rate was well maintained in the aged females.

C. Aging and Hypothalamic-Pituitary-Ovarian Function

The aged ovary cannot be considered in isolation from the rest of a system that is presumably also subject to aging to a greater or lesser degree. To elucidate this problem a few investigators [ASCHEIM, 1964; KROHN, 1955; ZEILMAKER, 1969] have replaced the ovaries of old rats or mice with those of young animals. This approach was reexamined recently by PENG and HUANG [1972], who made hypophyseal transplants from old to young animals. They concluded that defective reproductive function in aged female rats cannot be attributed merely to aging in the pituitary gland and/or ovaries but that the central nervous system must also be involved. This accords with LABHSETWAR's [1969] finding of a 2- to 3-fold increase in LH and FSH stores in the pituitary of aged female rats. On this evidence, LABHSETWAR [1970] has concluded that the primary lesion lies in the hypothalamus, since this organ regulates the release of these hormones. He notes that both ASCHEIM [1964] and ZEILMAKER [1969], who employed widely different approaches, reached a similar conclusion.

D. Ovarian Response to Exogenous Gonadotrophins

1. In Prepubertal Animals

In several species the ovary is capable of responding to exogenous gonadotrophins well before puberty. The level and quality of the response may vary widely according to species, age, and bodyweight. Thus, in some species, for example in the cow, the ovary is capable of responding grossly to follicle stimulating hormone within a few days of birth [MARDEN, 1953]; in others it gains the ability to respond only after some weeks; for example, rats [UMEZA et al., 1968] and mice [GATES and RUNNER, 1957] respond at about 3 weeks of age whereas in the rabbit the refractory period covers the first 10 weeks of life [ADAMS, 1953]. The onset of a gross follicular response to FSH preparations is dependent upon the appearance of antra, the timing of which has been examined for only a few species. In the rabbit, the appearance of antral follicles can be delayed by restricting feed intake. Very recently, it has been shown that the initial response to gonadotrophins in the rat ovary takes place at 6–8 days of age and is marked by development of the theca interna [GOLDENBERG et al., 1973].

In some species FSH treatment causes overt signs of estrus, and superovulation may occur as a result of the release of endogenous LH. However, in others, as exemplified by the rabbit, although signs of estrus were present, ovulation did not necessarily occur even when exogenous HCG or LH was given, thereby pointing to initial deficiencies at the ovarian level. It appears that FSH primed, immature animals could provide a particularly useful model for the study of ovulation. Hitherto, there has been a tendency to concentrate on the induction of ovulation for the production of eggs with the consequent neglect of the ovulation process itself. However, work in this area should be stimulated by the increasing interest in the practical application of the egg transfer technique, particularly in cattle, where the cost of adult stock is becoming prohibitive.

2. In Aging Animals

Several workers have reported that ovarian response to injected gonadotrophins declines with age. In the rabbit BEATTY [1958] found that the re-

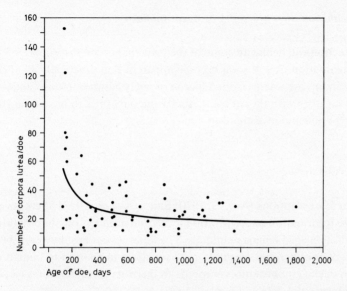

Fig. 2. Relation between number of corpora lutea and age of doe subjected to super-ovulation treatment. One dot equals one doe. The graph is plotted from regression coefficient $b_{y_c 6.4}$.

sponse to FSH, as measured in terms of the number of corpora lutea, 137–144 h p.c., was determined mainly by the doe's age, as depicted in figure 2. Whether counts of corpora lutea 6 days p.c. reflect accurately the ovulation rate may be queried, especially where the age span of the material is considerable and the full complement of eggs is not accounted for. However, a similar trend was noted by ADAMS [1970], who counted the number of ovulations at 60 h p.c. In many of his FSH treated aged does the number of ovulations barely exceeded that in young, untreated females, though in a few cases the response was still elevated by a factor of 3 (table I). Other workers have also recorded a much reduced superovulatory response in aged does [LARSON et al.,1973; MAURER et al., 1968; MAURER and FOOTE, 1971].

In the hamster the ability to respond to PMS appears to be quite well maintained, since the mean number of ovulations in aged females was increased 2 ½ times over controls [BLAHA, 1967]. Previously, ORTIZ [1955] had reported that the ovary of the senescent hamster was 'very reactive'. On the other hand, THORNEYCROFT and SODERWALL [1969 b] described it as 'refractory', though their senescent animals ovulated 74% as many ova as young animals in response to PMS.

II. Preimplantation Mortality in Aged Animals

This section will deal with some of the principal processes from fertilization to implantation. It will soon become apparent that practically all of our knowledge in this area stems from 3 species, namely hamster, mouse, and rabbit, which together with the rat are virtually the only ones to have been subjected to experimental investigation.

A. Fertilization

With a few exceptions [ADAMS, 1970; SPILMAN *et al.*, 1972], there is very little precise information on fertilization levels and even less on abnormalities of fertilization in aged female mammals. The latter aspect has, however, been the subject of considerable speculation, particularly in relation to human reproduction where circumstances combine to merit its consideration as a factor in developmental defects [AUSTIN, 1970].

In aged rabbits ADAMS [1970] reported that the mean proportion of eggs fertilized, 84%, though still relatively high, was much impaired in some individuals. For comparison, it may be noted that in the majority of young rabbits it is quite usual to find every egg fertilized, with fertilization failing completely in no more than 5% of cases. In this particular species, the position in aged females may be complicated by the occurrence of uterine lesions [ADAMS, 1965] that could interfere with preliminaries to fertilization, such as sperm transport and capacitation. Moreover, oviductal function may also deteriorate with age.

In an attempt to overcome these problems, ADAMS [1970] transferred 165 newly ovulated eggs recovered from 20 aged does (4–6 years old) to the oviducts of young recipients that had been artificially inseminated 12–14 h previously. Upon recovery 48 h after transfer, 83% of the 123 eggs examined were classified as fertilized. On first inspection, therefore, fertilization does not appear to have been improved in the 'young environment', suggesting that the failure could be attributable to inherently defective eggs ovulated by the old does. However, the validity of this conclusion is impaired because, unfortunately, in the control series, in which eggs from young does were similarly treated, only two thirds of the eggs were fertilized owing to poor fertilization in a few individuals. The problem of whether old animals do ovulate a proportion of eggs that are incapable of undergoing fertilization merits further investigation. The contribution of disturbances in the fertilization process, due either directly or indirectly to aging, to the production of abnormal zygotes is unknown.

B. Egg Pick-Up and Transport

In a series of 13 aged does, whose oviducts were flushed at autopsy 60 h p.c., only 62.5% of the expected eggs were recovered compared with 96.4% from young, control does [ADAMS, 1970]. Very similar results were obtained in the case of a second series of 20 aged does autopsied at 13.5–14.5 h p.c.; in this case 69% of the eggs were recovered in comparison with 88.9% from the control, young does (table III). The failure to recover eggs may be explained in at least 2 ways: (1) the eggs were never present in the tubes, owing to disturbances in ovulation or faulty ovum pick-up, and (2) accelerated transport to the uterus, which may arise through hormonal imbalance, tends to affect eggs as batches rather than as individuals, especially after 25 h p.c. [ADAMS,

Table III. Comparison of egg recovery, fertilization and cleavage in aged and young does

Group	Number of does	Number of ovulations	Egg recovery, %	Number of eggs transferred	Egg recovery, %	Proportion eggs, % fertilized	un-fertilized	Arrested cleavage number	%
Aged[1]	13	251	62.5			84.1	15.9	7	4.3
Young[2]	22	229	96.4			98.6	1.4	0	
Young[3]	114	3,659[4]				96.1	3.9	70	1.9
					In temporary recipient				
Aged[5]	20	248	69	165	74.5	82.9	17.1	10	9.8
Young	23	257	88.7	264	85.7	66.7	36.7	2	1.4

1 Fertilization *in situ;* egg recovery 60 h p.c.
2 Untreated.
3 Superovulated: mean age 222 ± 5 days.
4 This is the actual number of eggs recovered; at this level of stimulation it is impossible to count accurately the number of ovulations.
5 Eggs recovered 13.5–14.5 h p.c.; then transferred to a young estrous doe artificially inseminated 12–14 h previously.

1968]. Accelerated transport could not explain the results obtained shortly after ovulation, though delayed ovulation might.

In other species, too, it appears that tubal function may be impaired in aged females; for example, in the hamster [BLAHA, 1964] and in the mouse [TALBERT and KROHN, 1966], fewer eggs than expected were found in uterine flushings, 63–68 h after ovulation and on day 4, respectively. Based on a different method, namely egg counts in serially sectioned oviducts, CONNORS *et al.* [1972] also recorded significantly fewer eggs than expected in pregnant, senescent hamsters at 56 h p.c.

C. Incidence of Abnormal Eggs and Rate of Egg Development

An increased incidence of abnormal eggs in aged animals has been recorded in the hamster [BLAHA, 1964]; mouse [BOOT and MÜHLBOCK, 1954; TALBERT and KROHN, 1966]; rabbit [ADAMS, 1970] and rat [MAIBENCO and KREHBIEL, 1973]. BOOT and MÜHLBOCK [1954] appear to have been the first to observe a 'reduction both in the number and quality of ova' recovered from old animals. From 8 female mice, aged 19–23 months, that were autopsied 3 days p.c., they recovered only 18 eggs of which no fewer than 12 were classed as abnormal. Subsequently, TALBERT and KROHN [1966] recorded 13% grossly abnormal eggs recovered from the uteri of old mice on day 4 of pregnancy and 5% from young mice. The same workers also observed that a significantly higher proportion of the ova from the young mice had reached the blastocyst stage at the time of recovery (81 versus 58%; $p< 0.01$). However, the slower rate of egg development in the old mice was not an early expression of their impending death; on the contrary, the morulae appeared to survive as well as the blastocysts following transfer to young recipients. GOSDEN [personal commun.] has also observed a slower rate of cleavage among eggs recovered from aged mice.

In aged rats, MAIBENCO and KREHBIEL [1973] reported that 23 out of a total of 58 eggs examined histologically were abnormal; unfortunately no material from young animals was provided for comparison. Apparently in this species no attempt appears to have been made to examine eggs while fresh in tubal or uterine flushings of old animals.

In aged rabbits, the incidence of abnormal eggs, characterized by arrested cleavage, was more than double that found in young does, comprising 4.3 and 1.9%, respectively, of eggs examined at 60 h p.c. [ADAMS, 1970]. It seems especially significant that in a second series where eggs from old donors were transferred to young recipients prior to fertilization the incidence of abnormal cleavage was even higher (table III). This clearly suggests that the cause is to be sought within the egg; previously, other explanations incriminating the aging genital tract have been proffered.

In the hamster, where the eggs normally enter the uterus on the third day at the 8-cell stage [WARD, 1948], BLAHA [1964] observed an especially high proportion of retarded cleavage among eggs recovered from aged females at 63–68 h after ovulation. Thus, in 24 old females more than one sixth of the eggs (22/122) contained only 1–4 cells; in contrast only 2 out of 209 eggs recovered from 21 young hamsters were similarly retarded.

D. Implantation

1. Mouse

In the mouse, HARMAN and TALBERT [1970] found that the number of implantations, counted at autopsy 7 ½ days p.c., declined significantly after 9 months of age, and in mice more than 9 months old the proportion of animals with implants also fell (table IV). Histological examination of the ovaries showed that this decline was associated with degenerative changes of the corpora lutea. Mice killed at 12–13 months of age had no recognizable corpora lutea 7 ½ days p.c. though the number of ovulations observed in similar animals at 12 h p.c. was normal. TALBERT and KROHN [1966] examined their recipients on the 8th day of gestation in order to determine the number of im-

Table IV. Effect of maternal age on the numbers of corpora lutea of pregnancy (CLP) and implantation sites in mice examined on the 8th day of pregnancy

Age, months	Total number of females	Animals with implants number	%	Implants/ mouse mean ± SE	Animals with CLP number	%	CLP/mouse of mice with one or more CLP, mean ± SE
4–7	30	22	73.3	6.86 ± 0.80	26	86.7	10.2 ± 1.67
8–9	33	23	69.7	5.97 ± 0.73	25	80.7	9.8 ± 0.45
10–11	31	23	74.2	4.45 ± 0.62[1]	27	86.7	9.8 ± 0.68
12–13	29	8[2]	27.6	1.21 ± 0.40[3]	11[2]	37.9	7.9 ± 0.82
14–15	31	4[2]	12.9	0.61 ± 0.30[3]	7[2]	22.6	9.0 ± 0.69

1 Mean differs significantly from 4- to 7-month-old group, p < 0.02.
2 χ^2 test indicates distribution different from 4- to 7-month-old group, p < 0.001.
3 Mean differs significantly from 4- to 7-month-old group, p < 0.001.

plantation sites. Whereas very similar rates of survival were recorded in their young recipients, irrespective of whether the eggs came from young or old donors (61 and 63%), that of eggs obtained from young donors and transferred to old recipients was significantly lower (29%; p<0.01). Since resorbing embryos were rarely observed on the 8th day of pregnancy, it was concluded that most of the losses prior to this age were either due to failure of implantation or to very early death following implantation. Recently, GOSDEN [personal commun.] has shown that some of this loss can be prevented by treating the recipients with progesterone – a finding that is consistent with the reported early degeneration of corpora lutea [HARMAN and TALBERT, 1970]. In aged rabbits, on the contrary, reproductive efficiency was not improved by progesterone therapy [LARSON et al., 1973], a result not altogether unexpected in view of the fact that luteal function, as reflected in progesterone concentrations both in luteal tissue and peripheral plasma, appears to be well maintained in aged does [SPILMAN et al., 1972].

2. Hamster

THORNEYCROFT and SODERWALL [1969 a] concluded that the reduced litter size in senescent hamsters was not due to a reduction in ovulation rate but largely to a 7-fold increase in preimplantation deaths. This was also reflected in the pregnancy rate on day 8, which was 62.7% in senescent females aged 14–19 months and 100% in young females. The preimplantation period has been subjected to further analysis by CONNORS et al. [1972], who employed ORSINI's [1962] method to visualize the implantation sites 132 h after ovulation. As can be seen from table V their study indicates that the greatest loss occurs between 56 and 132 h after ovulation, i.e. when implantation normally occurs. Not only were significantly fewer implants present in the older uteri, namely 2.8 compared with 6.1 per horn in young females but, in addition, those that were present were smaller and less well developed. Earlier, BLAHA [1964] had found in old recipients of eggs from young females that 'most implantation sites were smaller than normal' when examined at laparotomy at 6–8 days of pregnancy. It has been suggested that the senescent ovary could be contributing to the mortality by secreting less progesterone [THORNEYCROFT and SODERWALL, 1969 b]. Support for this appears to come from BLAHA's [1970] findings that old hamsters that had received ovarian grafts from young females were more successful in maintaining transferred blastocysts than were their controls. On the other hand, BLAHA [1971] has subsequently reported that the level of plasma progesterone was normal in most old hamsters either with or without implantation sites.

Table V. The number of surviving ova during early pregnancy in young and old hamsters (means ± SE; number of observations in parentheses) after CONNORS et al. [1972]

Group	Number of corpora lutea/ovary	Number of ova/oviduct at 56 h	Number of implants/cornu at 132 h
Young	7.3 ± 0.14 (12)	6.6 ± 0.1 (12)	6.1 ± 1.0 (10)
Old	6.8 ± 0.19 (10)	4.9 ± 0.2 (10)	2.8 ± 1.5 (12)
Difference	0.5[1]	1.7[2]	3.3[3]

1 Difference not significant p < 0.05 (number of ovaries).
2 Difference significant p < 0.01 (number of oviducts).
3 Difference significant p < 0.01 (number of cornu).

3. Rat

Surprisingly little appears to be known about the incidence and distribution of embryo mortality in aged rats. Recently, it was reported that in females aged 18 months or more that were examined on days 6–9 of pregnancy: 'The average number of decidual reactions per uterine horn (5,6) was comparable to that in younger females' [MAIBENCO and KREHBIEL, 1973]. However, this finding refers specifically to animals with implants; the overall position is far less satisfactory since implantation apparently failed completely in quite a high proportion of the old animals.

Results obtained with semi-spayed rats are relevant to the present discussion in so far as removal of 1 ovary accelerates the decline in reproductive capacity owing to increased prenatal mortality [ADAMS, 1970]. Thus, in 2-ovary rats autopsied in their sixth pregnancy 62% of the eggs failed to survive to term, almost exactly double the loss experienced by the intact rats (table VI). It was estimated that slightly over half of the mortality occurred before implantation with a high proportion of the remainder taking place at or soon after implantation.

4. Rabbit

Up to 30 months of age, during which time 11 pregnancies were recorded, the proportion of eggs lost before implantation, 8–18%, was relatively constant, though possibly showing a tendency to rise with advancing parity [ADAMS, 1970]. Among older does, aged 4–5 years, there was considerable variability in the incidence of preimplantation mortality [ADAMS, 1964].

Table VI. Reproduction performance of semi-spayed and control rats in sixth pregnancy (six animals per group)

Group	Number of corpora lutea	Number of live fetuses	Number of moles	Number missing	Total mortality, %
Two-ovary	104	71	13	20	32
One-ovary	101	38	28	35	62

Table VII. Effect of age of recipient and donor on the survival to term of fertilized eggs

Group	Rabbit						Hamster[1]			Mouse[2]		
	recipients		eggs transferred		survival at term		num-ber of recip-ients	num-ber of eggs trans-ferred	sur-vival at term, %	num-ber of recip-ients	num-ber of eggs trans-ferred	sur-vival at term, %
	n^3	n^4	n^3	n^4	$\%^3$	$\%^4$						
Young-to-old	7	7	67	40	1.5	50	8	72	8.3	38	222	14
Young-to-young	27	7	161	40	33.5	40	8	63	49.2	30	157	48
Old-to-young	37	7	209	21	12.9	23.8	11	88	4.5	30	144	54

1 BLAHA [1964].
2 TALBERT and KROHN [1966].
3 ADAMS [1964, 1970].
4 MAURER and FOOTE [1971].

III. Egg Transfer Studies

A practical means of differentiating between losses attributable to defects within the egg as opposed to the environment is afforded by the egg transfer technique. Reciprocal egg transfer between young and old animals has been carried out in the hamster [BLAHA, 1964], mouse [TALBERT and KROHN, 1966], and rabbit [ADAMS, 1964, 1970; MAURER and FOOTE, 1971]. The main results of these studies are summarized in table VII. With one exception [MAURER and FOOTE, 1971] there is general agreement that old recipients provide a poor environment. However, there appears to be marked variation between species concerning the survival of eggs from old donors. The exceptional retention of egg viability in aged mice [TALBERT and KROHN,

1966], has now been confirmed by GOSDEN [personal commun.], who used CBA mice aged 10–16 months. Nevertheless in the mouse, too, the oocytes may ultimately deteriorate, as there is some evidence that donors aged over 600 days yielded less viable eggs [TALBERT and KROHN, 1966].

In discussing why so few eggs, 4.5%, from old donors developed in young recipients, BLAHA [1964] acknowledged that one sixth of the eggs transferred were manifestly abnormal at the time of transfer but pointed out that the majority appeared normal at that time. It was difficult to explain why, if it was the transfer process itself that had had a damaging effect, it should have affected disproportionately the eggs of old donors. Against this background and the known critical relationship between ovular maturity and endometrial progestational development in relation to fertility [NOYES and DICKMAN, 1960], BLAHA [1964] surmised: 'that ova from old females could differ in their rate of development and thus be less likely to implant normally in the young uterus'. Very recently another possibility, namely a delay in uterine sensitivity to blastocyst implantation in senescent animals, has been indicated [STOCKTON et al., 1973]. These workers found that late morulae or early blastocysts recovered 62–67 h after ovulation survived best in young recipients that were exactly synchronous, whereas with old recipients the best results were obtained 86–91 h after ovulation. Retarded transformation of the endometrium in aged animals may occur as a result of a reduced capacity of their uterine tissue to take up steroid hormones, as demonstrated experimentally [LARSON et al., 1972].

Also relevant are experimental studies concerned with the response of aged females to a decidualizing stimulus: observations on the hamster [BLAHA, 1967], mouse [FINN, 1966], and rat [MAIBENCO and KREHBIEL, 1973] indicate that the response is less 'efficient' in aged than in young animals, suggesting a decreased uterine responsiveness. However, according to LABHSETWAR [1970] the response was not diminished in rats, estimated to be 9–12 months old, in comparison with that in 2- to 3-month-old females.

IV. Conclusions

Although ovarian activity and endocrine function appear to be generally well maintained in the aging mammal, evidence is accumulating that egg quality does eventually deteriorate, as revealed in an increasing incidence of abnormal eggs and developmental failure. More important, however, is uterine failure since it tends to occur earlier in life. With advancing age and/or parity prenatal mortality occurs progressively earlier in pregnancy so that in aged animals the preimplantation component may assume considerable significance. In rodents a lack of coordination seems to develop within the reproductive system, culminating in implantation failure.

It is perhaps worth emphasizing that most of our knowledge on the subject of aging and reproduction stems from only 3 species, of which 2 are rodents. Clearly, there is a need to extend observations to a wider range of species.

Acknowledgment

I am grateful to Dr. R. Gosden, Marshall Laboratory, University of Cambridge, for giving me permission to quote from his unpublished work.

References

Adams, C.E.: Some aspects of ovulation, recovery and transplantation of ova in the immature rabbit; in Wolstenholme Mammalian germ cells, p. 198 (Churchill, London 1953).

Adams, C.E.: The influence of advanced maternal age on embryo survival in the rabbit. Proc. 5th Int. Congr. Anim. Reprod. A.I., Trento 1964, vol. 2, p. 305.

Adams, C.E.: The influence of maternal environment on preimplantation stages of pregnancy in the rabbit; in Wolstenholme and O'Connor Preimplantation stages of pregnancy, p. 345 (Churchill, London 1965).

Adams, C.E.: Ovarian response to human chorionic gonadotrophin and egg transport in the pregnant and part parturient rabbit. J. Endocrin. *40:* 101 (1968).

Adams, C.E.: Ageing and reproduction in the female mammal with particular reference to the rabbit. J. Reprod. Fertil. Suppl. *12:* 1 (1970).

Ascheim, S.: Résultats fournis par la greffe des ovaires dans l'étude de la régulation hypothalamo-hypophyso-ovarienne de la ratte sénile. Gerontologia, Basel *10:* 65 (1964).

Austin, C.R.: Ageing and reproduction: post ovulatory deterioration of the egg. J. Reprod. Fertil. Suppl. *12:* 39 (1970).

Beatty, R.A.: Variation in the number of corpora lutea and in the number and size of 6-day blastocysts in rabbits subjected to superovulatory treatment. J. Endocrin. *17:* 248 (1958).

Biggers, J.D.: Problems concerning the uterine causes of embryonic death, with special reference to the effects of ageing of the uterus. J. Reprod. Fertil. Suppl. *8:* 27 (1969).

Biggers, J.D.; Finn, C.E., and McLaren, A.: Long-term reproductive performance of female mice. II. Variation of litter size with parity. J. Reprod. Fertil. *3:* 313 (1962).

Blaha, G.C.: Effect of age of the donor and recipient on the development of transferred golden hamster ova. Anat. Rec. *150:* 413 (1964).

BLAHA, G.C.: Effects of age, treatment, and method of induction on deciduomata in the golden hamster. Fertil. Steril. *18:* 477 (1967).

BLAHA, G.C.: The influence of ovarian grafts upon young donors on the development of transferred ova in aged golden hamsters. Fertil. Steril. *21:* 268 (1970).

BLAHA, G.C.: Ovarian steroid dehydrogenase and plasma progesterone levels in aged golden hamsters. Anat. Rec. *169:* abstr., p. 279 (1971).

BOOT, L.M. and MÜHLBOCK, O.: The ovarian function in old mice. Acta physiol. pharmacol. neerl. *3:* abstr., p. 463 (1954).

COLLETT, M.E.; WERTENBERGER, G.E., and FISKE, V.M.: The effect of age upon the pattern of the menstrual cycle. Fertil. Steril. *5:* 437 (1954).

CONNORS, T.J.; THORPE, L.W., and SODERWALL, A.L.: An analysis of preimplantation embryonic death in senescent golden hamsters. Biol. Reprod. *6:* 131 (1972).

DÖRING, G.K.: The incidence of anovular cycles in women. J. Reprod. Fertil. Suppl. *6:* 77 (1969).

FINN, C.A.: The initiation of the decidual cell reaction in the uterus of the aged mouse. J. Reprod. Fertil. *11:* 423 (1966).

FRANCIS, W.J.A.: Reproduction at menarche and menopause in women. J. Reprod. Fertil. Suppl. *12:* 89 (1970).

GATES, A.H. and RUNNER, M.N.: Influence of prepubertal age on number of ova that can be superovulated in the mouse. Anat. Rec. *128:* 554 (1957).

GOLDENBERG, R.L.; REITER, E.O., and ROSS, G.T.: Follicle response to exogenous gonadotrophins; an estrogen-mediated phenomenon. Fertil. Steril. *24:* 121 (1973).

HARMAN, S.M. and TALBERT, G.B.: The effect of maternal age on ovulation, corpora lutea of pregnancy, and implantation failure in mice. J. Reprod. Fertil. *23:* 33 (1970).

JONES, E.C.: The ageing ovary and its influence on reproductive capacity. J. Reprod. Fertil. Suppl. *12:* 17 (1970).

KROHN, P.L.: Tissue transplantation technique applied to the problem of the ageing of the organ of reproduction; in WOLSTENHOLME and MILLAR Ciba Found. Colloq. on Ageing, vol. 1, p. 141 (Churchill, London 1955).

KROHN, P.L.: The reproductive lifespan. Proc. 5th Int. Congr. Anim. Reprod. A.I., Trento 1964, vol. 3, p. 23.

LABHSETWAR, A.P.: Age-dependent changes in the pituitary-gonadal relationship. II. A study of pituitary FSH and LH content in the female rat. J. Reprod. Fertil. *20:* 21 (1969).

LABHSETWAR, A.P.: Ageing changes in pituitary ovarian relationships. J. Reprod. Fertil. Suppl. *12:* 99 (1970).

LARSON, L.L.; SPILMAN, C.H.; DUNN, H.O., and FOOTE, R.H.: Reproductive efficiency in aged female rabbits given supplemental progesterone and oestradiol. J. Reprod. Fertil. *33:* 31 (1973).

LARSON, L.L.; SPILMAN, C.H., and FOOTE, R.H.: Uterine uptake of progesterone and estradiol in young and aged rabbits. Proc. Soc. exp. Biol. Med. *141:* 463 (1972).

MAIBENCO, H.C. and KREHBIEL, R.H.: Reproductive decline in aged female rats. J. Reprod. Fertil. *32:* 121 (1973).

MARDEN, W.G.R.: The hormone control of ovulation in the calf. J. agric. Sci. *43:* 381 (1953).

MAURER, R. R. and FOOTE, R. H.: Maternal ageing and embryonic mortality in the rabbit. I. Repeated superovulation, embryo culture and transfer. J. Reprod. Fertil. *25:* 329 (1971).

MAURER, R. R.; HUNT, W. L., and FOOTE, R. H.: Repeated superovulation following administration of exogenous gonadotrophins in Dutch-belted rabbits. J. Reprod. Fertil. *15:* 93 (1968).

NORRIS, M. and ADAMS, C. E.: Incidence of cystic ovaries and reproductive performance in the Mongolian gerbil, *Meriones unguiculatus.* Lab. Anim. *6:* 337 (1972).

NOYES, R. W. and DICKMANN, Z.: Relationship of ovular age to endometrial development. J. Reprod. Fertil. *1:* 186 (1960).

ORSINI, M. W.: Technique of preparation, study and photography of benzyl-benzoate cleared material for embryological studies. J. Reprod. Fertil. *3:* 283 (1962).

ORTIZ, E.: The relation of advancing age to reactivity of the reproductive system in the female hamster. Anat. Rec. *122:* 517 (1955).

PENG, M. T. and HUANG, H. H.: Ageing of hypothalamic-pituitary-ovarian function in the rat. Fertil. Steril. *23:* 535 (1972).

PETERS, H.: Migration of gonocytes into the mammalian gonad and their differentiation. Philos. Trans. roy. Soc. B *259:* 91 (1970).

SHARMAN, A.: The menopause; in ZUCKERMAN, MANDL and ECKSTEIN The ovary, vol.1, p. 539 (Academic Press, New York 1962).

SPILMAN, C. H.; LARSON, L. L.; CONCANNON, P. W., and FOOTE, R. H.: Ovarian function during pregnancy in young and aged rabbits: temporal relationship between fetal death and corpus luteum regression. Biol. Reprod. *7:* 223 (1972).

STOCKTON, B. A.; PARKENING, T. A., and SODERWALL, A. L.: Blastocyst transfer study in the senescent golden hamster. J. Reprod. Fertil. *32:* 145 (1973).

TALBERT, G. B.: Effect of maternal age on reproductive capacity. Amer. J. Obstet. Gynec. *102:* 451 (1968).

TALBERT, G. B. and KROHN, P. L.: Effect of maternal age on viability of ova and uterine support of pregnancy in mice. J. Reprod. Fertil. *11:* 399 (1966).

TANNER, J. M.: Trend towards earlier menarche in London, Oslo, Copenhagen, the Netherlands and Hungary. Nature, Lond. *243:* 95 (1973).

THORNEYCROFT, I. H. and SODERWALL, A. L.: The nature of the litter size loss in senescent hamsters. Anat. Rec. *165:* 343 (1969a).

THORNEYCROFT, I. H. and SODERWALL, A. L.: Ovarian morphological and functional changes in reproductively senescent hamsters. Anat. Rec. *165:* 349 (1969b).

UMEZU, M.; KODAMA, C., and TAKEUCHI, S.: The effects of PMS or HCG on the ovulation in female immature rats. Tohoku J. agric. Res. *19:* 50 (1968).

WARD, M. C.: The early development and implantation of the golden hamster, *Cricetus auratus,* and the associated endometrial changes. Amer. J. Anat. *82:* 231 (1948).

ZEILMAKER, G. H.: Effects of prolonged feeding of an ovulation inhibitor (Lyndiol) on ageing of the hypothalamic-ovarian axis and pituitary gland tumorigenesis in rats. J. Endocrin. *43:* XXI (1969).

Author's address: Dr. C. E. ADAMS, A. R. C. Unit of Reproductive Physiology and Biochemistry, 307 Huntingdon Road, *Cambridge CB3 0JQ* (England)

Aging Gametes. Int. Symp., Seattle 1973, pp. 249–264 (Karger, Basel 1975)

Prolonged Storage of Gametes in Relation to Fertility and Progeny Characteristics in Farm Animals

L.E.A. Rowson

Agricultural Research Council's Unit of Reproductive Physiology and Biochemistry, University of Cambridge, Cambridge

When considering the aging of the gametes it is necessary to define clearly the moment at which aging begins. In the case of the female gametes the event that is usually taken as the onset of aging is the time of ovulation [Austin, 1970]. The question is more complex as regards the male where, following spermatogenesis, there is the prolonged period of passage of the spermatozoa through the epididymis. Moreover, spermatogenesis continues following ligation of the vas deferens, and live spermatozoa can be recovered for many months from the part of the tract proximal to the testes. Igboeli and Rakha [1970] examined 6 bulls, one 5 months and five 5 years, after vasectomy and found that the operation did not affect spermatogenesis and that spermatozoa obtained from the cauda exhibited good activity. It appears, however, that in bulls the resorption of old spermatozoa takes place normally mainly in the cauda [Amann and Almquist, 1962]. In the vasectomized rhesus monkey Alexander [1972] showed that spermatozoa become agglutinated after vasectomy and are ingested by macrophages. She postulates the occurrence of an autoimmune response. All in all, it seems that for practical purposes it may be best to use the time of ejaculation as the moment at which aging of the male gamete begins.

In evaluating the end-effect that aging of gametes has on progeny numbers, it is necessary to take into consideration the age of the female animal. Adams [1964] has shown that the uterine environment is in this respect an important factor. He demonstrated that fertilized eggs taken from an old rabbit and transferred to a young one will lead to a consistently larger litter than the reciprocal procedure. The young rabbits that Adams used for this purpose were less than one year of age, and the aged rabbits were 4–5 ½ years old. He concluded from his experiments that the gametogenic function of the ovary in old rabbits outlasts the ability of their uterus to maintain pregnancy.

There can be little doubt that in farm animals most of the embryonic mortality is due to an abnormal uterine environment; and only some of it can be attributed to defects in the gametes themselves. Experiments on cows have shown that under natural mating conditions most eggs undergo fertilization. About 90–95% of cow eggs will commence normal development; yet, only about 55–60% of these eggs will continue developing to term. What then is responsible for the prenatal loss of 30–35% of embryos?

When considering the prenatal losses one is faced with the difficulty of deciding to what extent embryonic loss is due to genetic faults in the gametes themselves and how much of it is due to defective uterine environment. Some light has been thrown on this problem by the results of egg transplantation experiments in which the synchronization of estrus in the donor and the recipient animal had been examined. These experiments, which were carried out on cattle and sheep, have shown that it is absolutely essential to synchronize closely the estrus in the donor and recipient animal if pregnancy is to continue normally after egg transfer. In other words, despite the fact that one is introducing a perfectly normal zygote into the uterus, if the stage of the cycle of the donor and of the recipient differs, i.e., if they are 'out of phase', many zygotes will perish. Obviously, the uterine environment must be changing rapidly, and this leads to significant changes in the uterine secretion. In order to investigate this possibility, analyses are now being carried out on uterine secretion taken from sheep and cattle at intervals of 3–4 days during the cycle. This time interval was selected because it is known that if the donor and recipient animal are 'out of phase' by 3 days, then embryonic death will almost invariably occur following egg transfer (fig. 1).

Hormones play, of course, a pivotal role in influencing the uterine environment. In egg transplantation experiments on rabbits Beier et al. [1972] found that if a recipient rabbit is injected with estrogen during the luteal phase of the cycle, it is possible to 'reprogam' the uterine secretion in such a way that, although this recipient is 'out of phase', embryos can be successfully transferred into it. All this indicates that the composition of uterine secretion is a decisive factor in the survival of the embryo.

Quite apart from the effects of uterine secretion, there are other factors that influence the fertilization of the egg and the normal development of the embryo. Most important are the changes that occur in the gametes as part of the progressive aging process. These changes may be brought about in several ways, but in every case they render the gametes incapable of forming a nor-

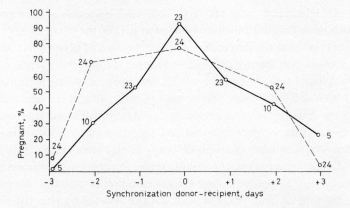

Fig. 1. The effect of the degree of synchronization of donor and recipient on pregnancy rate. The continuous line represents cattle in the present experiment; the dotted line represents sheep [Rowson and Moor, 1966]. The number of animals is given against each symbol.

mal and viable embryo after syngamy. The age of gametes can also influence profoundly the results obtained by artificial insemination (AI). AI must be performed at the right time in relation to ovulation and always with the fact in mind that the life span of spermatozoa in the female tract is relatively short in most of the domestic species, for instance, 1–3 days in cattle, sheep, and pigs [Dauzier and Winterberger, 1952; Du Mesnil du Buisson and Dauzier, 1955; Laing, 1945]; but in the horse a period of survival of more than 5 days has been recorded [Burkhardt, 1949; Day, 1942]. It must equally be borne in mind that the fertilizing capacity of spermatozoa is lost before motility ceases and that even when an aged spermatozoon has succeeded in penetrating an egg, abnormal development of the zygote and its subsequent death often results [Young, 1931].

I. Aging of Eggs

Efforts to study the behaviour of aging eggs in domestic animals have been hampered by the lack of reliable methods for detecting the exact time of ovulation. Nevertheless, there is now ample evidence that the period during which the female gamete retains its fertilizing ability after ovulation is relatively short: it probably does not exceed 24 h. Moreover, the adverse effect

that aging of the female gamete produces becomes progressively more pronounced with time. Fertilization during the latter part of the life of an egg results frequently in impaired development of the zygote, and delayed fertilization often leads to polyspermy or fragmentation of the embryo. Dziuk and
Polge [1962] found that, when the artificial insemination of gilts with fresh
semen had been delayed 8–20 h after ovulation, over 50% of the eggs were
abnormal; the abnormalities observed included eggs with polynucleated
blastomeres, eggs with incomplete nuclei, and eggs showing irregular division
or fragmentation. A similar situation develops in pigs after natural mating
has been delayed; under these conditions, many eggs become polyspermic
[Hancock, 1959]. The optimum time for insemination of pigs and sheep in
relation to the time of ovulation has been studied in detail by Hunter and
Dziuk [1968] and Dziuk [1970]. Another factor relating to abnormal development of aged eggs that merits attention is the possible involvement of abnormal, and in particular diploid, spermatozoa. Such spermatozoa have been
described both in the bull [Salisbury and Baker, 1966] and in the rabbit
[Beatty and Fechheimer, 1972].

Attempts have been made to preserve zygotes either by storing at low
temperature or by culturing *in vitro*. It has been possible to induce pregnancy
in sheep after storing fertilized eggs cooled to 8–10°C for up to 10 days. With
cultured eggs a difficulty was initially encountered in attempts to use 8-cell
eggs [Moor and Cragle, 1971], but later this was overcome, and zygotes can
now be successfully cultured to the blastocyst stage in both sheep and cattle.
Retransfer of such cultured embryos to recipient animals results in normal
pregnancies [Tervit *et al.*, 1972].

An interesting offshoot of the transfer experiments with *in vitro* cultured
embryos has been the finding that the rabbit oviduct can serve as a temporary
site for preservation and development of zygotes obtained from sheep, cattle,
and pigs. However, storing of sheep eggs prior to retransfer for too long,
namely 5 days or more, leads in many cases to abnormal development of the
conceptus. In such cases only the membranes develop, and the conceptus is
eventually expelled or resorbed. In the cow zygote similar changes can take
place even a day or so earlier. In a case where 2 cow eggs were left in the
rabbit for 4 days prior to retransfer to the recipient cow, she failed to calve;
when slaughtered she was found to be carrying a pair of dead twins with
deformities of the legs (fig. 2). On the other hand, storage of cow eggs in the
rabbit for up to 3 days has been highly successful. Retransfer of a pair of
such stored embryos into each of 8 recipient cows, resulted in the birth of
7 pairs of healthy twin calves.

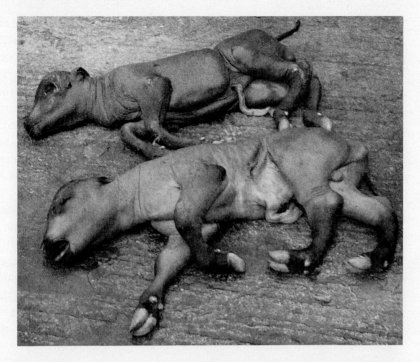

Fig. 2. Calves born with deformed legs, the eggs having been stored in a rabbit for a period of 4 days.

In vitro eggs cannot be stored for too long at a temperature of 37°C prior to transfer. In the case of 2 sheep carrying transferred eggs that had previously been cultured for 5 days, 1 of the 2 animals gave birth to a dead lamb, and the other produced a live lamb without a rectum. Stillbirth was also the result of some experiments that we performed in cattle with eggs that had been cultured too long prior to transfer. This emphasizes how extremely careful one would have to be in attempting to transfer human eggs. There is, of course, no reason to suppose that the abnormalities following transfer of cultured mammalian eggs were due to aging of the zygotes *per se*; it is more likely that these abnormalities were the result of abnormal development under conditions *in vitro*.

The main defect in the aged mammalian egg is undoubtedly the loss of the ability to prevent polyspermy, that is, the penetration of more than one spermatozoon. The mechanism responsible for this defect is not known at present. But relevant to this problem may be the observation that when one attempts to induce ovulation at a stage when the progesterone level in the animal is high, i.e., during the luteal phase of the estrous cycle, polyspermy often occurs. There are reports that a similar defect occurs as a result of elevated temperature [Austin and Braden, 1954]. When ewes were kept in a hot room at 35–40°C for a period of 6 h after estrus, the eggs recovered from these animals were found to be capable of undergoing fertilization, but the subsequent process of zygote segmentation was abnormal [Thwaites, 1967]. In another experiment ewes of varyng ages were placed in a hot room; such an exposure was again found to have a detrimental effect on egg development and embryonic survival, irrespective of the age of the ewes. Embryonic mortality reached 75–100% after the ewes had been subjected to 'heat stress' during the first 15 days of pregnancy; moreover, the weight and diameter of the corpora lutea of these animals were markedly reduced, and it was impossible to remedy this situation by progesterone administration [Thwaites, 1968 a, b]. Another investigation of a similar kind was conducted by Alliston and Ulberg [1961] who transferred embryos from donor ewes that had been kept at 32°C to recipient ewes at 20°C and found that this produced damage to the embryos. It appears from the results reported by Dutt et al. [1959] that as the age of the zygote increases the damage to the zygote from high environmental temperature becomes less marked.

II. Aging of Spermatozoa

The impressive growth of literature on the subject of sperm aging in farm animals is largely due to sustained efforts in extending for as long as possible the viability of spermatozoa in semen used for AI. Many of these efforts were specifically directed toward solving the difficulty of preventing sperm aging in semen used in AI and included extensive studies on effects exerted on spermatozoa by temperature, dilution, pH, and ionic composition of the semen and the diluting media. Many of these studies were also combined with observations on the metabolism of semen [Mann, 1964]. But it is still difficult to correlate the findings made with semen *in vitro* with the actual fertilizing potential of the semen as expressed in the so-called nonreturn or conception rate after AI. At the same time, it is possible to predict from certain changes observed in spermatozoa that they have suffered damage of the kind that must result in decreased fertility. Many of the physico-chemical changes that occur in semen under storage conditions *in vitro* are, moreover, irreversible. Some of them may result from improper handling of the semen after collection. For example, the too rapid cooling of freshly collected semen results in cold shock that inactivates spermatozoa irreversibly. Cold shock, which has been studied extensively, is known to result in the leakage of many protein constituents, including cytochrome c from spermatozoa and in a rapid loss of other intracellular sperm constituents, probably as a direct result of a general loosening of the surface structure of spermatozoa.

Of great practical importance is the fact that some of the deleterious effects, including cold shock, can be effectively prevented by the use of media containing protective agents. For this reason, bull semen is routinely diluted immediately after collection with media, such as the egg-yolk diluents. WIL-LETT [1950, 1953] compared the 'nonreturn rates' of cattle inseminated with semen that had been diluted with appropriate medium either 1:100 or 1:300 and reported that the nonreturn rate obtained with the 1:300 diluted semen was only 5.8% lower than that obtained with 1:100 diluted semen provided that the diluted semen was inseminated in both cases on the first day of storage. But when the diluted semen was used on the second day of storage, the decline in the nonreturn rate was 3.6% with the less diluted and 8.2% with the more diluted semen.

Even when properly diluted bull semen is stored at temperatures below room temperature, but above the freezing point, e.g. at 4–5°C one has to reckon with a progressive fall in fertility, something of the order of 2–3% during the first few days of storage and with accelerating decline during the subsequent days. For example, SALISBURY and FLERCHINGER [1967 a, b], who stored bull semen at 4–5°C, reported that when that semen was used for AI on the 2nd day of storage, the fertility was actually somewhat higher than that after the use of fresh semen, but thereafter the nonreturn rate began to fall, from 66.2% on day 2 to 54.4% on day 4, and to 39.4% on day 5 (as assessed on day 180 after AI).

The two main methods used routinely for storing bull semen in such a way as to prevent irreversible damage to spermatozoa, or at least to minimize it, are (1) careful cooling of semen after it has been diluted with a suitable protective medium containing, e.g., egg yolk or milk heat-treated to temperatures above 0°C (4 or 5°C), and (2) passing CO_2 through the suitably diluted and buffered semen. The treatment with CO_2 results in a reversible arrest of sperm motility and metabolism even at ordinary temperature so that there is no need to cool semen down to low temperatures, such as 4 or 5°C [VANDE-MARK and SHARMA, 1957]. Some further examples of the effect on fertility obtained with stored bull semen are provided by ANISOV [1968] who stored bull semen, diluted with a glucose-egg yolk-citrate medium, at 0°C prior to AI and recorded the following pregnancy rates: 70.5% after 12–14 h storage, 68.5% after 24–36 h, 60.0% after 36–48 h, and 47% after 48–72 h.

Effects of *in vitro* storage of semen on fertility have also been studied in domesticated animals other than cattle, in particular pigs. FIRST *et al.* [1963] noted that when boar semen was used for AI after storage for 6 and for 54 h and the sows slaughtered and examined 25 days later, there was evidence of a higher fertility rate in the sows inseminated with semen stored for 6 h than for those inseminated with semen stored for 54 h.

We still lack an adequate explanation for why fertility declines so much faster than motility when spermatozoa are stored prior to AI. SALISBURY and co-workers have argued that the DNA content of spermatozoa may be changing during the storage and that this affects fertility without affecting motility. Unfortunately, so many observations relating to the behavior of DNA in stored spermatozoa were made by using methods that depend on the use of the Feulgen technique for DNA determination. One of the earliest observations of this kind, made with bull semen, was that by LEUCHTENBERGER *et al.* [1955]; it was followed by other similar studies that indicated that the amount of Feulgen-positive material in sperm heads of bull spermatozoa may decrease by as much as 30% over a period of 5 days storage at 5°C [SALISBURY, 1965; SALISBURY and FLERCHINGER, 1967 a, b]. Of the many other studies concerned with this problem only a few need be mentioned here. For example, QUINN and WHITE [1968] extracted DNA from ram spermatozoa that had been frozen to –79°C, and subsequently incubated for 1 h at 37°C. They found that freezing alone had no effect on DNA, but if the spermatozoa were incubated after thawing for 1 h at 37°C, a change in DNA did occur. HANADA *et al.* [1968] also made some analyses of DNA in frozen-thawed spermatozoa and found that freezing alone had no effect on the DNA content but that the content decreased when the thawed material was stored for a further period of 3 days at 5°C. A reduction of the DNA content of spermatozoa was also reported by PAUFLER and FOOTE [1967] in bull semen stored in sealed ampoules at 5°C. When, however, BOUTERS and VAN NIEUWEHUYSE [1968] tried to correlate the DNA content of bull spermatozoa with fertility of the semen samples, they could find no such correlation. No change in the thermal denaturation behavior of DNA could be demonstrated by BERCHTOLD *et al.* [1971] in bull spermatozoa stored for periods up to 15 days. Studies on the effects of storage on the DNA content of spermatozoa have also been carried out by ANAND *et al.* [1966], ANAND and FIRST [1968], and SEGINA and NORMAN [1964]. In the end it became clear that the Feulgen technique alone is not suitable for assessing the DNA content of spermatozoa

Table I. The number of cows inseminated and the conception rate over 9 years by using semen frozen to –196 °C

Bull	1–4 weeks		1 year		2 years		4 years		9 years	
	first insemination	conception rate, %	first insemination	conception rate, %	first insemination	conception rate, %	first insemination	conception rate, %	first insemination	conception rate, %
S 3	105	67.6	124	64.5	142	66.2	133	63.2	126	57.9
S 14	104	65.4	148	59.5	156	62.8	143	60.8	129	58.1
Total	209	66.5	272	61.8	298	64.4	276	62.0	255	58.0

Data from STEWART [1964].

and that the results obtained by this method do not necessarily agree with results obtained by more sophisticated methods [GLEDHILL, 1970]. SALISBURY and HART [1970] had to admit that: 'The conflicting nature of these results when compared to those obtained by the Feulgen technique would suggest that either the latter method was unreliable or that it not only quantitates DNA but also reflects transitional states of the molecule.' Recently, BLACKSHAW and SALISBURY [1972] reported their findings on nuclear DNA of bull spermatozoa stored for up to 9 days, measured by 3 methods, (1) ultraviolet absorption, (2) Feulgen staining, and (3) acridine orange fluorescence. Their results confirm the now generally accepted view that DNA as such does not change during storage, and the variability observed after Feulgen staining is probably due to changes in the DNA-protein association.

When the method of freezing semen came into practice, it was first thought that even at –79°C some residual metabolic activity persisted and that that could perhaps explain the gradual decline in the conception rate achieved by use of such semen. For example, it was reported by STEWART [1964] that after a 9-year period of storage at –79°C the conception rate was 58.0% as compared with 66.5% after 1 year of storage (table I). It has to be remembered, however, that in the early days the storage cabinets had to be frequently opened for sorting and replacing the stock of semen samples so that the temperature in these cabinets may not have been always at –79°C. Both MIXNER [1968] and we conducted some further studies on the effects of storage at low temperatures on the fertilizing quality of bull semen. In Cambridge we have kept some bull semen samples at –79°C for 20 years, and we

Table II. The number of cows inseminated and conception rate with semen stored either at –79°C or at –196°C for a minimum period of 3 weeks

Bull	Solid carbon dioxide (–79°C)		Liquid nitrogen (–196°C)	
	first inseminations	conception rate, %	first inseminations	conception rate, %
F19	233	58.4	213	54.5
F20	215	60.5	205	65.4
F23	209	62.2	218	67.4
J30	205	52.7	203	59.6
A21	218	54.6	208	47.6
H11	220	61.8	204	66.2
	1,300	58.4	1,251	60.1

Data from Stewart [1964].

have found that the conception rate obtained with such semen after AI was only slightly reduced. With the present method of storing bull semen, that is, in liquid nitrogen at –196°C, it should be possible to preserve even more effectively the viability of bull spermatozoa (table II). We believe that freezing and storing of semen in the frozen state, particularly in liquid nitrogen, is at present the most effective method for preventing aging in spermatozoa. But there are several factors that can influence the 'freezability' of semen samples. It seems, for example, that bull semen collected during the summer months loses its fertilizing potential more quickly than semen collected during the cooler season [Salisbury, 1967]. Bulls seem to differ from each other also, and the semen from some bulls can be maintained in a frozen state much better than that from other bulls. It is of some interest to note that in semen with poorer keeping quality one often observes after thawing a higher proportion of dead spermatozoa and more structural damage, particularly to the sperm heads and the acrosomal membranes. Nowadays bulls are selected for AI not merely on the grounds of superior phenotype or genotype but also for the 'freezability' of their semen.

It is possible of course, that there may be other as yet unidentified causes of aging in stored spermatozoa, such as the formation of peroxides. It has been reported that the addition of catalase to semen has a beneficial effect on the keeping quality of spermatozoa so far as their fertilizing potential is concerned, but the amount of catalase that was used for that purpose was far in excess of what would be required for elimination of hydrogen peroxide

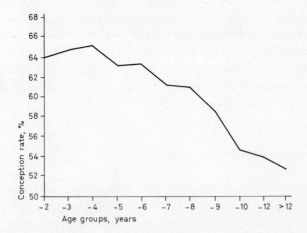

Fig. 3. Fertility of AI bulls in relation to age. Fertility is measured as conception rate at 3 months. Redrawn from Milk Marketing Board [1950].

[FOOTE, 1962]. There remains also the possibility that some lipid peroxide could be formed during storage. MROTEK *et al.* [1966] are of the opinion that there can be little, if any, lipid peroxide formed during storage of boar semen at 5°C. The whole question of lipid peroxidation has been recently reopened by the current study of JONES and MANN [private commun.].

A possible future approach to the study of the aging process in spermatozoa of farm animals could be based on results obtained with artificially inseminated heterospermic semen, fresh as well as aged. Heterospermic insemination has been already of considerable use in somewhat related studies, such as that by BEATTY *et al.* [1969], in which equal numbers of spermatozoa originating from bulls of different breeds were used for AI.

More remains to be learned about the influence that the age of the bull has on the fertility and progeny. In England this question, which is of considerable economic importance, received first serious attention in 1951 when the Milk Marketing Board [1950] reported that the conception rate after AI lowered when old bulls were used (fig. 3). The whole question has been reexamined by the Milk Marketing Board, and the main conclusion of that examination is that there is indeed a definite trend in dairy bulls to become less fertile as they advance in age but that no similar trend seems to exist in beef-breed bulls. It is unlikely that this conclusion will affect seriously the choice of bulls for AI. When bulls are selected for AI, prime consideration is given to their so-called genetic merits, rather than their age. In the USA, a similar investigation has been conducted by COLLINS *et al.* [1962] who found that the fertility of Holstein and Guernsey bulls declined with age by 0.50% per year and 0.31% per year, respectively. The extent to which the age of animals affects the morphology of spermatozoa still remains to be determined. It is, however, interesting to note that in inbred mice, the decline in fertility that occurs with advancing age, is accompanied by certain abnormalities in the sperm acrosomes [Beatty and Mukherjee, 1963].

III. Deep-Freezing of Mammalian Eggs

Now that egg transfer in farm animals such as sheep and cattle can be carried out by well established methods [Rowson, 1971], it becomes increasingly important in relation to practical problems, such as the production of twins in cattle [Rowson et al., 1971]. Therefore the question of preventing age-dependent changes in eggs is assuming great importance. Sheep or cow eggs represent a highly valuable commodity, much more difficult to secure than semen, and a method is urgently needed for long-term preservation of such eggs under conditions where aging could be reliably prevented. Preservation at temperatures above 0°C, although practicable, will not provide the solution to the problem of egg storage for the purpose of later transfer. What is needed is an uncomplicated and reproducible technique for deep-freezing of eggs, comparable in efficiency to the one in current use for storing semen.

Fortunately, there are several indications that the technique for storing eggs in a deep-frozen state can be developed on a large scale. The first step in that direction was taken when Whittingham [1971] announced that he succeeded in deep-freezing mouse blastocysts by using the so-called PVP medium. This particular medium we have found to be unsuitable. But more recently excellent results were obtained with a medium containing dimethylsulfoxide [Whittingham et al., 1972; Wilmut, 1972]. When the experiments with mouse eggs produced the desired result, work was initiated in our Unit's laboratory by Wilmut and co-workers including myself, on the problem of deep-freezing of fertilized cow eggs, and very recently we have succeeded in obtaining a live and apparently healthy calf from a cow that had received 2 eggs previously stored in liquid nitrogen (fig. 4).

In general, the whole question of how senescence affects the gametes of farm animals can be answered at present by saying that, to the best of our knowledge, senescence of gametes results in embryonic losses during the early stages of embryonic development rather than in changes in the progeny characteristics. But much more work in this area is required. We know, for

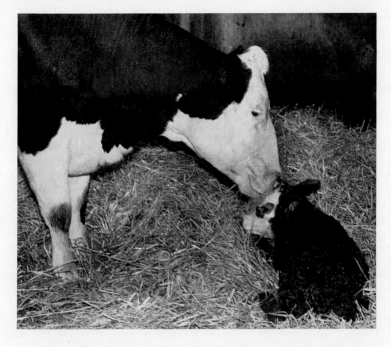

Fig. 4. The first calf ever to be born following deep-freezing at the blastocyst stage and transference to a host cow.

example, that in some cases the chromosomal make-up of embryos aborted by the domestic animals is abnormal, but there is no clear-cut evidence to suggest that these abnormalities have arisen as a direct result of gamete senescence.

References

ADAMS, C.E.: The influence of advanced maternal age on embryo survival in the rabbit. Proc. Int. Congr. Anim. Reprod. A.I., Trento 1964, p. 305

ALEXANDER, N.J.: Vasectomy. Long-term effects in the Rhesus monkey. J. Reprod. Fertil. *31:* 399 (1972).

ALLISTON, C.W. and ULBERG, L.C.: Early pregnancy loss in sheep at ambient temperatures of 70° and 90°F as determined by embryo transfer. J. anim. Sci. *20:* 608 (1961).

AMANN, R.P. and ALMQUIST, J.O.: Reproductive capacity of dairy bulls. VII. Morphology of epididymal sperm. J. Dairy Sci. *45:* 1516 (1962).

Anand, A.S. and First, N.L.: Effect of aging of boar semen on the DNA content of live and dead spermatozoa. Proc. Int. Congr. Anim. Reprod. A.I., Paris 1968, vol. 2, p. 1209

Anand, A.S.; Hoekstra, W.G., and First, N.L.: Effect of aging of boar spermatozoa on cellular loss of DNA. J. anim. Sci. 25: abstr., p. 917 (1966).

Anisov, A.A.: Conception rate of cows in relation to duration of semen storage and the time and number of inseminations. Zhivotnovodstvo. Mosk. 30/10: 68 (1968).

Austin, C.R.: Ageing and reproduction: post ovulatory deterioration of the egg. J. Reprod. Fertil. Suppl. 12: 39 (1970).

Austin, C.R. and Braden, A.W.H.: The reaction of the zona pellucida to sperm penetration. Austr. J. Biol. Sci. 7: 195 (1954).

Beatty, R.A.; Bennett, G.H.; Hall, J.G.; Hancock, J.L., and Stewart, D.L.: An experiment with heterospermic insemination in cattle. J. Reprod. Fertil. 19: 491 (1969).

Beatty, R.A. and Fechheimer, N.S.: Diploid spermatozoa in rabbit semen and their experimental separation from haploid spermatozoa. Biol. Reprod. 7: 267 (1972).

Beatty, R.A. and Mukherjee, D.P.: Spermatozoa characteristics in mice of different ages. J. Reprod. Fertil. 6: 261 (1963).

Beier, H.N.; Mootz, U. und Kuhnel, W.: Asynchrone Eitransplantation während der verzögerten Uterussekretion beim Kaninchen. Proc. Int. Congr. Anim. Reprod. A.I., Munich 1972.

Berchtold, M.; Salisbury, G.W., and Graves, C.N.: Ageing phenomena in spermatozoa. V. Thermal denaturation characteristics of deoxyribonucleic acid isolated from fresh and aged bovine spermatozoa. J. Dairy Sci. 54: 1536 (1971).

Blackshaw, A.W. and Salisbury, G.W.: The effect of storage in vitro on the DNA content of bull semen. Austr. J. Biol. Sci. 25: 175 (1972).

Bouters, R. and Van Nieuwenhuyse, E.: The relation between the Feulgen DNA content and fertilizing capacity of A.I. bulls. Vlaams diergeneesk. T. 37: 472 (1968).

Burkhardt, J.A.: Sperm survival in the genital tract of the mare. J. agric. Sci. 39: 201 (1949).

Collins, W.E.; Inskeep, E.K.; Dreher, W.H.; Tyler, W.J., and Casida, L.E.: Effect of age on fertility of bulls in artificial insemination. J. Dairy Sci. 45: 1015 (1962).

Dauzier, L. and Winterberger, S.: Duration of the fertilising ability of ram spermatozoa in the genital tract of the ewe and duration of fertility of the ovum after ovulation. C.R. Soc. Biol. 146: 660 (1952).

Day, F.T.: Survival of spermatozoa in the genital tract of the mare. J. agric. Sci. 32: 108 (1942).

Du Mesnil du Buisson, F. and Dauzier, L.: Distribution and resorption of semen in the genital tract of the sow: spermatozoal survival. Ann. Endocrin., Paris 16: 413 (1955).

Dutt, R.H.; Ellington, E.F., and Carlton, W.W.: Fertilization rate and early embryo survival in sheared and unsheared ewes following exposure to elevated air temperature. J. anim. Sci. 18: 1308 (1959).

Dziuk, P.: Estimation of optimum time for insemination of gilts and ewes by double mating at certain times relative to ovulation. J. Reprod. Fertil. 22: 277 (1970).

Dziuk, P.J. and Polge, C.: Fertility of swine after induced ovulation. J. Reprod. Fertil. 4: 207 (1962).

FIRST, N.L.; STRATMAN, F.W., and CASIDA, L.E.: Effect of sperm age on embryo survival in swine. J. anim. Sci. *22:* 135 (1963).

FOOTE, R.H.: Survival of bull sperm in milk and yolk extenders with added catalase. J. Dairy Sci. *45:* 907 (1962).

GLEDHILL, B.L.: Enigma of spermatozoal deoxyribonucleic acid and male fertility. A review. Amer. J. vet. Res. *31:* 539 (1970).

HANADA, A.; NAGASE, H.; YAMASHITA, S., and IRIE, S.: DNA content of bull spermatozoa after freezing and thawing and its relation with fertility rate. Bull. nat. Inst. Anim. Ind., Chiba *18:* 77 (1968).

HANCOCK, J.L.: Polyspermy of pig ova. Anim. Prod. *1:* 103 (1959).

HUNTER, R.H.F. and DZIUK, P.J.: Sperm penetration of pig eggs in relation to the timing of ovulation and insemination. J. Reprod. Fertil. *15:* 199 (1968).

IGBOELI, G. and RAKHA, A.M.: Bull testicular and epididymal functions after long-term vasectomy. J. anim. Sci. *31:* 72 (1970).

LAING, J.A.: Observation on the survival time of the spermatozoa in the genital tract of the cow and its relation to fertility. J. agric. Sci. *35:* 72 (1945).

LEUCHTENBERGER, C.; WEIR, B.R.; SCHRADER, F., and MURMANIS, L.: The deoxyribonucleic acid (DNA) content of repeated seminal fluids and fertile and infertile men. J. Lab. clin. Med. *45:* 851 (1955).

MANN, T.: The biochemistry of semen and of the male reproductive tract (Methuen, London 1964).

Milk Marketing Board: The bulls age and his conception rate. Rep. Prod. Div. Milk Market. Board *1:* 31 (1950).

MIXNER, J.P.: Fertility of bull semen frozen for twelve years. Proc. Int. Congr. Anim. Reprod. A.I., Paris 1968, p. 188.

MOOR, R.M. and CRAGLE, R.G.: The sheep egg: enzymatic removal of the zona pellucida and culture of eggs *in vitro*. J. Reprod. Fertil. 27: 401 (1971).

MROTEK, J.J.; HOEKSTRA, W.G., and FIRST, N.L.: Effect of boar semen senility on peroxidation of semen lipids. J. anim. Sci. *25:* 688 (1966).

PAUFLER, S. and FOOTE, R.H.: Influence of light on nuclear size and deoxyribonucleic acid content of stored bovine spermatozoa. J. Dairy Sci. *50:* 1475 (1967).

QUINN, P.J. and WHITE, I.G.: A spectral analysis of ram sperm DNA after cold shock and deep freezing. Proc. Int. Congr. Anim. Reprod. A.I., Paris 1968, p. 242.

ROWSON, L.E.A.: Egg transfer in domestic animals. Nature, Lond. *233:* 379 (1971).

ROWSON, L.E.A.; LAWSON, R.A.S., and MOOR, R.M.: Production of twins in cattle by egg transfer. J. Reprod. Fertil. *25:* 261 (1971).

ROWSON, L.E.A. and MOOR, R.M.: Embryo transfer in the sheep: the significance of synchronizing oestrus in the donor and recipient animal. J. Reprod. Fertil. *11:* 207 (1966).

SALISBURY, G.W.: Ageing phenomena in gametes. J. Geront. *20:* 381 (1965).

SALISBURY, G.W.: Aging phenomena in spermatozoa. III. Effect of season and storage at −79° to −88°C on fertility and prenatal losses. J. Dairy Sci. *50:* 1683 (1967).

SALISBURY, G.W. and BAKER, F.N.: Nuclear morphology of spermatozoa from inbred and line-cross Hereford bulls. J. anim. Sci. *25:* 476 (1966).

SALISBURY, G.W. and FLERCHINGER, F.H.: Aging phenomena in spermatozoa. I. Fertility and prenatal losses with use of liquid semen. J. Dairy Sci. *50:* 1675 (1967a).

Salisbury, G.W. and Flerchinger, F.H.: Aging phenomena in spermatozoa. II. Estrous cycle length after unsuccessful insemination with spermatozoa of varying age. J. Dairy Sci. *50:* 1679 (1967b).

Salisbury, G.W. and Hart, R.G.: Gamete aging and its consequences. Biol. Reprod. Suppl. *2:* 1 (1970).

Segina, M.R. and Norman, C.: Age-related changes in the DNA of bovine sperm. Proc. Int. Congr. Anim. Reprod. A.I., Trento 1964, p. 276.

Stewart, D.L.: Observations on the fertility of frozen semen stored at –79° and –196°C. Proc. Int. Congr. Anim. Reprod. A.I., Trento 1964, p. 617.

Tervit, H.R.; Whittingham, D.G., and Rowson, L.E.A.: Successful culture *in vitro* of sheep and cattle ova. J. Reprod. Fertil. *30:* 493 (1972).

Thwaites, C.J.: Embryo mortality in the heat stressed ewe. J. Reprod. Fertil. *14:* 5 (1967).

Thwaites, C.J.: Age and heat tolerance in sheep. Int. J. Biomet. *2:* 209 (1968a).

Thwaites, C.J.: Embryo mortality in the heat stressed ewe. Proc. Int. Congr. Anim. Reprod. A.I., Paris 1968b, resume, p. 79.

VanDemark, N.L. and Sharma, U.D.: Preliminary fertility results from the preservation of bovine semen at room temperatures. J. Dairy Sci. *45:* 438 (1957).

Whittingham, D.G.: Survival of mouse embryos after freezing and thawing. Nature, Lond. *233:* 125 (1971).

Whittingham, D.G.; Leibo, S.P., and Mozut, P.: Survival of mouse embryos frozen at –196°C and –269°C. Science *178:* 411 (1972).

Willett, E.L.: Fertility and livability of bull semen diluted at various levels to 1:300. J. Dairy Sci. *33:* 43 (1950).

Willett, E.L.: Decline in fertility of bull semen with increase in storage tome as influenced by dilution rate. J. Dairy Sci. *36:* 1182 (1953).

Wilmut, I.: Effect of cooling rate, warming rate, cryoprotective agent and stage of development on survival of mouse embryos during freezing and thawing. Life Sci. *2:* part II, p. 1071 (in press, 1972).

Young, W.C.: Functional changes undergone by spermatozoa during their passage through the epididymis and vas deferens in the guinea-pig. J. exp. Biol. *8:* 151 (1931).

Author's address: Dr. L.E.A. Rowson, Agricultural Research Council's Unit of Reproductive Physiology and Biochemistry, University of Cambridge, *Cambridge CB2 3EZ* (England)

Aging Gametes. Int. Symp., Seattle 1973, pp. 265–277 (Karger, Basel 1975)

Effects of Long-Term Storage of Human Spermatozoa in Liquid Nitrogen [1]

KEITH D. SMITH, DANIEL R. STULTZ and EMIL STEINBERGER

Program in Reproductive Biology and Reproductive Endocrinology, The University of Texas Medical School at Houston, Texas Medical Center, Houston, Tex.

The information available concerning the physiologic aging of the human male gamete in either the female or the male reproductive tract is limited. The freezing of spermatozoa to delay aging and to preserve fertility has been studied actively by animal breeders. Less extensive investigations of the effect of freezing on human spermatozoa have been conducted.

The first report of effects of cold on spermatozoa was that of SPALLANZANI [1776], who noted that spermatozoa became immotile after exposure to freezing temperatures and regained motility after warming. Ninety years later MANTEGAZZA [1866] reported that spermatozoa resisted freezing to –15°C and predicted the feasibility of frozen sperm banks in the future. In 1897, DAVENPORT reported the survival of spermatozoa after freezing at –17°C. Over 40 years elapsed before the next published observation. JAHNEL [1938] observed some spermatozoal motility after thawing semen samples frozen at –79, –196, and –269°C. SHETTLES [1940] confirmed the survival of spermatozoa after freezing semen at –269.5°C. Although survival never exceeded 10%, he could detect no structural change in spermatozoa after thawing. Although these studies established the feasibility of preserving spermatozoa in the frozen state, the survival was insufficient to warrant practical application.

Subsequent to SHETTLE's [1940] report several investigators focused on details of the technique of freezing spermatozoa and investigated various physical parameters. HOAGLAND and PINCUS [1942] utilized liquid nitrogen and observed the survival of 20–40% of original motility in foamed semen specimens. One sample that was frozen as a smear on cellophane retained

1   This study was supported in part by grants from the Ford Foundation and the Population Council.

67% of its original motility. PARKES [1945] froze semen in capillary tubes with inside diameters of 0.15, 0.5 and 1 mm at temperatures of –20, –79, and –196°C and observed optimal survival in those samples frozen in the largest tubes at either –79 or –196°C. He concluded that the volume frozen was the limiting factor in spermatozoal survival.

None of these methodological modifications yielded a technique of freezing satisfactory for practical application. In 1949, POLGE *et al.* reported the protective action of glycerol on spermatozoa; this was the first firm basis for the development of frozen sperm banks for animal breeders and for humans.

I. Development of Human Sperm Banks Utilizing Solidified CO_2

In the early 1950s, SHERMAN and BUNGE [1953] re-evaluated PARKES' [1945] data and concluded that the volume of semen frozen was not the limiting factor in spermatozoal survival. Since larger volumes freeze at slower rates, they suggested that the rate of freezing was the important parameter. They studied the effect of the rate of freezing on the recovery of spermatozoal motility by employing 4 procedures, each yielding a different rate of freezing. The slowest rate was provided by dry ice and resulted in the highest survival (67% of original motility). These investigators determined that a 10-percent concentration of glycerol provided superior protection to spermatozoa, and they emphasized the need to add the glycerol dropwise in order to prevent toxicity. Semen, frozen by this procedure, retained not only motility but also fertilizibility, as evidenced by conceptions in 3 women inseminated with donor semen, frozen and stored in a dry ice chest [BUNGE and SHERMAN, 1953]. The following year, BUNGE *et al.* [1954] reported normal progeny from the first three conceptions, an additional pregnancy and the establishment of a frozen sperm bank.

TYLER and SINGHER [1956] collected split ejaculates from oligospermic men and froze the portion containing the highest concentration of spermatozoa. The wives were inseminated with several thawed semen samples plus a single fresh sample. Pregnancies were reported in 3 women, all of whom failed to conceive from prior inseminations with single, fresh split ejaculates. Unfortunately, this procedure made it impossible to determine whether fresh or frozen semen produced the conceptions. Two problems were noted. Many specimens from oligospermic men with low initial spermatozoal motility showed an unacceptable rate of motility after thawing. In addition, many specimens with fairly good initial motility did not survive the freezing and thawing procedures well enough to warrant their use.

KEETTEL *et al.* [1956] summarized the results of inseminations with semen from the first human sperm bank [BUNGE *et al.*, 1954] and compared these results with those obtained with fresh semen. Frozen semen was employed in 26 women, each of whom was inseminated 3 times a cycle for as long as 7 menstrual cycles. Nine pregnancies (34.6%), all occurring during the first two cycles, resulted. Fresh semen was utilized in 20 women, resulting in conceptions in 11 (55%), 8 of whom were women who failed to conceive with frozen semen. Additional pregnancies resulting from insemination with human semen frozen and stored in dry ice were reported by Japanese investigators [IIZUKA and SAWADA, 1958; SAWADA, 1959, 1964] and by FERNANDEZ-CANO *et al.* [1964].

II. Development of Human Sperm Banks Utilizing Liquid Nitrogen

In 1962, SHERMAN reported an improved technique, freezing semen samples in liquid nitrogen vapor and storing the samples under the surface of liquid nitrogen. Utilizing this technique, PERLOFF *et al.* [1964] reported the first successful pregnancies after artificial insemination with human semen frozen and stored in liquid nitrogen. Subsequently, STEINBERGER and PERLOFF [1965] reported preliminary observations on the clinical use of a human sperm bank employing liquid nitrogen for freezing and storage.

BEHRMAN and ACKERMAN [1969] and BEHRMAN and SAWADA [1966] suggested a modification of SHERMAN's [1962] technique by employing a semen expander (glycerol-egg yolk-citrate mixture) to dilute the semen sample by 50% and freezing samples at a slower rate. Most investigators have used either SHERMAN's rapid freeze or BEHRMAN's slower freeze techniques, although modifications of the glycerol concentrations have been employed. Motility of spermatozoa after thawing (postthaw motility) varied from 50 to 70% of original motility. FREUND [1967], employing a semen expander composed of tissue culture media, glycerol, and egg yolk and an extremely slow freezing rate requiring over 10 h for completion, reported no loss of spermatozoal motility. This report has not been confirmed.

Two studies attempted to compare the techniques of SHERMAN and of BEHRMAN. TRELFORD and MUELLER [1969] reported that the rapid-freeze technique resulted in survival of 44% of original motility compared to 21% for the slower procedure. However, they modified both techniques, employing 7.5% glycerol instead of 10% in the rapid-freeze procedure and eliminating the semen expander in the slower freeze procedure and replacing it with 7.5% glycerol. Friberg and Nilsson [1971] divided semen samples into 4 aliquots. Two were pretreated with 10% glycerol and 2 were pretreated with glycerol-egg yolk-citrate semen expander. One sample from each pretreatment group was frozen by the rapid freeze technique, and the other sample from each group was frozen by the slow freeze technique. No differences in postthaw motility were detected in any of the 4 aliquots. However, ultrastructural studies demonstrated wrinkling of the acrosome in samples pretreated with 10% glycerol but not in samples pretreated with semen expander. Despite the wrinkling of the acrosome, *in vivo* survival of spermatozoa in cervical mucus 24 h after insemination was better in samples pretreated with 10% glycerol. These reports suggest that if there are any differences between these 2 techniques they are slight. Perhaps more extensive investigations employing more sensitive parameters will detect important differences between these techniques.

The effect of freezing and thawing on the fertility of spermatozoa is more difficult to evaluate than are the effects of freezing and thawing on motility. Fertility requires motility of spermatozoa; yet motility does not insure fertility. A comparison of results of artificial inseminations with fresh or frozen semen is one way to evaluate the efficacy of sperm banking. Behrman [1971] reported conception rates of 72% (796 of 1,188 cases) with fresh semen and 52% (104 of 200 cases) with frozen. Carlborg [1971] noted pregnancy rates of 80% with fresh semen and 30–50% with frozen. In older studies in which dry ice storage was used [Keettel *et al.*, 1956] fresh semen also appeared to produce higher rates of conception.

The length of time frozen semen samples may be stored and maintain both motility and fertility has not been established. In Behrman's [1971] series the oldest fertile specimen was stored for 33 months. Sawada and Ackerman [1968] observed fertility in a specimen stored 315 days and satisfactory motility in a specimen stored 1,401 days. Sherman [1972] recently reported no loss of motility in semen samples stored for 10 years in liquid nitrogen and in 3 of these specimens he demonstrated fertility. No details concerning the insemination procedures or the clinical evaluations of the recipients and their husbands were provided in any of these publications.

Sherman [1973] summarized the results of pregnancies from frozen semen and reported 686 conceptions, resulting in 564 normal children, 7 abnormal children and 50 spontaneous abortions. Results of the conceptions in 65 women were not available, nor was any estimate of failure rate. This sum-

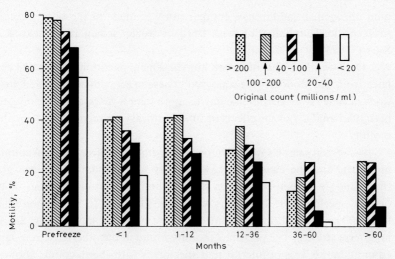

Sperm count, millions/ml	Prefreeze motility		Storage time, months								
			<1		1–12		12–36		36–60		>60	
	N	SE	N	SE	N	SE	N	SE	N	SE	N	SE
< 20	18	4.3	14	3.8	15	4.0	8	4.6	6	1.0	20	0.0
20– 40	59	2.0	42	2.2	75	1.6	42	2.3	34	1.5	19	1.8
40–100	186	0.7	221	0.7	259	1.0	78	1.8	38	3.3	10	4.5
100–200	197	0.6	278	0.9	270	1.0	43	2.1	35	1.9	10	6.4
> 200	73	1.0	110	1.7	98	1.7	23	3.4	15	2.3	0	–

N = Number of specimens; SE = standard error of the mean.
Reprinted by permission of the Editor, Journal of the American Medical Association.

Fig. 1. Comparison of means of prefreeze and postthaw motility of semen samples grouped on the basis of sperm count and related to time of storage in liquid nitrogen. N = Number of specimens; SE = standard error of the mean. Reprinted by permission of the Editor, Journal of the American Medical Association.

mary, compiled from published reports and from a survey questionnaire that SHERMAN sent to investigators maintaining frozen sperm banks, confirmed the efficacy of artificial insemination with semen stored in a frozen sperm bank but provided no information on conception rates or comparison with use of fresh semen.

Recently, SMITH and STEINBERGER [1973] published the results of a systematic study of the motility and fertility of semen specimens after storage in liquid nitrogen. In addition, a comparison was made of the results obtained from artificial insemination with fresh or frozen semen [STEINBERGER and SMITH, 1973].

Data on 1,764 vials of frozen human semen, partitioned from 533 ejaculates from 207 donors were analyzed. These specimens were stored for periods of time ranging from one day to more than 8 years, a storage range that permitted analysis of the effects of time in storage on recoverable (postthaw) motility.

All semen samples were grouped according to prefreeze sperm counts or motilities, and the mean postthaw motility was calculated for each group (fig. 1 and 2). In figure 1, semen samples are grouped on the basis of their original sperm count. Specimens with counts from 40 to 100 million/ml and from 100 to 200 million/ml retained the best postthaw motility (fig. 3a) after long-term storage. The postthaw motility found in the other groups is depicted in figure 3b. It is of interest that specimens with sperm counts above 200 million/ml retain good postthaw motility during the first year and then undergo a marked decline.

Correlation of original motility with survival after various times in storage is illustrated in figure 2. Specimens with prefreeze motility above 60% had better postthaw motility than those with prefreeze motility below 60%. The mean survival of the latter group was never as high as 20% at any time after thawing.

Common procedure in the past has been to report postthaw motility in terms of percent recovery (postthaw motility divided by the prefreeze motility and multiplied by 100). The percent recovery versus time in storage is illustrated in figure 4. The freezing and thawing process resulted in a loss of approximately half of the prefreeze motility. No additional significant loss in percent recovery occurred in samples stored for 3 years. Through the remainder of the study a continued decline in percent recovery was observed.

It should be emphasized that individual semen specimens may vary considerably from these means. In fact, the oldest samples in this study were stored 8 years 3 months, and had postthaw motilities of 50%, identical to that found in aliquots from the same ejaculates shortly after freezing. Conversely, occasional samples with prefreeze sperm counts and motilities in the range that would be expected to have good postthaw recovery (counts between 40 and 200 million/ml and motilities above 60%), demonstrated unacceptable postthaw motility. No single factor or combination of factors analyzed was a significant indicator in predicting the percent recovery in individual semen samples. Even different specimens from the same donor occa-

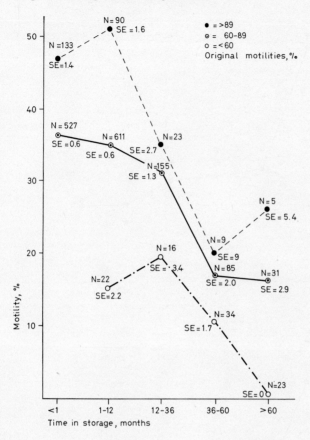

Fig. 2. Comparison of means of prefreeze and postthaw motility of semen samples grouped on the basis of original motility and related to time of storage in liquid nitrogen. N = Number of specimens; SE = standard error of the mean. Reprinted by permission of the Editor, Journal of the American Medical Association.

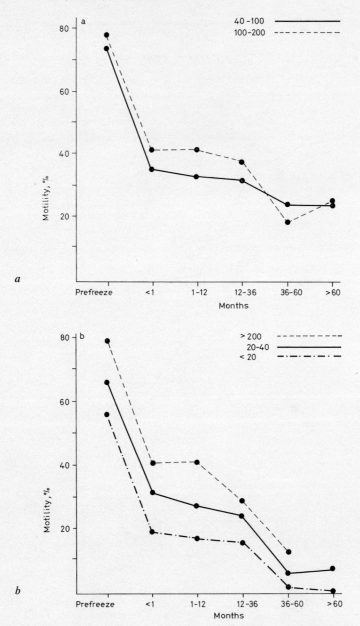

Fig. 3. Division of data from figure 1 into semen samples with sperm counts resulting in better (a) and poorer (b) postthaw motility after various times in storage. N and SE levels are the same as those in figure 1.

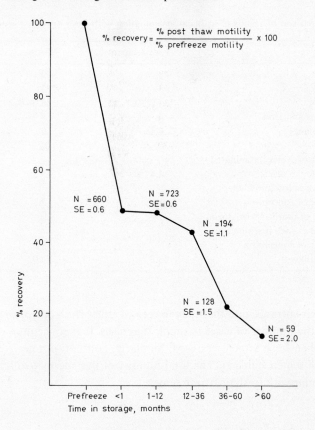

$$\% \text{ recovery} = \frac{\% \text{ post thaw motility}}{\% \text{ prefreeze motility}} \times 100$$

Fig. 4. Relation of percent recovery of all samples to time in storage in liquid nitrogen. N = Number of specimens; SE = standard error of the mean. Reprinted by permission of the Editor, Journal of the American Medical Association.

sionally demonstrated varied postthaw motility. Additional study is necessary to define parameters that will predict adequate postthaw motility and fertility of semen stored in liquid nitrogen.

III. Comparison of Fertility of Fresh and Frozen Semen

Artificial insemination was performed in a group of women who together with their husbands requested this procedure. All husbands were either azoospermic or severely oligospermic. The patients were assigned alternately

Table I. Comparison of results of artificial insemination with fresh or frozen semen

	Fresh semen	Frozen semen
Cases	48	59
No pregnancy	13	23
Pregnancy	35 (73%)	36 (61%)
Spontaneous abortion	4	7
Tubal pregnancy	1	0
Live births	30	29
Mean number of cycles inseminated for pregnancy to occur	4.4	5.3
Mean numbers of inseminations during cycle of conception	1.9	2.1
Total number of motile spermatozoa inseminated at each insemination during cycle of conception (mean in millions)	69.0	74.0

at the time of their entrance into the study to receive either fresh or frozen se-men. Although the number of cases is small, it appears that conception oc-curred earlier when fresh semen was used. Similarly, conception rates were higher with fresh semen (table I). The total number of live spermatozoa in-seminated is similar with fresh or frozen semen.

IV. Commercial Sperm Banking

Several commercial sperm banks have been established recently. Their primary purpose is to store semen of men who are contemplating vasectom-ies. The depositor purchases 'fertility insurance' after he deposits several se-men samples in a commercial sperm bank. This 'insurance policy' is esta-blished on the premise that if the man wishes to have children at some future time, he may retrieve his own frozen semen. In addition, sperm banks may provide a ready source of donor semen for physicians performing artificial insemination. The concept of 'fertility insurance' probably is premature un-less extensive explanation is provided to the prospective depositor concern-ing the inability of the bank to guarantee the fertility or even the motility of semen specimens after long-term storage. TYLER [1973] has commented that less than 1% of patients that are offered free, prevasectomy 'fertility insur-ance' express any interest in semen storage.

Table II. Range of sperm counts in a group of fertile men requesting vasectomy as a contraceptive measure compared to previous report of sperm counts in fertile men

Sperm counts (millions/ml)	Percent of 1,000 subjects [MacLeod, 1951]	Percent of 503 prevasectomy subjects
<20	5	14
20–40	12	18
40–60	12	17
60–80	14	15
80–100	13	10
>100	44	26

During the past year we have been evaluating semen from men with proven fertility who are about to undergo vasectomy. In table II the sperm counts on this group of patients is compared to the group of fertile men reported by MacLeod [1951]. In the prevasectomy subjects a greater proportion had sperm counts below 20 million/ml with a corresponding drop in those with counts above 100 million/ml. This study raises questions about the success of 'fertility insurance', since approximately 40% of this large sample of men requesting vasectomy have sperm counts in the ranges expected to have poorer postthaw motility (fig. 3b).

The inability of commercial sperm banks to guarantee fertility of semen specimens after long-term storage and the apathy of potential depositors raise doubts about the need of 'fertility insurance'. The future of commercial sperm banks may reside in their ability to provide short-term storage of a wide range of donor semen specimens.

V. Conclusion

Aging of the male gamete can be delayed by freeze preservation in liquid nitrogen. Although successful pregnancies resulted from artificial insemination with semen specimens stored in liquid nitrogen, the rate of conception was lower than when fresh semen was employed. The process of freezing and thawing resulted in a loss of approximately 50% of the original motility. After 36 months of storage in liquid nitrogen a further gradual loss of postthaw motility occurred. The best mean long-term survival (over 3 years) was found in semen specimens with sperm counts between 40 and 200 million/ml and prefreeze motility above 60%. Additional studies are necessary to determine the longevity of semen in the frozen state, to improve existing techniques and to evaluate possible genetic repercussions. Until these aims are realized, human sperm banks might best be utilized for short-term preservation of donor semen.

References

Behrman, S.J.: Freeze preservation of human spermatozoa in liquid nitrogen vapor. Schweiz. Z. Gynäk. Geburtsh. 2: 307 (1971).

Behrman, S.J. and Ackerman, D.R.: Freeze preservation of human semen. Amer. J. Obstet. Gynec. 103: 654 (1969).

Behrman, S.J. and Sawada, Y.: Heterologous and homologous inseminations with human semen frozen and stored in a liquid-nitrogen refrigerator. Fertil. Steril. 17: 457 (1966).

Bunge, R.G.; Keettel, W.C., and Sherman, J.K.: Clinical use of frozen semen. Fertil. Steril. 5: 520 (1954).

Bunge, R.G. and Sherman, J.K.: Fertilizing capacity of frozen human spermatozoa. Nature, Lond. 172: 767 (1953).

Carlborg, L.: Some problems involved in freezing and insemination with human sperm; in Ingelman-Sundberg and Lunel Current problems in fertility, p. 23 (Plenum Publishing, New York 1971).

Davenport, C.B.: Experimental morphology. I. Effect of chemical and physical agents upon protoplasm, p. 244 (Macmillan, London 1897).

Fernandez-Cano, L.; Menkin, M.F.; Garcia, C.-R., and Rock, J.: Refrigerant preservation of human spermatozoa. I. Factors influencing recovery in euspermic semen: clinical applications. Fertil. Steril. 15: 390 (1964).

Freund, M.: Complete recovery of motile human spermatozoa after dilution, freezing and storage at –196°C for 24 months. Fed. Proc. 26: 335 (1967).

Friberg, J. and Nilsson, O.: Motility and morphology of human sperms after freezing in liquid nitrogen; in Ingelman-Sundberg and Lunel Current problems in fertility, p. 17 (Plenum Publishing, New York 1971).

Hoagland, H. and Pincus, G.: Revival of mammalian sperm after immersion in liquid nitrogen. J. gen. Physiol. 25: 337 (1942).

Iizuka, R. and Sawada, Y.: Successful inseminations with frozen human semen. Jap. J. Fertil. Steril. 3: 241 (1958).

Jahnel, F.: Über die Widerstandsfähigkeit von menschlichen Spermatozoen gegenüber starker Kälte. Klin. Wschr. 17: 1273 (1938).

Keettel, W.C.; Bunge, R.G.; Bradbury, J.T., and Nelson, W.O.: Report of pregnancies in infertile couples. J. amer. med. Ass. 160: 102 (1956).

MacLeod, J.: Semen quality in one thousand men of known fertility and in eight hundred cases of infertile marriage. Fertil. Steril. 2: 115 (1951).

Mantegazza, P.: Fisiologia sullo sperma umano. Rendi Ist. Lombardo 3: 183 (1866).

PARKES, A.S.: Preservation of human spermatozoa at low temperatures. Brit. med. J. *ii:* 212 (1945).

PERLOFF, W.H.; STEINBERGER, E., and SHERMAN, J.K.: Conception with human spermatozoa frozen by nitrogen vapor technic. Fertil. Steril. *15:* 501 (1964).

POLGE, C.; SMITH, A.U., and PARKES, A.S.: Revival of spermatozoa after vitrification and dehydration at low temperatures. Nature, Lond. *164:* 666 (1949).

SAWADA, Y.: Studies on the freezing preservation of human spermatozoa. Jap. J. Fertil. Steril. *4:* 1 (1959).

SAWADA, Y.: The preservation of human semen by deep freezing. Int. J. Fertil. *9:* 525 (1964).

SAWADA, Y. and ACKERMAN, D.R.: Use of frozen human semen; in BEHRMAN and KISTNER Progress in infertility, p. 731 (Little, Brown, Boston 1968).

SHERMAN, J.K.: Preservation of bull and human spermatozoa by freezing in liquid nitrogen vapour. Nature, Lond. *194:* 1291 (1962).

SHERMAN, J.K.: Long-term cryopreservation of motility and fertility of human spermatozoa. Cryobiology *9:* 332 (1972).

SHERMAN, J.K.: Current perspectives. Synopsis of the use of frozen human semen since 1964: state of the art of human semen banking. Fertil. Steril. *24:* 397 (1973).

SHERMAN, J.K. and BUNGE, R.G.: Observations on preservation of human spermatozoa at low temperatures. Proc. Soc. exp. Biol. Med. *82:* 686 (1953).

SHETTLES, L.B.: The respiration of human spermatozoa and their response to various gases and low temperatures. Amer. J. Physiol. *128:* 408 (1940).

SMITH, K.D. and STEINBERGER, E.: Survival of spermatozoa in a human sperm bank: effects of long-term storage in liquid nitrogen. J. amer. med. Ass. *223:* 774 (1973).

SPALLANZANI, L.: Opuscoli di Fisica. animale e vegetabile. Opuscolo II. Osservazione e sperienze intorno ai vermicelli spermatici dell'uomo e degli animale (Modena 1776).

STEINBERGER, E. and PERLOFF, W.H.: Preliminary experience with a human sperm bank. Amer. J. Obstet. Gynec. *92:* 577 (1965).

STEINBERGER, E. and SMITH, K.D.: Artificial insemination with fresh or frozen semen: a comparative study. J. amer. med. Ass. *223:* 778 (1973).

TRELFORD, J.D. and MUELLER, F.: Observations and studies on the storage of human sperm. Canad. med. Ass. J. *100:* 62 (1969).

TYLER, E.T.: The clinical use of frozen semen banks. Fertil. Steril. *24:* 413 (1973).

TYLER, E.T. and SINGHER, H.O.: Male infertility. Status of treatment, prevention and current research. J. amer. med. Ass. *160:* 91 (1956).

Authors' address: Dr. KEITH D. SMITH, Dr. DANIEL R. STULTZ and Dr. EMIL STEINBERGER, Program in Reproductive Biology and Reproductive Endocrinology, The University of Texas Medical School at Houston, 6400 West Cullen Street, Texas Medical Center, *Houston, TX 77025* (USA)

Aging Gametes. Int. Symp., Seattle 1973, pp. 278–299 (Karger, Basel 1975)

Influence of Age on Avian Gametes

F.W. Lorenz

Department of Animal Physiology, University of California, Davis, Calif.

I. The Ovary and Ova

Special features of the natural history of avian gametes are obviously related to the typical reproductive patterns of this class of homeothermic vertebrates. The avian female ovulates sequentially, once each day until the clutch is completed; she immediately proceeds to invest each ovum with nutritive and protective coverings of albumen, membranes and shell, and oviposits as soon as this process is completed, at about the time of the next ovulation.

As a result the avian ovary (it is unpaired in most species) resembles that of no other vertebrate. The large, yolk filled ovules of an active ovary so distend the follicles that they somewhat resemble a cluster of grapes except that no two are of the same size. Instead, a hierarchy exists, from microscopic size to almost that of the yolk of a laid egg, and one can readily determine the order in which they will be ovulated by their relative sizes. Such an ovary also contains one or more empty (discharged) follicles. These form no obvious corpora lutea and are completely resorbed within 2–3 days in most species. They do exert controlling influences on subsequent ovulations, ovipositions, and behavior, however, either through hormonal secretion or through action of their abundant neural supply or both, a subject that is beyond the scope of this paper but has recently been reviewed elsewhere [GILBERT and WOOD-GUSH, 1971].

Immediately after ovulation the ovum descends into the oviduct and within a few minutes passes through the infundibulum, where fertilization occurs, and reaches the albumen secreting segment. The first albumen to be secreted forms the chalaziferous layer; some fluid passes through the vitelline membrane; protein from the same albumen remains behind, investing the original vitelline membrane with multiple thin layers [BELLAIRS *et al.*, 1963], effectively thickening and strengthening it severalfold. Both the resulting change in the characteristics of the vitelline membrane and the presence of gross albumen are considered to be effective blocks to penetration of spermatozoa, and the effective fertilizable life of the ovum is thus considered to be limited to within a few minutes after ovulation.

II. Parthenogenesis

Regardless of the above mechanism, however, there is another that definitively terminates fertilizability shortly thereafter. Within 4–5 h after ovulation, if the ovum has not been fertilized, parthenogenic cleavages are usually initiated with the production of a few or many blastomeres. Blastomere formation in unfertilized eggs has long been recognized; they were first described by OELLACHER [1872] and have been discussed and pictured subsequently by several investigators, some of whom considered them to be abortive parthenogenesis and some mere fragmentation of the blastodisc. OLSEN [1941] described the process at some length in his Ph.D. dissertation but omitted this discussion from subsequent publications based on his graduate research. He spoke of it as fragmentation that usually begins at the margin of the blastodisc and is initiated by furrows 'which closely resemble true cleavage furrows' and produce 'small pieces that in surface view closely resemble true cell formation'. He proposed that this fragmentation should be considered to be an abortive type of parthenogenesis since nuclei were found in some of the cell-like bodies; he also observed divisions of some of the larger fragments with corresponding nuclear divisions.

KOSIN [1945] also described this process and revived the previous controversy concerning its nature; he referred to it as 'abortive parthenogenesis' and demonstrated mitosis occurring in unfertilized eggs but, at that time, was convinced that such parthenogenic cell divisions could not occur much past oviposition. Considerably more prolonged development was subsequently demonstrated in turkeys by OLSEN and MARSDEN [1953] and confirmed more rigorously the following year [OLSEN and MARSDEN, 1954]. Ultimately these investigators succeeded in hatching parthenogenic poults and developed a line with a high incidence of parthenogenesis. Also similar results were subsequently obtained with certain strains of chickens.

What is of importance to the present discussion is that a type of fragmentation or abortive development usually occurs in unfertilized blastodiscs that grades imperceptably into a much more extensive development and may even lead to viable young. OLSEN and MARSDEN [1954] described the condition of eggs they believed destined to show parthenogenic development when incubated. This type of development, which may be called the 'parthenogenic pattern', is essentially similar to that of the more common pattern except that blastomere formation has been more extensive; the entire blastodisc is packed with blastomeres and these ordinarily contain nuclei that stain well with hematoxylin, whereas the stainability of nuclei in the more usual blastomeres varies from intense to no staining. In a survey of 158 eggs from virgin hens made here, 75% contained various numbers of blastomeres, of which about half had at least a few with well-staining nuclei; in the remainder, the nuclei were either not apparent or appeared to be degenerate and failed to stain. Seven blastodiscs had the parthenogenic pattern; of these, 5 were from 2 hens, a considerably higher incidence of parthenogenic development than that reported by OLSEN [1966] based on macroscopic examination after several days incubation. In figure 1 are shown 3 blastodiscs from virgin hens with different degrees of blastomere development. Figure 1c is an example of the parthenogenic pattern as described by OLSEN and MARSDEN [1954].

Parthenogenic development has been described as a reaction to 'over-ripeness' in unfertilized ova. The incidence of spontaneous development has been shown to depend in part on heredity and to be subject to striking increase through selection [OLSEN et al., 1968]. However, parthenogenesis has also been increased through the agency of fowl-pox virus [OLSEN and POOLE, 1962], which is of interest in the present context because observations in the author's laboratory strongly suggest that insemination (under conditions to be described below) that results in a high incidence of abnormal embryonic development also increases the incidence of the parthenogenic pattern which, at the very least, complicates interpretation of 'fertility' data under these conditions. Unfortunately, the key experiment to determine whether or not blastodiscs with this pattern are truly parthenogenic in the presence of spermatozoa has not yet been performed. SARVELLA [1971] observed a large increase in what she called parthenogenic development (apparently blastoderms without embryos) after AI with heavily irradiated semen (20,000 rads) in a parthenogenic but not in a nonparthenogenic line of chickens. Her results are strong presumptive evidence that defective spermatozoa can induce parthenogenesis, but no such interpretation can be accepted as conclusive without a demonstration of the lack of genetic material from the spermatozoa in the embryo.

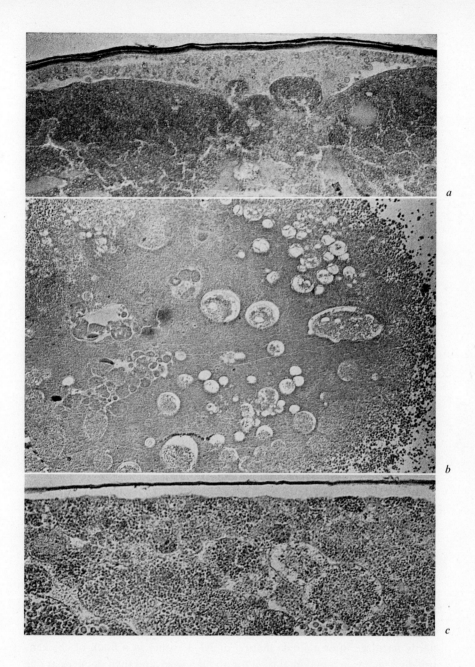

Fig. 1. Unincubated blastodiscs from virgin hens showing various degrees of abortive parthenogenic development. *a–c* × 250. *a* Blastodisc with small cluster of blastomeres in center; cross section. *b* Blastodisc with clusters of blastomeres; frontal section. *c* Blastodisc entirely converted into close-packed blastomeres many of which show nuclei; cross section.

III. Spermatozoa in the Oviduct; the Sperm-Host Glands

Before discussing this circumstance further the physiology of avian spermatozoa must be considered with special reference to their behavior in the
oviduct and to the effects of senescence on fertilizing capacity. Central to
these considerations is the presence of storage organs, the 'sperm-host
glands' in the uterovaginal region and in the infundibulum [BOBR et al., 1962,
1964 a, b; FUJII and TAMURA, 1963] in which spermatozoa survive and retain
fertilizing capacity for several days or weeks. How they accomplish this, considering the short life spans of avian spermatozoa in vitro (see below) is one
of the important problems of avian reproductive physiology. When present
in large numbers spermatozoa are found in these glands packed side by side
in compact bundles with heads all pointed toward the blind end of the gland.
So far as can be judged from biopsy material they are usually immotile in the
glands, but occasionally a bundle may be observed in vigorous motion with all
the tails waving in unison.

As a result of mating or intravaginal artificial insemination (IVAI) spermatozoa are deposited in the vagina, from whence a few penetrate the uterovaginal junction and are carried rapidly to the infundibulum unless a descending egg blocks the way. These are immediately capable of fertilizing, and
the next yolk may be so fertilized even if ovulated almost simultaneously with
the AI. Some of these spermatozoa may enter glands in the infundibulum
where they are preserved with full functional capacity for a considerable period. Only a few spermatozoa are ordinarily found in these glands after natural mating, however, and more often than not, none after IVAI [BOBR et al.,
1964 b]. By far the larger numbers of spermatozoa, in either event, enter the
uterovaginal glands where they are likewise stored with retention of full functional capacity and from where they leave from time to time to ascend the
oviduct to the site of fertilization.

IV. Fertility and Embryo Normality

As a result of the functions of these glands a succession of eggs is ordinarily fertilized after a single mating or AI. Fertility in a flock of chickens
usually remains at a maximal level for about a week and then declines as one
bird after another becomes infertile, with the last fertile egg from the average
hen laid about 12 days after IVAI [LORENZ and OGASAWARA, 1968; VAN
KREY et al., 1966]. In turkeys these periods are over twice as long, usually ap-

proaching 3 weeks for maximum fertility and about 34 days during the early part of the breeding season [OGASAWARA and FUQUA, 1972].

Remarkably, the apparent fertility of the first egg ovulated after semen deposition is somewhat lower than in subsequent eggs [LORENZ, 1950]. However, this is largely due to the presence of abnormal embryos[1] that have developed so little they cannot be distinguished from infertile eggs except by microscopic examination (see below). MUNRO and KOSIN [1945] called these 'preoviposital dead embryos' but they are not necessarily dead; about half are capable of further development though all but very few die during the first few days in the incubator [LORENZ and OGASAWARA, 1968].

Abnormal embryos of other types are also frequently found in the first egg after insemination, as demonstrated by the following grouped data. Among 141 first eggs laid on days 1 and 2 only after AI (and excluding hard eggs in utero at the time of AI) in a number of experiments, 90 were fertile and of these 56.7% were abnormal; 26.0% of the abnormal embryos were preovipositally dead. In contrast, among 294 second and third eggs laid during the first week after AI in the same experiments, 267 were fertile and of these only 18.7% were abnormal; just 1 embryo, or 0.35% of the abnormal was preovipositally dead. Additional eggs in both groups showed the retardation on candling after a day of incubation that is characteristic of the embryos with some developmental potential described in the preceding paragraph.

The large excess of infertiles among the first-laid eggs may or may not have been a real effect; it was doubtless made up in part at least of eggs ovulated prior to the AI. The difference in incidence of embryonic abnormalities, on the other hand, is unquestionable and striking. At least 2 physiological differences may have been involved in these results. The first and most obvious is the difference in spermatozoan age, but what may be more important is a difference in behavior of the spermatozoa in the oviduct. Spermatozoa fertilizing the first-laid eggs had ascended directly to the infundibulum after AI, but before ovulation of subsequent eggs all spermatozoa free in the oviduct had been swept out by the first, and, consequently, fertilizing spermatozoa must have entered and been released from host glands.

That the incidence of embryo abnormality also increases progressively with time after insemination has long been recognized [see LORENZ, 1969 for review]; a high percentage of the last fertile eggs are also of the kind that can only be detected microscopically.

---

1   This effect has a parallel in mammalian ova as described by SALISBURY and HART [1970].

V. Causes of Abnormal Embryos

What the cause or causes are of the temporally related embryonic failures have been the source of some speculation [LORENZ, 1966, 1969] on little or no concrete evidence. The situation is complicated by a further observation made in my laboratory [LORENZ and OGASAWARA, 1968; VAN KREY et al., 1966], and subsequently confirmed with other species elsewhere, that insemination under circumstances that lead to greatly augmented numbers of spermatozoa at the site of fertilization lead also to a large increase in the incidence of embryonic abnormalities.

In these experiments we introduced semen directly into the anterior oviduct via laparotomy and a hypodermic needle through the oviduct wall (intramagnal insemination or IMAI). The introduced semen floods the infundibulum and tremendous numbers of spermatozoa engorge the infundibular glands. Ordinarily none migrates distally past the uterovaginal junction and enters the uterovaginal glands, so we have used this technique in conjunction with IVAI to compare the potentialities of the 2 groups of glands for functional preservation of spermatozoa. We found that in chickens the life span of spermatozoa in the infundibular glands is appreciably longer than in uterovaginal glands [VAN KREY et al., 1966] although in turkeys their life span is shorter [OGASAWARA et al., 1970; OGASAWARA and FUQUA, 1972]. The prolonged life span in chickens is clearly shown in the values presented in table I. With fresh untreated semen in dosage of 0.05 ml, IMAI produced high fertility that lasted through 3 weeks and was still appreciable during the fourth week, and a few fertile eggs were produced during the fifth. Following IVAI, by contrast, fertility dropped appreciably in the second week and was negligible during the third and fourth weeks.

The prolonged fertility following IMAI appears to be due largely to the greatly increased number of sperm stored. Their life span was shortened by decreasing the number inseminated [LORENZ et al., 1969]. Reducing the dose to 0.0005 ml (table I) yielded a fertility curve essentially similar to that for IVAI with 0.05 ml and at the same time reduced the number of spermatozoa stored in infundibular glands approximately to the number stored after IVAI (table II).

Most interesting in the present context, IMAI strikingly increased the number of abnormal embryos, as described above, especially during the first few days after insemination. The doubled incidence of abnormal embryos during the first week following IMAI shown in table I is typical of earlier results [LORENZ and OGASAWARA, 1968; VAN KREY et al., 1966].

Table I. Fertility and incidence of abnormal embryos after intravaginal (IVAI) and intramagnal (IMAI) artificial insemination with semen treated in various ways

Semen dose and treatment	IVAI, interval after AI (days)				IMAI, interval after AI (days)				
	2–8	9–15	16–22	23–29	2–8	9–15	16–22	23–29	30–36
Fresh, untreated, 0.05 ml									
Number of eggs	255	238	243	137	149	203	210	201	169
Fertile eggs, %	96.5	68.5	10.7	2.2	96.0	95.6	87.6	40.3	4.7
Abnormal embryos, %[1]	15.4	28.1	61.5	66.7	31.2	31.9	48.4	74.1	100.0
Fresh, untreated, 0.0005 ml[2]									
Number of eggs					119	138	146	106	
Fertile eggs, %					99.2	78.3	26.7	7.5	
Abnormal embryos, %					15.6	24.3	59.0	100.0	
Stored 24 h at 5°C, 0.05 ml[3]									
Number of eggs	26	24	27		18	24	28	20	
Fertile eggs, %	46.2	8.3	3.7		100.0	95.8	57.1	5.0	
Abnormal embryos, %[1]	33.3	50.0	–		11.1	13.1	50.0	–	
Stored 48 h at 5°C, 0.05 ml[3]									
Number of eggs	25	27			9	14	20	18	
Fertile eggs, %	16.0	3.7			100.0	92.9	35.0	0	
Abnormal embryos, %[1]	50.0	–			11.1	38.5	42.9	–	
90 min. at 40°C, 0.05 ml[3]									
Number of eggs	36	29	34		28	32	32	31	
Fertile eggs, %	22.2	10.3	0		100.0	93.8	59.4	6.4	
Abnormal embryos, %[1]	25.0	66.7			10.7	20.0	47.4	–	
150 min. at 40°C, 0.05 ml[3]									
Number of eggs	45	35			26	31	33		
Fertile eggs, %	8.9	0			84.6	77.4	21.2		
Abnormal embryos, %[1]	0	–			13.6	29.2	42.9		
Cold shock, 0.05 ml									
Number of eggs	33	30	36		20	29	29	28	33
Fertile eggs, %	75.8	30.0	2.8		100.0	100.0	82.8	17.9	0
Abnormal embryos, %[1]	57.5	50.0	–		25.0	13.8	54.2	100.0	–

1 Given as a percentage of fertile eggs.
2 Semen diluted 1 : 100 with Lakes diluent; 0.05 ml diluted semen injected.
3 Semen diluted 1 : 1 with phosphate buffer; 0.10 ml diluted semen injected.

Table II. Incidence of spermatozoa in uterovaginal and infundibular sperm-host glands after IVAI and IMAI with semen treated in various ways

Semen dose, treatment, and oviduct site	IVAI		IMAI	
	1 day after AI	8 days after AI	1 day after AI	8 days after AI
Fresh, untreated, 0.05 ml				
Uterovaginal junction	69,45,40 29,23	22,21,1,0	13,10,9 9, 1	17,0,0,0
Infundibulum	+,+,0,0,0	0,0,0,0	++++,++++ ++++,++++ +++	++++,+++ +++,++
Fresh, untreated, 0.0005 ml				
Uterovaginal junction			0,0,0	1,0,0
Infundibulum			++,+,0	+,0,0
Stored 24 h at 5°C, 0.05 ml				
Uterovaginal junction	50		0	
Infundibulum	0		+	
Stored 48 h at 5°C, 0.05 ml				
Uterovaginal junction	0		0	
Infundibulum	0		++	
Held 90 min. at 40°C, 0.05 ml				
Uterovaginal junction	0	5	0	15
Infundibulum	0	0		
Held 150 min. at 40°C, 0.05 ml				
Uterovaginal junction	0	0	1	
Infundibulum	0	0	++	+

Figures for the uterovaginal junction are percentages of glands in a single longitudinal section [OGASAWARA *et al.*, 1966]. Since empty glands in the infundibulum are not easily identified with certainty, the density of spermatozoa was estimated by scoring: ++++ represents a maximal accumulation, many glands containing spermatozoa in close-packed bundles; + indicates very few glands containing usually single spermatozoa. Each number or score is the datum for the corresponding site in a single bird. See also footnotes to table I.

Attempts to determine the proximal cause of this increased incidence have only yielded results that fail to rule out either of 2 hypothetical mechanisms, and it begins to seem likely that both are operative. These possibilities are (1) that the extraordinarily large number of spermatozoa at the site of fertilization may interfere in some way with normal fertilization, and (2) that depositing semen directly in the anterior oviduct bypasses effective mechanisms in the uterovaginal glands and/or the uterovaginal junction that normally prevent large numbers of abnormal spermatozoa from reaching the infundibulum. COHEN [1967, 1969] has presented theoretical reasoning supporting the latter hypothesis, whereas FOFANOVA [1964] presented some evidence in support of the former, although this evidence was based on sperm numbers of a different order of magnitude from that encountered here.

The earliest evidence from my laboratory was obtained with grossly abnormal spermatozoa and tended to support the second hypothesis [OGASAWARA et al., 1966]. Semen was investigated from low-fecundity cocks that produced very little fertility by IVAI, yet the few fertile eggs that were produced all hatched. When spermatozoa from the same cocks were deposited in the uterus (i.e., in the posterior oviduct but anterior to the junction) there was a severalfold increase in fertility but at the same time such a large increase in embryonic mortality that few if any more chicks were hatched.

The results of the dosage-reduction experiment, in contrast, support the sperm-number hypothesis, because this treatment not only reduced the numbers of spermatozoa in infundibular glands (table II) and the duration of fertility, but also the numbers and distribution of embryonic abnormalities, almost exactly to what was observed after IVAI (table I).

Following these results additional experiments were performed with spermatozoa damaged in various ways and then inseminated both IV and IM in equivalent doses of 0.05 ml. Semen samples were diluted 1:3 in phosphate buffer and held for 24, 48, and 168 h at 5°C, incubated for 90 and 150 min at 40°C, or subjected to 'cold shock' as described by MANN and LUTWAK-MANN [1955], a treatment that kills few cock spermatozoa (in contrast to results with some other species) but does induce a high percentage of bent midpieces. These treatments were intended to increase the numbers of abnormal spermatozoa so that use of treated samples could be compared with the results previously obtained from semen of the low-fecundity cocks described above.

The results, recorded in table I, however, were quite different. Fertility following IVAI was severely impaired by all treatments, though to different degrees, depending on the severity of the treatment. The incidence of embryonic abnormalities was increased. The numbers of embryos involved are small because of the low fertility, but consistency of the effect is convincing.

Fertility following IMAI was reduced much less, and, in fact, except with the most severely treated sample (150 min at 40°C), remained superior to results with fresh spermatozoa by IVAI. More surprisingly, embryo abnormalities were actually decreased and, except with cold-shocked spermatozoa, were actually fewer during the first week than by either insemination route with fresh semen.

The results of one additional treatment, 168 h at 5°C, are not recorded in table I because very few birds were inseminated. No fertile eggs were laid following IVAI with semen, but of 15 eggs laid by 2 hens during 2 weeks following IMAI 73.3% were fertile, and of these only 18.2% were abnormal embryos, so that results even with these severely damaged spermatozoa were consistent with those of the other treatments.

As shown in table II, the various treatments consistently reduced the numbers of spermatozoa stored in the host glands. Thus, numbers of spermatozoa apparently played a role in all of these results. However, the role abnormalities of spermatozoa play in induction of embryonic abnormalities is not ruled out. Quite possibly the spermatozoa best able to induce normal embryos were also best able to withstand the insult of all of the treatments except perhaps that of cold shock. These results do demonstrate that moderate damage to spermatozoa affects their ability to enter the uterovaginal glands and/or to penetrate the uterovaginal junction and ascend the oviduct more than it does their ability to survive in the infundibular glands and to fertilize. Quite likely a major mechanism for screening defective spermatozoa resides in the uterovaginal region.

These results must be considered together with the observations mentioned above on embryo abnormality at the beginning and end of the fertile period after natural mating or IVAI. Abnormality at the end of the fertile period can certainly not be due to excessive numbers of spermatozoa, and it seems unlikely that enough would ascend the oviduct after such inseminations to produce a sufficient excess for that effect at the beginning. To be sure, FOFANOVA's [1964] conclusions, based on such data, were that both excessive and deficient spermatozoal numbers cause abnormal development, but it

---

Fig. 2. Disorganized cellular development in certain eggs following IMAI, compared with normal embryonic development. *a* Normal unincubated embryo showing 1-cell-thick ectodermal and entodermal layers; cross section, × 41. *b–d* Random cellular proliferation with large and small nucleated cells investing the entire blastodiscs. A few cells have apparently begun organization into a blastoderm in *c* and *d* while in *b* the entire cell mass appears to have attempted to form an atypical multilayered blastoderm. These eggs were incubated for 20 h after being laid; however, most likely no development occurred in the incubator. The blastodiscs were less than half as large as that in *a* and were grossly indistinguishable from blastodiscs of infertile eggs; cross section, × 250.

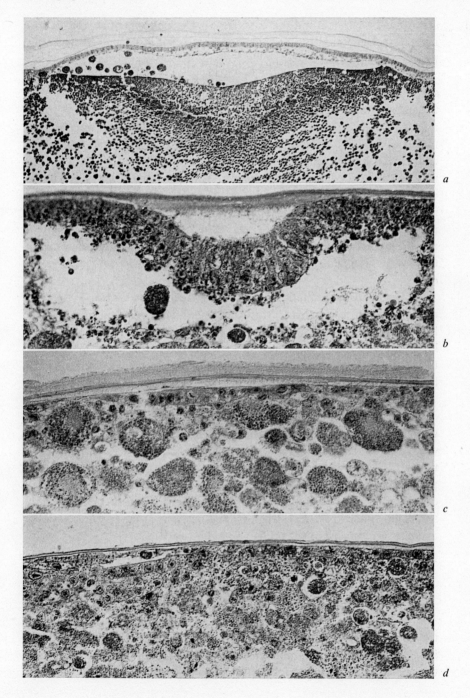

seems more likely that in these cases both were due to spermatozoal abnormalities, congenital at the beginning and senescent at the end of the fertile period.

Thus, the conclusion seems inescapable that both excessive numbers and spermatozoal abnormalities of more than one kind have been responsible for the embryonic abnormalities that appear to be related to insemination techniques and the resulting temporal fertility patterns. The mechanisms that may be involved, however, are entirely a matter of speculation. Senescence could cause damage to DNA but could also result in depletion of the acrosomal enzymes. The latter would interfere with penetration but might do so only partially in a way that might induce or favor parthenogenic development. Large amounts of acrosomal enzymes from excessive numbers of spermatozoa might be even more effective in the latter process; the possibility of polyspermy must also be recognized. No evidence for any of these possibilities has yet been adduced; key experiments to test them are very much needed.

Microscopic examination of the abnormal embryos has also yielded little evidence on mechanisms. Most of the embryos so examined appear to have undergone rapid and uncoordinated cell development with minimal cellular organization, as illustrated in figure 2, but considerable numbers of blastodiscs indistinguishable from that of figure 1c were also observed. (The latter were not counted as fertile.) None of these was able to develop perceptibly during the first day in the incubator, yet other abnormal embryos did develop, albeit slowly. Whether or not the initial development of the latter were like those in figures 2b and c has not been determined.

To recapitulate briefly, the avian ovum has an extraordinarily short fertilizable life whereas the spermatozoon has a long functional life in the reproductive tract of the female. Accordingly, investigations of the possibility of extending spermatozoan life *in vitro* have been active (though currently seeming to wane in interest) whereas investigations of the postovipositional ovum *as a gamete* have been nil.

VI. The Whole Egg

Nevertheless, age changes in the entire ovum and its covering layers, i.e., the whole egg, do deserve brief mention. These changes and factors influencing them were subjects of much research up to a few years ago, because of their potential roles during incubation of fertile eggs and because of the im-

portance of eggs as marketable food items. But interest has waned and research has almost completely ceased with the cessation of the practice of cold
storage of market eggs and the development of methods for increased speed
and improved methods of handling. Much of the earlier research, described
briefly below has been extensively reviewed by Romanoff and Romanoff
[1949] and by Gilbert [1967, 1971].

Immediately after an egg is laid, as it cools below the body temperature
of the hen its contents undergo slightly more thermal contraction than does
the capacity of the shell. The difference is made up by an abrupt separation of
the two shell membranes forming a small 'air cell', almost always at the blunt
end of the egg. This air cell grows progressively larger subsequently as a result of evaporation of moisture through the thousands of pores in the egg
shell. In an incubating egg it is penetrated by the chick's beak shortly before
hatching and supplies the first breathed air. In market eggs its size (determined by candling) is sometimes used to estimate the age of the egg, but because of the great dependence of evaporation rate on temperature, humidity,
and the presence of shell coatings such as mineral oil, air-cell size is almost
useless for this purpose. Because, however, egg deterioration is also partly
dependent on these parameters, as described below, air-cell size yields a
somewhat better estimate of egg quality.

Egg white is deposited in the oviduct on the descending yolk in a seemingly homogeneous mass with a stiff jelly-like consistency. By the time the egg
is laid, somewhat more than 20 h later, the white is present in distinct layers,
alternately jelly-like and liquid, and differing greatly in dry-matter content.
The innermost layer is jelly-like and most concentrated; it is continuous with
the chalazae that anchor the yolk to the middle thick layer. Surrounding the
innermost layer are liquid, thick, and liquid layers, from the yolk outward
progressively less concentrated in dry matter. As the egg ages, further
changes occur: the dry-matter concentration of the several layers tends to
equalize and the jell structure weakens; eventually the entire egg white may
liquify.

The mechanisms of these changes are known in some detail but some of
the most interesting questions remain unanswered. Egg white is a mixture of
a number of well-defined proteins with characteristic biological activities [see
Feeney and Allison, 1969, for review] plus small amounts of glucose, salts,
and other crystalloids. One protein, ovomucin, is secreted in continuous submicroscopic fibers that are responsible for the gel structure of the white. The
egg rotates as it passes down the oviduct so that the ovomucin fibers are deposited over the yolk in a spiral envelope. Very soon some of the earlier de-

posited white liquifies, freeing the yolk which, because of density differences, presumably no longer rotates with the egg. The relatively few remaining ovomucin fibers in the newly liquified white that remain attached both to the yolk and the middle, thick-white envelope thus become twisted to form the chalazae. The outer liquid layer is formed after the egg enters the uterus from the protein-free fluid that penetrates the shell membrane by osmosis and dissolves a portion of the original thick layer.

Break-up of the ovomucin fibers, resulting in liquefaction of the thick layer after laying, involves conjugation of ovomucin with another egg-white protein, lysozyme [HAWTHORNE, 1950]. There is some, albeit incomplete and very preliminary, evidence from my laboratory that the rapid initial lique-faction leading to formation of the inner liquid layer may also involve this conjugation, but whether so or not, there are distinct differences between the reaction and the nature of the secretions that form these 2 layers.

When anterior and posterior segments of the magnum were isolated with ligatures and secretion stimulated by inserting paraffin pellets, egg white was harvested from the 2 segments that was initially similar in appearance but very different in subsequent history. When sealed in tubes and incubated, the egg white from the anterior segment liquified within an hour, leaving only fragments of cloudy jell that appeared somewhat like an untwisted chalaza. That from the posterior magnum remained essentially unaltered, stiff enough to retain the shape of the oviduct it had displayed when first harvested.

In intact eggs the egg white from the anterior oviduct liquifies before oviposition, as already stated, and at a pH of about 7.6; that from the poste-rior magnum, by contrast, requires days, weeks, or months to liquify, de-pending in part on temperature, and the process is strongly favored by elevat-ed pH. Egg white pH normally rises to as high as 9.7 within a few days at room temperature because of loss of CO_2 through the egg-shell pores. Coat-ing eggs with mineral oil reduces increase in pH by reducing CO_2 loss and used to be used extensively to retard or prevent thick white liquifaction (as well as moisture loss) in stored eggs. If oil was applied too soon after the eggs were laid, and pH was thus held too low, a reverse process occurred; the ovo-mucin fibers aggregated and gave a cloudy appearance to the egg white.

Other biochemical factors are involved in the egg white thinning pro-cess, but unfortunately these have not been adequately followed up. Ovomu-cin is sensitive to reductive cleavage, and sulfhydral groups generated by ovalbumin during incubation may contribute to thinning of the thick white [see FEENEY and ALLISON, 1969 for review]. There is also evidence of an inter-action of glucose and protein in the egg white that contributes to thinning.

This interaction may also involve liberation of reducing compounds. In a recent study REINKE *et al.* [1973] clearly separated the effects of reducing agents and pH on egg-white thinning.

Changes in the yolk are simpler. As soon as it reaches the magnum it starts to absorb moisture by osmosis from the enveloping egg white and this process continues during the storage life of the egg. The vitelline membrane is reinforced and strengthened by layers of egg white proteins, deposited presumably through ultra-filtration during passage of water and cystalloids into the yolk. Shortly after oviposition the resulting yolk has sufficient strength to maintain much of its rounded shape when placed on a flat surface. But as egg white thinning progresses the vitelline membrane weakens, doubtless by the same process, and this, together with membrane stretching and lowered viscosity of the yolk contents through water absorption, weakens the yolk so that it progressively flattens and eventually ruptures spontaneously when placed on a flat surface.

VII. Semen Storage Above Freezing

As stated above, attempts to extend the functional life of avian spermatozoa have been an active field of research. Storage of chicken and turkey semen has been investigated both above and below freezing, but in spite of much research neither approach has been notably successful. This has led to the concept that avian spermatozoa are especially fragile, but it seems more likely that the difficulty lies in the fact that more is expected of them than of those of species, such as the bull, that are more successfully stored. Mammalian spermatozoa are introduced into the female at a time calculated to permit fertilization very shortly thereafter, but avian spermatozoa are expected to remain viable and fertilizable for several days: at least a week in chickens and over twice as long in turkeys. If the fertility of the first egg ovulated after insemination only were considered, the storability of avian semen would not appear so poor.

Nevertheless, the technology of avian semen storage got off to a slow start, and long after bull-semen storage was an important commercial operation cock semen was considered incapable of being stored for as much as a few hours. The first breakthrough was the discovery of a 12° C temperature optimum for storage of sperm in undiluted semen; earlier investigations had been done at temperatures much closer to freezing. The second was the discovery that moderate dilution (ca. 1: 3) would allow storage at 2–4°C.

The role of the diluent composition, long an active field of research, has been extensively reviewed [LAKE, 1966; LORENZ, 1969]; several criteria have been established with varying degrees of certainty. The presence of both buffering and chelating agents aid in maintaining fertilizing capacity of spermatozoa stored at 2°C whereas both Cl⁻ and Ca⁺⁺ are damaging and should be kept as low as possible or omitted from semen diluents.

Moderate hypertonicity has been reported to reduce plasmolysis of the midpiece and thus aid in maintaining fertilizing capacity during storage, but this finding has not been confirmed by all investigators and, in any event, there appears to be an interaction between diluent composition and optimum osmolarity. In one experiment with turkey semen [GRAHAM and BROWN, 1971] fertility was unaffected within a considerable range of osmolarity, but any appreciable departure from isotonicity with the seminal plasma significantly increased the proportion of abnormal embryos.

The value of glycolysable carbohydrates during storage is unproven although such substances, especially fructose, are widely used in semen diluents. However, fructose apparently does enhance fertilizing capacity of stored cock spermatozoa if added shortly before insemination [WILCOX and SHAFFNER, 1958]. Avian spermatozoa do metabolize these sugars and, in fact, they appear to be necessary to supply the energy for motility in the absence of O_2. However, independent investigations have suggested that fertilizing capacity is prolonged by reducing metabolism during storage; the 2°C storage temperature itself does that; also addition of the metabolic inhibitor 2-ethyl-5-methylbenzimidazole is beneficial, as is also dissolved CO_2, which inhibits motility. Thus, very likely, the only favorable function of carbohydrate may be to help spermatozoa resume motility.

It seems strange that more efforts have not been made to put all the above criteria together. LAKE [1960] designed a rather complex diluent for cock spermatozoa in which glutamate is the major chelating agent and also does most of the buffering. This diluent maintains fertilizing capacity for a day or two, but its advantage may be largely in avoiding Cl⁻. Other successful diluents are less complex. The CO_2 diluent studied by HARRIS and HOBBS [1968] was simply $NaHCO_3$, Na citrate, and citric acid with added antibiotics that exert a chelating action. Metabolic inhibition exerted by citrate may also play a role in this diluent. WILCOX and SHAFFNER [1958] used a simple phosphate buffer with antibiotics; they stored semen diluted 1:10 and then centrifuged and reconstituted it to the original concentration in fresh buffer with fructose added as described above just before insemination.

A completely independent series of experiments [PROUDFOOT, 1972] has led to some observations on the role of atmospheric pressure and composition on maintenance of fertilizing capacity of undiluted semen held at 10–15°C. An atmosphere of pure O_2 was beneficial, but storage in O_2 under high pressure (21 atmospheres) for 7 h completely abolished the fertilizing capacity. CO_2 under the same conditions was also lethal to cock spermatozoa, but 7 h under either N_2 or air at 21 atmospheres enhanced both motility and fertilizing capacity. These results are not easy to fit into a present conceptual framework; they should be repeated and extended.

VIII. Frozen Storage of Semen

The present status of frozen storage of avian semen is even less advanced. Although the initial breakthrough for freezing semen – the discovery by POLGE et al. [1949] of the protective action of glycerol – was made with cock semen, little further progress has been made. The problem remains, largely at least, the one immediately recognized by these authors, the inhibiting effects of glycerol on fertilizing capacity (whether frozen or not) even while protecting against the lethal effects of freezing.

An important part of the inhibiting effect of glycerol is exerted within the vagina, for thawed glycerol-containing semen deposited above the uterovaginal junction does produce fertile eggs [ALLEN, 1958]. This observation has no immediate practical value, however; penetrating the uterovaginal junction with the inseminating cannula is traumatic and usually interrupts egg production, and laparotomy, even though rapid and nonstressful under local anesthesia, is still too slow and laborious to be economically feasible.

At least 8% glycerol is necessary to protect cock sperm from damage during freezing, and this must be reduced to below 2% before any fertility can be obtained by IVAI. POLGE's [1951] original method was to dialyse the thawed mixture. However, an unacceptable amount of spermatozoan degeneration occurs during the necessary hours at room temperature. Glycerol removal by centrifugation also causes an unacceptable amount of (presumably mechanical) damage to spermatozoa already weakened by freezing and thawing and, indeed, no satisfactory method of glycerol removal has yet been devised.

Most investigations of the technology of freezing and thawing have used spermatozoan motility and morphology as an end point, since fertility results have been so uniformly poor, but this approach may be self-defeating. HARRIS et al., [1971] have pointed to severe damage of the cytoplasmic membranes and acrosomes in frozen and thawed cock spermatozoa while the axonemal complex remained intact. In general the favored techniques have paralleled those used for mammalian sperm but are of a different order of magnitude. Dilution is of the order of 1:2 or 1:4 only but is nevertheless done stepwise to avoid the shock of too rapid change in glycerol concentration. Equilibration and measured cooling rate are performed, but the whole process is relatively rapid, usually being completed in an hour or less [HARRIS, 1968]. Usually the diluted semen has been cooled thus to 0°C before plunging it into CO_2 or LN_2 (–79 or –196°) but LAKE [1968] cooled it to –22°C at 1°C per min before the rapid cooling phase.

Ironically the avian species for which semen storage would have considerable commercial importance, the turkey, has been the subject of relatively little semen-storage research, and the parameters worked out so far for chicken semen have proved to be almost entirely inapplicable. So far no method has been developed that allows nonfreezing storage for even as much as a few hours, or any fertility with frozen storage at all. All the problems with chicken semen appear to be present, only amplified, and there are doubtless others as well.

Apparently turkey spermatozoa are severely damaged by temperatures below 15°C, diluted or undiluted, and are much more sensitive than chicken spermatozoa to cold shock. My colleague, Dr. OGASAWARA, has been making an intensive study of freezing parameters without success as yet with IVAI though he has produced some fertility by IMAI, which points again to glycerol removal as one important factor. BROWN and GRAHAM [1971] have pointed to the considerable toxicity of glycerol for turkey sperm (greater than for chicken sperm) and studied other agents of which ethylene glycol appears most promising, but have not reported fertility tests with this agent.

References

ALLEN, T.E.: The storage of fowl semen at low temperatures. Proc. Austr. Soc. anim. Prod. *2:* 118 (1958).

BELLAIRS, R.; HARKNESS, M., and HARKNESS, R.D.: The vitelline membrane of the hen's egg: a chemical and electron microscopical study. J. Ultrastruct. Res. *8:* 339 (1963).

BOBR, L.W.; LORENZ, F.W., and OGASAWARA, F.X.: The role of the uterovaginal junction in storage of cock spermatozoa. Poultry Sci. *41:* 1628 (1962).

BOBR, L.W.; LORENZ, F.W., and OGASAWARA, F.X.: Distribution of spermatozoa in the oviduct and fertility of domestic birds. I. Residence sites of spermatozoa in fowl oviducts. J. Reprod. Fertil. *8:* 39 (1964a).

BOBR, L.W.; OGASAWARA, F.X., and LORENZ, F.W.: Distribution of spermatozoa in the oviduct and fertility in domestic birds. II. Transport of spermatozoa in the fowl oviduct. J. Reprod. Fertil. *8:* 49 (1964b).

BROWN, K.I. and GRAHAM, E.F.: Effect of some cryophylactic agents on turkey spermatozoa. Poultry Sci. *50:* 832 (1971).

COHEN, J.: Correlation between sperm 'redundancy' and chiasma frequency. Nature, Lond. *215:* 862 (1967).

COHEN, J.: Why so many sperms? An essay on the arithmetic of reproduction. Sci. Progr. *57:* 23 (1969).

FEENEY, R.E. and ALLISON, R.G.: Evolutionary biochemistry of proteins. Homologous and analogous proteins from avian egg whites, blood sera, milk and other substances (J. Wiley & Sons, Chichester 1969).

FOFANOVA, K.A.: Morphologic data on polyspermy in chickens. Zhur. Obschei. Biol. *25:* 22 (1964). See also Fed. Proc. Suppl. *24:* T 239 (1965).

FUJII, S. and TAMURA, T.: Location of sperms in the oviduct of the domestic fowl with special reference to storage of sperms in the vaginal gland. J. Fac. Fish. anim. Husb. Hiroshima Univ. *5:* 145 (1963).

GILBERT, A.B.: Formation of the egg in the domestic chicken; in McLAREN Advances in reproductive physiology, vol. 2, p. 111 (Logos Press and Academic Press, London 1967).

GILBERT, A.B.: Egg albumen and its formation; in BELL and FREEMAN Physiology and biochemistry of the domestic fowl, vol. 3, p. 1291 (Academic Press, New York 1971).

GILBERT, A.B. and WOOD-GUSH, D.G.M.: Ovulatory and ovipository cycles; in BELL and FREEMAN Physiology and biochemistry of the domestic fowl, vol. 3, p. 1353 (Academic Press, New York 1971).

GRAHAM, E.F. and BROWN, K.I.: Effect of osmotic pressure of semen extenders on the fertility and hatchability of turkey eggs. Poultry Sci. *50:* 836 (1971).

HARRIS, G.C., jr.: Fertility of chickens inseminated intraperitoneally with semen preserved in liquid nitrogen. Poultry Sci. *47:* 384 (1968).

HARRIS, G.C., jr. and HOBBS, T.D.: Effects of freezing point depression and fluid to gas ratio on fertility of fowl spermatozoa stored in CO_2 extenders. J. Reprod. Fertil. *16:* 389 (1968).

HARRIS, G.C., jr.; THURSTON, R.J., and CUNDALL, J.: Changes in ultrastructure of the chicken spermatozoon due to freeze-thaw. Poultry Sci. *50:* 1584 (1971).

HAWTHORNE, J.R.: The action of egg white lysozyme on ovomucin. Biochim. biophys. Acta *6:* 28 (1950).

KOSIN, I.L.: Abortive parthenogenesis in the domestic chicken. Anat. Rec. *91:* 245 (1945).

LAKE, P.E.: Studies on the dilution and storage of fowl semen. J. Reprod. Fertil. *1:* 30 (1960).

LAKE, P.E.: Physiology and biochemistry of poultry semen; in McLAREN Advances in reproductive physiology, vol. 1, p. 193 (Logos Press and Academic Press, London 1966).

LAKE, P.E.: Observations on freezing fowl spermatozoa in liquid nitrogen. Proc. 6th Int. Congr. Anim. Reprod. Artif. Insem., Paris 1968, vol. 2, p. 1633.

LORENZ, F.W.: Onset and duration of fertility in turkeys. Poultry Sci. *29:* 20 (1950).

LORENZ, F.W.: Behaviour of spermatozoa in the oviduct in relation to fertility; in HORTON

SMITH and AMOROSO Physiology of the domestic fowl, vol. 39 (Oliver & Boyd, Edinburgh 1966).

LORENZ, F.W.: Reproduction in domestic fowl; in COLE and CUPPS Reproduction in domestic animals, p. 569 (Academic Press, New York 1969).

LORENZ, F.W.; BENNETT, E.B., and REYNOLDS, M.E.: An effect of sperm numbers on abnormal development of avian embryos. Proc. 2nd Ann. Meet., Soc. for the Study of Reproduction, Davis 1969, p. 14 (Abstract).

LORENZ, F.W. and OGASAWARA, F.X.: Distribution of spermatozoa in the oviduct and fertility in domestic birds. VI. The relation of fertility and embryo normality with site of experimental insemination. J. Reprod. Fertil. 16: 445 (1968).

MANN, T. and LUTWAK-MANN, C.: Biochemical changes underlying the phenomenon of cold-shock in spermatozoa. Arch. Sci. Biol. 39: 578 (1955).

MUNRO, S.S. and KOSIN, I.L.: Proof of the existence of pre-oviposital embryonic deaths in chickens and their bearing on the relation between 'fertility' and hatchability. Canad. J. Res. Ser. D 23: 129 (1945).

OELLACHER, J.: Die Veränderungen des unbefruchteten Keimes des Hühnereies im Eileiter und bei Bebrütungsversuchen. Z. wiss. Zool. 22: 181 (1872).

OGASAWARA, F.X. and FUQUA, C.L.: The vital importance of the uterovaginal sperm-host glands of the turkey hen. Poultry Sci. 51: 1035 (1972).

OGASAWARA, F.X.; FUQUA, C.L., and LORENZ, F.W.: A comparison of insemination routes on fertility in the domestic turkey. Poultry Sci. 49: 1422 (1970).

OGASAWARA, F.X.; LORENZ, F.W., and BOBR, L.W.: Distribution of spermatozoa in the oviduct and fertility in domestic birds. III. Intrauterine insemination of semen from low-fecundity cocks. J. Reprod. Fertil. 11: 33 (1966).

OLSEN, M.W.: Maturation, fertilization and early cleavage in the egg of the domestic fowl; thesis, Faculty of the Graduate School of the University of Maryland (1941).

OLSEN, M.W.: Frequency of parthenogenesis in chicken eggs. J. Hered. 57: 23 (1966).

OLSEN, M.W. and MARSDEN, S.J.: Embryonic development in turkey eggs laid 60–224 days following removal of males. Proc. Soc. exp. Biol. Med. 82: 638 (1953).

OLSEN, M.W. and MARSDEN, S.J.: Development in unfertilized turkey eggs. J. exp. Zool. 126: 337 (1954).

OLSEN, M.W. and POOLE, H.K.: Further evidence of a relationship between live fowl pox virus and parthenogenesis in turkey eggs. Proc. Soc. exp. Biol. Med. 109: 944 (1962).

OLSEN, M.W.; WILSON, S.P., and MARKS, H.L.: Genetic control of parthenogenesis in chickens. J. Hered. 59: 41 (1968).

POLGE, C.: Functional survival of fowl spermatozoa after freezing at −79°C. Nature, Lond. 167: 949 (1951).

POLGE, C.; SMITH, A.U., and PARKES, A.S.: Revival of spermatozoa after vitrification and dehydration at low temperatures. Nature, Lond. 164: 666 (1949).

PROUDFOOT, F.G.: Effects of high pressure gases on the motility and fertilizing capacity of avian spermatozoa stored in vitro. J. Reprod. Fertil. 31: 367 (1972).

REINKE, W.C.; SPENCER, J.V., and TRYHNEW, L.J.: The effect of storage upon the chemical, physical and functional properties of chicken eggs. Poultry Sci. 52: 692 (1973).

ROMANOFF, A.L. and ROMANOFF, A.J.: The avian egg (J. Wiley & Sons, Chichester 1949).

SALISBURY, G.W. and HART, R.G.: Gamete aging and its consequences. Biol. Reprod. Suppl. 2: 1 (1970).

SARVELLA, P.: Frequency of parthenogenesis in chickens after insemination with irradiated sperm. Radiat. Res. *46:* 186 (1971).

VAN KREY, H.P.; OGASAWARA, F.X., and LORENZ, F.W.: Distribution of spermatozoa in the oviduct and fertility in domestic birds. IV. Fertility of spermatozoa from infundibular and uterovaginal glands. J. Reprod. Fertil. *11:* 257 (1966).

WILCOX, F.H. and SHAFFNER, C.S.: The effect of different handling methods and added fructose on the fertilizing ability of chicken spermatozoa after storage. Poultry Sci. *37:* 1353 (1958).

Author's address: Dr. F.W. LORENZ, Department of Animal Physiology, University of California at Davis, *Davis, CA 95616* (USA)

Aging Gametes. Int. Symp., Seattle 1973, pp. 300–329 (Karger, Basel 1975)

The Effects of Preovulatory Overripeness of Human Eggs on Development

Seasonality of Birth

P. H. JONGBLOET

Huize 'Maria Roepaan', Institute for Observation and Treatment of
Mentally Retarded, Ottersum

It has been established in amphibians as well as in mammals that various teratological effects and chromosomal aberrations result from preovulatory and postovulatory aging of the egg. At present we have good reason to think that similar detrimental phenomena occur also in man [ARRATA and IFFY, 1971; INGALLS, 1972; JONGBLOET, 1969, 1970]. High risk conceptions, such as those immediately following parturition, abortion, or interruption of oral contraception, or those due to failure when the calendar rhythm method is used may affect the outcome of pregnancy, the fitness of the newborn child, and adolescent development [JONGBLOET, 1971 c].

In man a clear distinction between the preovulatory and postovulatory time intervals is not easy to establish precisely in either prospective or retrospective examinations. Epidemiological study, therefore, of seasonal birth curves in infants and patients with various psychic or somatic aberrations or combinations of them may prove helpful in clarifying the matter.

In mammals, such as rats and cattle, in spite of a polyestric pattern, a definite seasonal variation in the fecundity rate has been reported [HUNTINGTON, 1938; STEINBACH and BALOGUN, 1971]. A polyestric pattern, too, is the rule in many nonhuman primates but, contrary to expectation, the monthly distribution of conceptions does not show a uniform distribution. In *Macacus rhesus*, by far the majority of conceptions occur during one particular quarter of the year. Upon examining the ovaries after laparotomy HARTMAN [1932] discovered that the almost complete sterility of the rhesus female in certain seasons is due to her failure to ovulate. Increased irregularity of the menstrual cycle, nonovulating bleedings, low hormonal activity, and periods of amenorrhea have been found to coincide with these periods of sterility [NOMURA *et al.*, 1972].

In man, too, the monthly distribution of births shows seasonal ups and downs, and a typical curve with 2 peaks and 2 valleys is the rule. In north-western Europe one notices a birth curve with a broad peak in 'winter' (from February to May), a dip during 'spring' (June, July and August), a smaller peak in 'summer' (only September) and a broad valley in 'autumn' (from October to December). For different countries in Europe these peaks and valleys show only small shifts, and the variation in amplitude of the fluctuations is minimal.

To explain this seasonality of birth in man HUNTINGTON [1938] believed that a 'basic animal rhythm', caused a greater number of conceptions to occur in spring. FITT [1941], on the other hand, suggested there is an 'internal seasonal biological rhythm', based on endocrine rhythm. In 1971 we put forward the suggestion that the two-peaked birth curve shows only the effect of the competition between polyestrus and mono- or diestrus. Polyestrus seems to be an autonomous self-regulating system, not subject to seasonally defined meteorological factors. Again, monoestrus or diestrus is fundamentally influenced by meteorological factors.

In figure 1, based on data gathered by TIMONEN et al. [1964], it can be seen that a decrease in the incidence of endometrial hyperplasia, i.e., a normalization of the ovulatory pattern coincides with an increase in conceptions resulting in birth. Again, an increase in the incidence of endometrial hyper-

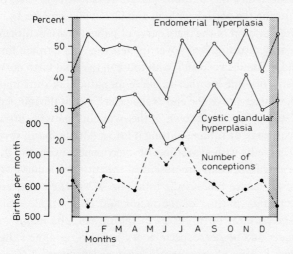

Fig. 1. Monthly variations in relative frequencies of endometrial hyperplasia and cystic glandular hyperplasias in Helsinki beside the monthly variations in the number of conceptions [TIMONEN et al., 1964].

plasia, i.e., an increase of anovulatory cycles, coincides with a decrease in conceptions. This same tendency was noticed in the 4 succeeding years. Moreover, these ups and downs of the reproduction rate and the inverse alternations of the hyperplasia frequency seemed to return each year in nearly the same months. Seasonality of incidence of amenorrhea and endometrial hyperplasia has also been demonstrated by ENGLE and SHELESNYAK [1934] and KIRCHOFF [1937]. In short, in man, too, there seems to be a striking correlation between fecundity, i.e., the biological ability to conceive, bear, and give birth to a child, and a seasonally alternating pattern of ovulatory and anovulatory cycles.

It is our hypothesis that just at the times of the cyclic breakthrough from anovulatory to ovulatory cycles and of the breakdown vice versa (indicated by arrows in fig. 2 A), the ovulation may be hampered. The preovulatory phase of the cycle, therefore, can be lengthened, i.e., preovulatory or intrafollicular overripeness. Of course, it is only to be expected that these phenomenon will occur more frequently during particular phases of reproductive life, at least in a not insignificant number of women.

Consequently an increase of pathological conceptions (fig. 2 B, broken line), might occur at the moment of passing from 'winter' to 'spring' and from 'spring' to 'summer'. In the same way, but much less so because of the smallness of its conception peak, the same phenomenon may be expected at the beginning and at the end of the 'autumn' period. As a matter of fact, this will be less frequent during the periods of high and low ovulation rate.

In a graphic representation of the birth curve of patients with malformations caused by ovopathy resulting from overripeness (fig. 2 C, broken line), the fluctuations would no doubt keep step with those in the total birth curve; but they should differ from one another in curve amplitude. A shift might also be expected at the outset and at the end of the peaks, i.e., at the moments of the breakthrough and of the breakdown of the ovulatory pattern, broadening the 'pathological' peak or rather splitting it into a double-hump surge.

A birth curve of patients with symptoms of overripeness ovopathy thus will show some typical features that are absent in the total birth curve. Although the 'pathological' curve follows the total one, a 3-peaked or even a 4-peaked curve, due to the splitting of the major and minor peaks, takes the place of the 2-peaked total birth curve. In the former, the major and minor peaks are broader and higher, especially at the flanks, and the valleys are deeper and narrower. This phenomenon is sketched in figure 2 C.

Epidemiological examination of the birth curves of pathological progeny could prove to be a useful method for studying the teratological effects of

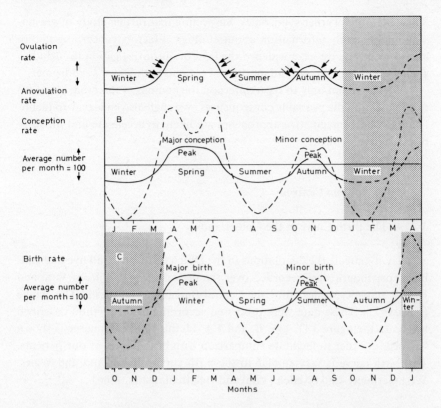

Ovulation rate

Anovulation rate

Conception rate

Average number per month = 100

Birth rate

Average number per month = 100

Fig. 2. A Ovulation and anovulation rate per month of year. *B* Conception rate per month of year. *C* Birth rate per month of year. Normal (——) and pathological (– – –) conception and birth rate as deviation from average number (100). For further explanation see text.

preovulatory overripeness of the egg. In fact, since springtime – and perhaps autumn as well – seems to promote sexual intercourse, postovulatory or intratubal delay of fertilization may be expected to be less at this time. This epidemiological examination moreover makes it possible, we hope, to keep developmental malformations caused by overripeness ovopathy separate from those caused by genetic and peristatic factors, respectively genocopies and phenocopies, and perhaps from those caused by spermatopathy.

In this paper the month of birth of all patients with anencephaly in the Netherlands between 1951 and 1968 is studied. For patients with chromosomal aberrations we could find neither a representative population nor a random sample. For this reason we extended our 1971 investigation of Down,

Klinefelter, and Turner syndromes. Suspecting that further study of seasonality might supply information about etiological factors concerning pathological offspring, we have widened the field of our investigation to include a
greater number of fathers and mothers of patients with Down's syndrome.

We intend not only to try to interpret the findings of this study, but also
to comment on the probable consequences. We shall also endeavor to identi-
fy areas where imaginative approaches are likely to accelerate and intensify
research development.

I. Patients and Controls

A. The Birth Curve in the Netherlands

To investigate the fluctuations in the Dutch birth curve, all live and still-
births per month were recorded over the period 1951–1968 from Vital and
Health Statistics, collected by the Central Bureau of Statistics in The Hague
[CBS, 1971]. These data were processed according to the method described
below. In the figure 3 D, 4 A, B, and 5 A–D, this total birth curve is shown
hatched, in order to facilitate comparison with birth curves of our patients.
This birth curve is very similar to the birth curves of England and Wales,
West Germany, and Sweden [Vital and Health Statistics, 1966].

1. The Birth Curve of Patients with Anencephaly
We were able to calculate the number of anencephalic births per month
from the Vital Statistics of the CBS [1971] in The Hague. The resulting
statistics gave a population of 5,166 anencephalics, that is, 1.19‰ of all
births. These data were processed as will be described and are listed in
table I. In figure 3 A–C the resulting curves are compared with the corresponding total birth curves. In figure 3 D the curve of all the anencephalics over the
period 1951–1968 is compared with the total birth curve over the same
period. Statistical probability analysis is not relevant here since we compared
the total population of anencephalics to the one of all births.

2. The Birth Curve of Patients with Down's Syndrome
In our institute for the mentally retarded, 529 patients have in the course
of the years been registered as suffering from Down's syndrome. Almost all
these patients were more than 1 year old when registered. There are other
similar institutes in this part of the country, and not all patients undergo med-

Table I. Month of birth of 5,166 patients with anencephaly in three 6-year periods: 1951–1956; 1957–1962; 1963–1968

	Numbers per month	Correction to the length of month	Index not smoothed	Index smoothed by the formula $\frac{a+2b+c}{4} = b'$
1951–1956				
January	226	221.9	128.5	117.7
February	183	197.5	114.4	120.3
March	218	214.0	123.9	124.9
April	234	237.4	137.5	130.6
May	217	213.0	123.4	116.3
June	138	140.0	81.1	93.1
July	153	150.2	87.0	83.1
August	136	133.5	77.3	79.1
September	127	128.8	74.6	73.5
October	119	116.8	67.6	73.8
November	145	147.1	85.2	84.4
December	175	171.8	99.5	103.2
Total	2,071	2,072.0	1,200.0	1,200.0
Average per month	172.58	172.67	100	100

	Numbers per month	Correction to the length of month	Index not smoothed	Index smoothed by the formula $\frac{a+2b+c}{4} = b'$
1957–1962				
January	185	181.6	125.4	112.9
February	141	152.5	105.3	114.3
March	179	175.7	121.3	119.6
April	186	188.7	130.3	122.4
May	159	156.1	107.8	110.6
June	138	140.0	96.7	98.5
July	137	134.5	92.9	91.3
August	122	119.8	82.7	85.3
September	118	119.7	82.7	81.5
October	115	112.9	78.0	80.0
November	116	117.7	81.3	84.1
December	141	138.4	95.6	99.5
Total	1,737	1,737.6	1,200.0	1,200.0
Average per month	144.75	144.8	100	100

Table I. (Continued)

	Numbers per month	Correction to the length of month	Index not smoothed	Index smoothed by the formula $\dfrac{a+2b+c}{4} = b'$
1963–1968				
January	124	121.7	107.4	103.8
February	125	134.9	119.0	115.3
March	134	131.5	116.0	119.8
April	143	145.1	128.0	122.2
May	135	132.5	116.9	117.1
June	119	120.7	106.5	106.1
July	109	107.0	94.4	94.4
August	95	93.3	82.3	89.6
September	111	112.6	99.3	88.4
October	84	82.5	72.8	80.2
November	85	86.2	76.0	76.6
December	94	92.3	81.4	86.5
Total	1,358	1,360.3	1,200.0	1,200.0
Average per month	113.17	113.36	100	100

ical examination. Some 40–60% die during their first year of life without entering a hospital, and often no medical help is sought at all. Consequently, this is not a random sample of the total population of patients with Down's syndrome in our district. Once again we prepared this material (table II) in the manner adopted for the other statistics and produced a birth curve, fig. 4 A, in order to compare it to the total one.

3. The Birth Curve of Patients with Klinefelter's Syndrome

Our material consists of 540 cases of Klinefelter's syndrome, karyotyped as 47,XXY, from the United Kingdom, Denmark, West Germany [JONG-BLOET, 1971 a], Dutch, and Belgian sources. Mosaics were excluded (table III). These data were processed in the usual way. The curve obtained is compared to the total birth curve for the Netherlands in figure 5 A.

4. The Birth Curve of Patients with Turner's Syndrome (table IV)

From Swedish, British [JONGBLOET, 1971 a], Dutch, and Belgian sources we tabulated data on month of birth of 392 patients with Turner's syndrome (224 with 45,X karyotype and 168 with mosaicism: 46XX/45X and structural

Table II. Month of birth of 529 patients with Down's syndrome

	Numbers per month	Correction to the length of month	Index not smoothed	Index smoothed by the formula $\dfrac{a+2b+c}{4} = b'$
January	57	55.96	126.9	111.5
February	43	46.41	105.2	111.6
March	49	48.10	109.0	107.8
April	47	47.68	108.1	107.5
May	47	46.14	104.6	107.5
June	49	49.71	112.7	105.9
July	42	41.23	93.5	94.4
August	35	34.36	77.9	88.2
September	45	45.65	103.5	93.5
October	40	39.27	89.0	91.1
November	36	36.52	82.8	85.4
December	39	38.29	86.8	95.8
Total	529	529.32	1,200.0	1,200.2
Average per month	44.8	44.11	100	100

aberrations of the X chromosome). In figure 5 B the birth curve of 224 patients with 45,X karyotype is shown and in figure 5 C that of all the 392 Turner syndrome patients; both of these are compared with the curve for all births in the Netherlands.

5. The Birth Curves of Parents of Children with Down's Syndrome

The month of birth of 369 mothers and 369 fathers of children with Down's syndrome, registered over a number of years in our institute, was analyzed and graphed (table V; fig. 5 D).

II. Methods

On the basis of the material collected we prepared birth curves. In these curves the number of births per month, expressed in index numbers, are set out against the successive month. The number per month was first corrected for the varying length of the month according to the formula: $30,433/X = Y$ (X = number of days in the month concerned; for February, X = 28.2; Y = corrected number of birth in the month concerned). In order to facilitate com-

Table III. Month of birth of 540 patients with Klinefelter's syndrome

	JONGBLOET [1971][1]	Present material[2]	Total number per month	Correction to length of month	Index not smoothed	Index smoothed by the formula $\dfrac{a+2b+c}{4} = b'$
January	20	16	36	35.3	78.3	97.6
February	36	17	53	57.2	126.9	111.3
March	32	20	52	51.0	113.2	118.2
April	32	21	53	53.8	119.4	116.9
May	33	20	53	52.0	115.4	107.2
June	21	14	35	35.5	78.8	88.4
July	18	19	37	36.3	80.6	80.7
August	23	15	38	37.3	82.8	87.5
September	28	18	46	46.7	103.6	99.7
October	28	22	50	49.1	108.9	101.7
November	20	18	38	38.5	85.4	96.6
December	26	23	49	48.1	106.7	94.3
Total	317	223	540	540.8	1,200.0	1,200.1
Average per month			45.0	45.07	100	100

1 COURT-BROWN *et al.* [1964]; FRØLAND [1967]; NIELSEN and FRIEDRICH [1969]; TÜNTE and NIERMANN [1968].
2 Amsterdam (36, Bijlsma); Ghent (13, Matton-vanLeuven; 4, Orye); Groningen (4, Gouw); Leyden (1, Pearson); Louvain (97, van den Berghe); Nijmegen (30, Hustinx; 31, Kirkels); Ottersum (7, van Kempen).

parison of the seasonal patterns, this corrected number was converted to a standard index (100 equals the average number of births per month). This standard index (100) is the number that would be obtained if no seasonal variation existed.

In the 'pathological' curves the graph has been smoothed in order to avoid random irregularities (e.g., prematurity and postmaturity) as much as possible. Therefore, the formula $a+2b+c/4 = b'$ was used (where b is the index of the month concerned and a and c the indices of the preceding and the succeeding month, respectively). For reasons mentioned above a statistical comparison of the anencephaly population is unnecessary; statistical probability analyses of the birth curve of Down's, Klinefelter's, and Turner's syndromes and of parents of children with Down's syndrome are not possible because these groups are not random samples of the populations concerned.

Table IV. Month of birth of 392 patients with Turner's syndrome

	45, X		Structural aberrations of X chromosome and mosaicism		Total number per month	Correction to length of month	Index not smoothed	Index smoothed by the formula $\dfrac{a+2b+c}{4} = b'$
	JONGBLOET [1971][1]	present material[2]	JONGBLOET [1971][1]	present material[2]				
January	9	9	4	7	29	28.5	87.1	100.2
February	7	16	5	7	35	37.8	115.5	108.0
March	6	8	9	15	38	37.3	114.0	109.1
April	6	10	6	8	30	30.4	92.9	100.5
May	7	17	2	8	34	33.4	102.0	105.2
June	8	18	6	8	40	40.6	124.0	108.5
July	4	11	6	7	28	27.5	84.0	95.5
August	3	12	4	11	30	29.5	90.1	94.7
September	10	12	3	12	37	37.5	114.6	97.1
October	2	8	3	10	23	22.6	69.0	87.1
November	8	12	1	10	31	31.4	95.9	92.9
December	5	16	2	14	37	36.8	110.9	101.2
Total	75	149	51	117	392	392.8	1,200.0	1,200.0
Average per month					32.67	32.73	100	100

1 COURT-BROWN *et al.* [1964]. LINDSTEN [1963].
2 Amsterdam (6/2, Bijlsma); Ghent (7/10, Matton; 21/16 Orye); Groningen (7/9, Gouw); Leyden (9/1, Pearson); Louvain (66/58, van den Berghe); Nijmegen (19/11, Hustinx; 13/9, Kirkels); Ottersum (1/3, van Kempen).

III. Results and Discussion

A. Anencephaly

Comparison of the birth curves of infants with anencephaly registered during 3 successive 6-year periods with those of total births in the corresponding periods, regularly show up the same indicative deviations (fig. 3 A–C). These curves are as anticipated and expressed in our sketch in figure 2, the expected birth curve of patients with symptoms of preovulatory overripeness ovopathy; the fluctuations of the anencephaly births markedly follow those of the total births, but the former have a much larger amplitude than the latter. Furthermore, the major peak clearly widens, splitting into a double-hump surge, and the valleys narrow.

Table V. Month of birth of 369 mothers and 369 fathers of patients with Down's syndrome

	Mothers				Fathers			
	numbers per month	correction to the length of month	index not smoothed	index smoothed by the formula $\frac{a+2b+c}{4} = b'$	numbers per month	correction to the length of month	index not smoothed	index smoothed by the formula $\frac{a+2b+c}{4} = b'$
January	37	36.3	118.1	107.0	40	39.3	127.6	112.6
February	31	33.5	108.9	110.3	33	35.6	115.5	112.8
March	33	32.4	105.4	112.1	29	28.5	92.5	108.9
April	39	39.6	128.8	119.5	41	41.6	135.1	114.6
May	36	35.3	114.8	113.5	30	29.5	95.8	101.4
June	29	29.4	95.6	94.0	24	24.3	78.9	90.5
July	22	21.6	70.2	92.5	34	33.4	108.5	93.1
August	42	41.2	134.0	105.2	24	23.6	76.6	86.1
September	25	25.4	82.6	96.4	25	25.4	82.5	85.9
October	27	26.5	86.2	81.9	32	31.4	102.0	98.0
November	22	22.3	72.5	78.5	32	32.5	105.5	98.1
December	26	25.5	82.9	89.1	25	24.5	79.5	98.0
Total	369	369.0	1,200.0	1,200.0	369	369.6	1,200.0	1,200.0
Average per month	30.75	100	100		30.8	100	100	

These anencephaly curves are all the more important as they take into account every registered case in the whole of the Netherlands during these three 6-year periods. In other words 2 entire populations are compared. With respect to anencephaly there is no danger of diagnostic confusion and, even if not every case were registered, it would probably not affect the distribution in time, i.e., it would not change the shape of the peaks and valleys.

Again, a certain distortion is inevitable when the material of 6 different years is combined into one graph. This obviously applies even more to an 18-year curve (fig. 3 D). NORRIS and CHOWNING [1962] drew attention to the fact that the seasonal distribution of births in a general population may vary appreciably from year to year in a particular country. We are convinced that the explanation of their findings must be sought in meteorological factors exerting their influence on the hypothalamo-hypophyseal-ovarian axis. For this reason it is only to be expected that the periodic increase and decrease of normal and pathological progeny will vary from year to year as a result of early or late onset of spring weather. Of course, a geographically restricted

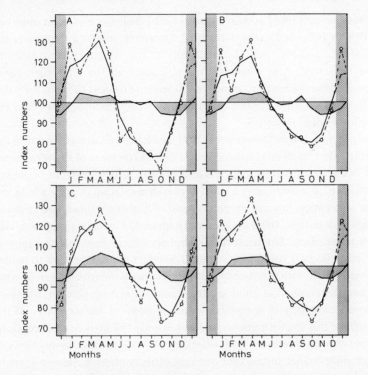

Fig. 3. Anencephaly in the Netherlands. *A* 1951–1956; *B* 1957–1962; *C* 1963–1968; *D* 1951–1968. – – – = Absolute numbers corrected to length of month and indexed. ——— = Curve smoothed by the formula: a + 2b + c/4 = b′. Hatched area: total births in the Netherlands in the corresponding periods.

area such as the Netherlands provides the advantage of homogeneous meteorological conditions, offset somewhat by the necessarily smaller numbers of a particular pathological condition. Combining the material of different years always takes place at the expense of exactness in graphical representation. A comparison of the anencephaly and the total birth curves in figure 3 D with those in figure 3 A–C demonstrates the validity of our view. Another reason for loss of definition in the graphs is the rather high frequency of anencephalics from pregnancies having lasted either shorter or longer than the normal 280 days after the last menstrual period [MILIC and ADAMSONS, 1969].

As a matter of fact, this very marked relationship between seasons and births of infants with anencephaly agrees with previous observations concerning congenital malformations of CNS in the Netherlands by DE GROOT

[1965], HAMERSMA [1966] and OVERBEKE [1971]. This has also been observed in the British Isles, in France, Germany, Denmark, Finland, Hungary, the USA, Canada, and Australia. In practically all investigations seasonality of birth was observed. And wherever comparisons with the total birth curve were possible, the fluctuations occurred at the same time as those in the pathological curve, only the greater amplitude is more obvious, and often the double-hump surge is seen.

In a previous paper [JONGBLOET, 1971 c] we have drawn attention to the fact that in other 'high-risk' conceptions a definite increase of malformations of the CNS arises in adolescent girls and primiparous women, in premenopausal women, in women after a short conception interval or after a long unintended conception interval, in prediabetic or diabetic women and in many other high-risk groups. In all these cases an increased incidence of anovulatory cycles takes place. The present anencephaly curves now seem to suggest that a meteorological stimulus is required to effect a breakthrough to ovulation or vice versa, with a possibility of preovulatory overripeness ovopathy. We believe therefore, that good grounds exist for stating that preovulatory overripeness ovopathy is acceptable as an etiology of anencephaly, all the more so since this malformation satisfies not only the high-risk conceptions mentioned above [criterion VII, JONGBLOET, 1971 c] but also many other criteria providing further support for our view of its etiology. Criterion I: anencephaly does not occur, or occurs only very rarely familially; criterion II: it frequently occurs in both monozygotic twins of equal size, but oftener in only the smaller one of such a twinpair; criterion III: it is often accompanied by a multiplicity of congenital malformations; criterion V: it is frequently characterized by hypogonadism; criterion VI: it is often a symptom of a maternal constitutional factor that manifests itself in a suboptimal reproductive history; criterion VIII: it is relatively more frequently accompanied by complications of pregnancy, parturition, and neonatal life. Only criterion IV, the accompaniment by nonspecific chromosomal aberrations, was not fulfilled. However, it must be understood that no comprehensive examination for chromosomal aberrations in anencephaly has been performed for the obvious reason that a very large number of infants with this malformation are stillborn or die soon after birth. In the literature concerning spontaneous abortion material, however, the association of malformations of the CNS with various chromosomal aberrations is often mentioned.

As a matter of fact, other factors, too, might cause anencephaly and thus affect the features of the anencephaly birth curve. Preovulatory overripeness ovopathy caused by other than the mentioned meteorological phenomena, e.g., stress or drugs, hampering or postponing the ovulation process, has to be considered. At first glance these factors are restricted neither to season nor to specific months in such a way that they could influence or even change the course of an anencephaly birth curve.

Of course, postovulatory overripeness is another possible cause of anencephaly. Lack of data, however, concerning both increased and decreased coital frequency due to the time of the year and the difference in age groups limits us to nothing better than an intelligent guess at the possible effects of intratubal aging of the egg in an anencephaly birth curve. Genocopies and phenocopies, or even spermatopathy, the latter suggested by BORDAHL [1971], could possibly also cause anencephaly. One cannot easily imagine how genetic factors could produce similar seasonal fluctuations. In fact genetic distribution, for example of ABO blood types, does not seem to be influenced by exogenous factors such as month of birth [COHEN, 1968]. Nevertheless, some interaction between genotype and unknown exogenous factors linked to seasonal variations cannot be excluded for the time being. The effects finally of peristatic factors and of spermatopathy (if they have any influence at all on the anencephaly birth curve) are unanswered questions.

If we assume that among other causes overripeness ovopathy could produce anencephaly as well as other malformations of the CNS, we are then suggesting the possibility that a very broad range of brain dysfunction may originate in this way. It is not without interest that BARRY and BARRY [1961, 1964] reviewing 7 separate investigations, as well as HARE and PRICE [1968], HARE et al. [1972], and DALÉN [1968] found evidence for a connection between season of birth and the major psychoses. These studies demonstrate convincingly that, with a single exception here and there, an excess of schizophrenic (and to a smaller extent of manic-depressive) patients were born more frequently in some months of the year and less often in others. These curves in fact are similar to the ones drawn for anencephaly, although the magnitude of the fluctuations seems less marked. Therefore, we believe that deviating birth curves in certain types of psychoses point to developmental organic defects of the brain. Apart from this, data from the literature concerning season of birth in patients with epilepsy, cerebral palsy, and chronic aggressive delinquency indicate a connection similar to the ones above. A number of studies dealing with mental retardation [FITT, 1941; KNOBLOCH and PASAMANICK, 1958; LANDER et al., 1964; ORME, 1962, 1963, 1965; DE SAUVAGE NOLTING, 1954], make it clear that the seasonal distribution of births also differed from the one that would be expected in the same region. Disagreement about the choice of both materials and time of fluctuations, however, could well arise, the more so since other factors such as the 'age-group position effect' [DOORNBOS, 1971; WILLIAMS, 1964] has to be considered. More research is required in order to arrive at a general agreement on this point.

All the same it is not unreasonable to speculate that a good many cases of what are considered to be psychopathologic, mental retardation, minimal brain dysfunction, or partial defects originate from an early brain maldevelopment due to overripeness ovopathy. It is outside the scope of this paper to show that quite a lot of these defects satisfy many other criteria for overripeness ovopathy as well. We would be the first to admit, however, that there are still many missing links in our epidemiological knowledge of these infirmities.

B. Down's Syndrome

Further registration of Down syndrome patients in our institute since our last publication [JONGBLOET, 1971 a], increasing the number from 441 to 529, did not bring about any fundamental changes in the deviation features of the Down syndrome curve (fig. 4 A). The characteristic pattern of the birth curve to be expected with our seasonal overripeness hypothesis is seen once again. The Down syndrome curve follows the total one, but a 3-peaked curve comes about owing to the double-hump surge superimposed on the flanks of the total birth peak, and the peaks and valleys differ in curve amplitude.

Although we see no reason to assume that our registered patients would greatly differ from the total Down syndrome population, our material still relates to a relatively small group whose selection does not fulfill statistical requirements and, therefore, may influence the features of our Down syndrome curve. A comparison with other groups of Down syndrome patients is for this reason most important.

We were able to draw a birth curve of 2,730 Down syndrome patients (fig. 4 B), listed by KÖNIG [1959], for the greater part from Denmark and the rest from various other European countries. We compared these data with the total birth curve in the Netherlands. A comparison was also made of 1,192 Down syndrome patients in Sweden [LANDER et al., 1964] with a control group from the Swedish Bureau for Vital Statistics (fig. 4 C). In these 3 northwestern European curves, apart from some small irregularities, the same features are seen (fig. 4 A–C). Sometimes a certain anteposition of the

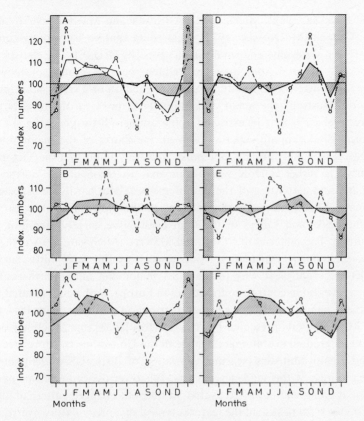

Fig. 4. Down's syndrome. *A* The Netherlands, 529 cases. *B* Denmark including European group, 2,730 cases. *C* Sweden, 1,192 cases. *D* Australia (Victoria), 1,134 cases. *E* United States (Michigan), 2,431 cases. *F* Canada (Quebec), 2,398 cases. – – – = Absolute numbers corrected to length of month and indexed. —— = Curve smoothed by the formula: $a + 2b + c/4 = b'$. Hatched area: total births in the corresponding countries.

Down syndrome peaks and valleys is faintly apparent, possibly as a consequence of a shorter pregnancy duration, which seems to be the rule for children with Down's syndrome. Processing of birth curves of 3 British groups of Down syndrome patients [EDWARDS, 1961; GREENBERG, 1963; LECK, 1966] was impossible because either the number of patients was too small or they were grouped in 3-month periods. However, the same deviations from the expected fluctuations are present.

Furthermore, we have investigated different groups of patients with Down's syndrome from non-European countries: Victoria, Australia [COLL-

MAN and STOLLER, 1962], Michigan, USA [STARK and MANTEL, 1967], and Quebec, Canada [McDONALD, 1972]. These data enabled us to draw comparable Down syndrome and total birth curves (fig. 4 D–F). The statistical value of this material, too, may be doubted, because groups of Down syndrome patients very seldom represent a population or a random sample. In Victoria, Australia the major and minor birth peaks in the total birth curve are reversed as may be expected in the southern hemisphere (fig. 4 D). The typical double hump superimposed on the flanks of the major total birth peak is seemingly absent. One must, however, admit that the Victoria birth curve is rather narrow when compared to those of the northern hemisphere, and a splitting of the pathologic peak can hardly be expected in this case. Furthermore, the fluctuations in the Down syndrome curve follow the peaks and valleys of the total birth curve, largely exceeding it in amplitude. The material of STARK and MANTEL (Michigan, USA [1967]) needs a preliminary explanation with respect to the total birth curve (fig. 4 E). It is not clear why in the USA major and minor birth peaks have been reversed in contrast to the curves in Europe, both being situated in the northern hemisphere. The seasonal distribution of births from 1847 to 1933 in Massachusetts presented by HUNTINGTON [1938] (fig. 24) clearly demonstrates a gradual evolutionary change in the United States. More recent Vital and Health Statistics (seasonal Variation of Birth, USA 1966) show that the progress of this tendency persists. Whatever the cause of this phenomenon, it is of great interest to us that, in spite of a changed pattern of major and minor birth peaks, all the features typical of a preovulatory overripeness birth curve are present once again (fig. 4 E). Strangely enough the total birth curve in Canada differs from the one of the USA, and is similar to those of Europe. Here again (fig. 4 F), we notice a double-hump surge superimposed on the flanks of the major total birth peak. The peaks and valleys, however, do not show the usual amplitudes.

All the samples of Down syndrome patients studied here in fact concern only the surviving trisomy-21 conceptuses. We know that a great many more Down syndrome conceptuses die *in utero* ending in spontaneous abortions or stillbirths. Another fraction of them die during neonatal life. Seasonality of spontaneous abortions [McDONALD, 1971] and of stillbirths [JANERICH *et al.*, 1971; SLATIS and DE CLOUX, 1967] has also been established. Therefore, for further analyses one has to check the course of the conception curve of subcategories with special attention to the trisomy-21 embryos dying *in utero*. To sum up, despite the fact that most authors, arranging their material in a different manner, deny all temporal or seasonal clustering in births of Down syndrome patients, we maintain that in all the material accessible to us the general trend is in agreement with the seasonal overripeness hypothesis. On the other hand, using data from the literature, we have come to the conclusion [JONGBLOET, 1971 c] that Down's syndrome largely satisfies all diagnostic criteria for overripeness ovopathy. Consequently, it would be but logical to accept that preovulatory overripeness of the egg could cause Down's syndrome. This theory is in accordance with the very recent determinations of meiotic errors leading to Down's syndrome by quinacrine-fluorescent variants of the 21st chromosome [MUTTON, 1973; ROBINSON, 1973]. In 7 patients with standard trisomy 21 the error could be localized. In 6 of them it occurred at first meiotic division, i.e., during the ripening phase of the egg, and in the remaining case at the second meiotic division, i.e., after penetration by the spermatozoon. As a matter of fact experiments with amphibians supply evidence that errors at both the first and second meiotic divisions may be possible consequences of preovulatory overripeness (MIKAMO, 1968).

We have no longer any doubt that both anencephaly and Down's syndrome answer the requirements of our seasonal overripeness hypothesis. However, comparing anencephaly curves with those of Down syndrome patients, we see immediately that the former have a greater amplitude than the latter. If these deviations are due exclusively to meteorological seasonal factors that affect the hypothalamo-hypophyseal-ovarian axis, we should expect the amplitude of the respective birth curves to deviate to the same degree. From an epidemiological view there are more differences between these 2 conditions and, therefore, the fluctuations in anencephaly would have to be enlarged by an additional factor or those of Down's syndrome would have to be leveled. Of the five other factors mentioned previously as being capable of affecting the birth curve amplitude, none was shown to enlarge the anencephaly fluctuations, and several can be excluded in the case of Down's syndrome: first of all, phenocopies, because peristatic factors after fertilization cannot possibly be the cause of aneuploidy in all cells of an organism; second, genocopies, because hereditary passing on of a 21-chromosome translocation from either parent includes less than 4% of the total Down syndrome population [WAHRMAN and FRIED, 1971]. Finally, nothing indicates that preovulatory overripeness due to other than meteorological influences, postovulatory overripeness, and spermatopathy introduces an interfering seasonal distortion in the Down syndrome curve. For lack of data we can only speculate; we think that leveling of the latter must be attributed to aneuploid spermatozoa. Spermatogenesis would then be less likely to be susceptible to meteorological factors than would ovogenesis.

This view is corroborated by EMME's [1960] conclusion that female mammals are more sensitive to photoperiodic influences than are males. This means that a Down syndrome population ought to be subdivided, separating the maternal trisomy-21m cases from the paternal trisomy-21p cases. The 21m curve would then tend to resemble the anencephaly curve, whereas the 21p curve would tend to take the shape of the total birth curve. Combining these 2 populations would necessarily bring about a leveling of both peaks and valleys. Later, we propose to show that there is more than one reason for our view that there is a contribution on the part of the father. This explains our interest in a birth curve of patients with 47, XYY karyotype.[1] This condition is almost certainly the result of nondisjunction in the male parent, except in a small number of patients in which this karyotype may arise from mitotic nondisjunction after fertilization. A birth curve of XYY patients, therefore, would supply decisive information concerning the absence or presence of seasonality in spermatopathy.

C. Klinefelter's Syndrome

Our series of Klinefelter syndrome patients with 47,XXY karyotype has now been extended from 317 to 540 cases. The new birth curve (fig. 5 A) continues to show a double-hump surge, superimposed on the flanks of the major total birth peak, and other exagerations of the expected seasonal fluctuations, all fitting in with the seasonal overripeness hypothesis.

Admittedly, our data were obtained from the Netherlands, Belgium, England, Denmark, and Germany, but as we have said, the total birth curves in these countries do not differ greatly. The selection problem is a real one because the only patients who receive medical attention from the clinician do so as a consequence of serious inborn defects (infertility, mental retardation or psychopathological illness). The Klinefelter syndrome is one of the most frequent chromosomal aberrations, and the symptoms are by no means always obvious. Furthermore, there is no way of determining in how many patients the Klinefelter condition may be associated with either 47,XmXmY or 47,XmXpY karyotype caused by either ovopathy or spermatopathy.

Fully aware of the inevitable unreliability, but lacking a better alternative, we may compare our Klinefelter syndrome curve with the anencephaly

---

1   Inquiries at the above-mentioned cytogenetic centers did not supply large enough numbers to justify a birth curve.

curve. Here also a leveling of the fluctuations is noticeable, although not as pronounced as in the Down syndrome curves. There is no point in assessing here a leveling effect by genocopies or phenocopies, since a 47,XXY karyotype is under consideration. Preovulatory overripeness due to other phenomena than the described meteorological ones and postovulatory overripeness certainly require further exploration. We lack as yet the means to assess with exactitude whether our curves have been affected by them. Knowing, however, that spermatopathy doubtless plays a part in causing Klinefelter's syndrome, we realise that a leveling effect can be expected here also. Unfortunately, the numbers of verified cases of 47,XmXmY and of 47,XmXpY are very small. It is obviously important to study the birth curves of these 2 groups of Klinefelter syndrome patients in order to detect any differences in seasonality.

D. Turner's Syndrome

The seasonal character of the birth curve of 224 patients with 45,X Turner's syndrome is suggested in figure 5 B. The same can be said of figure 5 C relating to 392 patients with the same karyotype with mosaics and structural aberration of the X chromosome. In both figures splitting of the major birth peak into a double-hump surge and fluctuations that strikingly deviate from the normal can be seen. The numbers per month however are rather small. The same remarks apply to selection in both Turner's and Klinefelter's syndromes. Again the possibility may not be excluded that factors other than meteorological influences have an effect on the shape of the birth curve. In contrast to Klinefelter's syndrome there is no proof from either study to indicate that spermatopathy plays a part here.

Next to neurological deficiencies, such as epilepsy and mental retardation, personality and character disorders appear in association with sex chromosome anomalies with abnormally high frequency [PFEIFFER, 1971; SCHULZ and HIENZ, 1969; ZÜBLIN, 1969]. There have been unsuccessful attempts to connect these abnormalities to the excess or the missing chromosome. If the birth curves of patients with Klinefelter's and Turner's syndromes continue to show features corresponding to those demanded by the seasonal overripeness hypothesis, we might have to revise our thinking on the etiology of a number of concomitant symptoms. For, as has been said above, deviations from the expected fluctuations have also been observed in cases of psychoses, disturbed aggressive behavior, epilepsy, mental retardation, and so on. It is

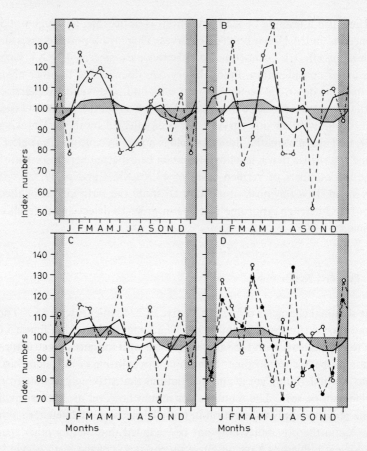

Fig. 5. A Klinefelter's syndrome, 540 cases (47,XXY). *B* Turner's syndrome, 224 cases (45,X). *C* Turner's syndrome, 392 cases (45,X; mosaicism and structural aberrations). *D* 369 mothers (●), and 369 fathers (○) of Down syndrome patients. – – – = Absolute numbers corrected to length of month and indexed. —— = Curve smoothed by the formula: $a + 2b + c/4 = b'$. Hatched area: total births in the Netherlands from 1951 to 1968.

then but logical to look for the causes of neurological and psychopathological disturbances elsewhere, i.e., not in the sex chromosomes. Overripeness ovopathy would serve to explain why both cerebral dysfunctions and chromosomal aberrations, although often occurring by themselves, are seen in combination more frequently than chance would warrant. A wide variety of organic cerebral defects, with their inevitable effects on psychic functions, should then not be exclusively attributed to sex chromosome abnormalities, but rather to a fundamental disorder within the plasm of the egg cell (and maybe even of the spermatozoon).

E. Parents of Children with Down's Syndrome

The greater data on mothers and fathers of patients with Down's syndrome only emphasized the seasonality feature (fig. 5 D) already clearly seen in our 1971 curves. The remarks concerning the sample of children with Down's syndrome apply equally to their parents. The double-hump surges, however, and the deviations from the expected birth curves invite investigation as to the possibility of a constitutional factor predisposing to either pathological oogenesis or pathological spermatogenesis that lead to trisomic progeny. This predisposing constitutional factor, present either in the mother or in the father, might itself be caused by preovulatory overripeness, since one of the most fundamental consequences of overripeness ovopathy seems to be a defect of the gonads. WITSCHI et al. [1957], after having studied overripeness of the egg in amphibians, came to the conclusion that germ plasm proves highly susceptible to even slight damage. The primordial germ cells soon exhibit degenerative features, multiply slowly, and enter the gonadal folds only in small numbers if at all. Consequently, constitutional defects in the ovaria could well bring about instability in the hypothalamo-hypophyseal-ovarian axis whereby exogenous meteorological influences would have a greater effect on the endogenous ovulation rhythm than would otherwise be the case. A gradual transition from normality in gonads (with a normal menstrual cycle) to dysgenesis (with menstrual irregularities), to gonadal agenesis (with primary amenorrhea) would not be contrary to expectation in the presence or absence of chromosomal aberrations [JONGBLOET, 1971 b].

The deviations from the expected birth curve presented here and data from the literature [JONGBLOET, 1971 c] cause us to suspect the presence of a maternal constitutional factor in mothers who have given birth to one or more children with Down's syndrome. Similar deviations in the male parent birth curve furnish further support for the view that one or more constitutional factors must be present in the male gonads. But this is not all. First, dermatoglyphic stigmata, including higher occurrence of simian crease, seem to differ significantly in number from those of a control group [KAPLAN and ZSAKO, 1970; PRIEST, 1969]. Second, in fathers as well as in mothers a higher frequency of electroencephalographic abnormalities is found [UOHASHI,

1970]. Finally, we are faced with the problem that a small or even a moderate paternal age effect cannot be ruled out [LILIENFELD, 1969].

F. General Considerations

Evidently further studies of seasonality would promote important research on the etiology of congenital malformations with and without chromosomal aberrations. The possible effect of time of birth on the subsequent destiny of the individual is an enigma that has perplexed man for thousands of years. To the first agricultural civilizations of Assyria, Babylon, and ancient Egypt, the 12 constellations of the zodiac probably meant at first no more than a division of the year into months. Their great familiarity with the workings of nature may well have led them to connect constellations (or months) of birth with inborn defects. It is not farfetched to think that these constellations acquired their mythological significance in this way. When the will of the gods was thought to be revealed in these constellations, priests were probably asked to interpret the signs of the heavens. The understandable misinterpretations that resulted therefrom should not induce modern science to reject the possibility of a real connection.

BOLK [1902] and VAN EYK [1904] in the Netherlands were struck by the high incidence of fatal tuberculosis among people born in wintertime. This lead WOLDA [1927, 1929] to undertake investigations in Dutch sanatoria. He found that chances of survival of tuberculosis patients were smaller when their dates of birth fell on the total birth curve peaks. This tended to confirm what had already been suspected by BOLK [1902], namely that the time of conception bears some definite relation to the fitness of the individual. These historical considerations would not deserve mention if similar epidemiological phenomena had not later on been detected in cancer studies. An additional reason for bringing up this matter is the recently rekindled interest in cell-mediated immunology in connection with tuberculosis as well as with cancer. As a result of his own investigations and those of others, DE SAUVAGE-NOLTING [1968] came upon a seasonality of birth in cancer patients. In more than 16,600 cancer cases from the Netherlands he found highly significant differences in the number of birth dates, January being the highest and June the lowest. The seasonal fluctuations seemed to be independent of the organ affected as mammary carcinoma, intestinal cancer, and pulmonary carcinoma all followed the same pattern. In material from other countries he found the same significant seasonal variation. Moreover, in Australia a reversed seasonal variation was found in cancer-prone children, but in 321 cases, all immigrants from the northern hemisphere, there was a seasonal distribution of birth-date frequency similar to that in the northern hemisphere.

The increased risk of contracting these diseases by persons born in certain months of the year, prompts the question: What is the connection between time of birth (or conception) and biological fitness? The answer perhaps may be hidden in overripeness ovopathy, which results in a faulty development of the thymus and consequently of the thymus-dependent humoral and cell-mediated immunologic systems. Anomalous development of the organs arising from the third and fourth pharyngeal pouch, resulting in hypoplasia or aplasia of the thymus, rather strikingly meet the criteria required of overripeness ovopathy as an etiology [JONGBLOET, 1968, 1971c]. The so-called III–IV pharyngeal pouch, or Di-George syndrome(s), is often characterized by a defective cell-mediated immunity and at least some weakness in antibody response [LISCHNER, 1972]. It is conceivable that in these and in other conditions, apart from the absence or the hypoplasia of the thymus, there may be a defect in the T cells that prevents them from carrying out their normal functions.

This idea, which implies injury to the immunological system as a consequence of ovopathy, provides a framework of answers to many of the questions we are dealing with. It would do more than explain merely seasonality of births in patients suffering and dying from tuberculosis and malignancies. Many other epidemiological facts concerning cancer become understandable when considered in the context of ovopathy. Apart from an increase of malignancy in patients with congenital malformations – criterion III – [BOAZ et al., 1971; MILLER, 1969; MILLER et al., 1969; WERTELECKI et al., 1970], with nonspecific chromosomal aberrations – criterion IV – [HOLLAND et al., 1962; KOBAYASHI et al., 1968; MILLER, 1971; MILLER et al., 1969; VAN DEN BERGHE et al., 1972] and from pregnancies in which there was a threatened abortion – criterion VIII – [STEWART and DRAPER, 1968], an increase was also noticed in high-risk conceptions – criterion VII – [STARK and MANTEL, 1969; STEWART et al., 1958]. STEWART et al. [1958] drew attention to the existence of an excessive increase of malignancy in children from primiparous and premenopausal mothers. Because of the finding that the frequency of both leukemia and Down's syndrome increases in children of mothers over 40 years old, they question the generally supposed cause-and-effect relationship. They hold the view that both diseases derive from a common factor, not that mongolism simply predisposes to leukemia. We not only agree with this view but go even further and think that this 'common factor' can be identified as over-

ripeness ovopathy. This would be a good explanation of how a nondisjunction or a disturbance of the immunological system or both are caused.
MENSER and PURVIS-SMITH [1969] think that there is a 'common prenatal
teratological cause' that produces both leukemia and abnormal dermatoglyphs, seen frequently together. Overripeness ovopathy provides the probable explanation of why leukemia (and neoplasia) occur not only with
dermatoglyphic stigmata but also with other congenital malformations,
especially chromosomal aberrations. The abnormally high infection rate in
children with Down's syndrome and the very high mortality rate during
their first year of life are in themselves reasons to believe in the existence of
an injured immunological system. Persistence of the Australia antigen has
been imputed to a poor T lymphocyte response due to abnormalities in the
lymphocyte itself [BLUMBERG et al., 1971; DUDLEY et al., 1972; GIUSTINO
et al., 1972]. And this is the reason why we think that overripeness ovopathy
causing damage to the immunological system is a common etiological origin
of the very heterogeneous group of patients who are unable to eliminate
the Australia antigen. These are patients with chronic hepatitis, lepromatous
leprosy, leukemia or lymphoma as well as Down's syndrome, mental retardation, or psychiatric diseases. Even though the examination of the birth curve
of all these groups is by no means complete, seasonality of birth was seen
in some.

   To sum up, we maintain that the study of birth curves holds an important clue to the understanding of the physiology and the pathology of brains,
gonads, and immunological defense mechanisms, to name but a few of the
systems liable to be affected. All this invites further study of the basic facts
that support the seasonal overripeness hypothesis insofar as it deals with the
seasonal alternating ovulatory and anovulatory pattern in women. Most information is likely to be gained where anovulatory cycles are more frequent,
i.e., in adolescent girls and primiparous mothers, in premenopausal women,
in cycles after abortion, childbirth, or interruption of oral contraceptives, in
women who conceive with difficulty, or in whom ovulation rhythm is upset
owing to endocrinological imbalance or drug treatment. We would also like
to see continued epidemiological research into the seasonality of these and
other kinds of pathological conditions.

   To conclude, the birth curves of children with inborn errors from known
genetic origin, from known peristatic factors, and from known spermato-
pathic origin are of special importance because they could help to clarify the
phenomena studied here.

   This research will prove rewarding because of the prevention that may become possible as a result. We do not subscribe to the view that definite seasons are especially suitable for conception. This goes contrary to the repeated advice given by the editorial staff of the British Medical Journal [1958, 1962]. We do have a strong conviction that many reproductive casualties can be prevented by guarding against conceptions carrying a high-risk because of overripeness-ovopathy.

Summary

The existence of a seasonal alternation of ovulatory and anovulatory cycles in animal species and in man led me to advance a verifiable seasonal overripeness hypothesis. At the moments of the seasonally dependent cyclic breakthrough from anovulatory to ovulatory periods and of the breakdown from ovulatory to anovulatory periods an undue interference could occur during the ripening phase of the egg with preovulatory overripeness as a consequence.

In a graphic representation of a birth curve of patients with malformations caused by preovulatory overripeness ovopathy, features differing from those in the total birth curve must be expected. The fluctuations of the former naturally follow those of the latter with these exceptions: they exceed them in amplitude; the major (and often the minor) birth peak will split into a double-hump surge, thus giving rise to a 3- or 4-peaked birth curve in clear contrast to the 2-peaked total curve.

The month of birth of all children born with anencephaly in the Netherlands between 1951 and 1968 was analyzed. Additional data from patients suffering from Down's, Klinefelter's, and Turner's syndromes and of parents of children suffering from Down's syndrome were similarly processed. In all these analyses a 3-peaked birth curve was manifested, giving support to the view that preovulatory overripeness is a possible etiology. Also preovulatory overripeness resulting from other than meteorological factors, postovulatory overripeness, spermatopathy, genocopies, and phenocopies, was considered wherever it could be of importance. The findings in mothers and fathers of Down syndrome patients induced the author to postulate a constitutional factor predisposing to preovulatory overripeness ovopathy and to spermatopathy.

Studies of the birth curve of patients show that many characteristics of human beings are highly dependent on the condition of the egg (and the spermatozoon) at the time of conception. Thus, intelligence, personality, progeny, and resistance to infections and malignancies could all be involved. Finally, the urgency of further research is stressed, especially in connection with the inherent possibilities of future prevention.

Acknowledgments

My thanks are due to J.B. Bijlsma (Amsterdam), Dr. M. Matton-van Leuven (Ghent) and Dr. E. Orye (Ghent), W.L. Gouw (Groningen), Dr. P. Pearson (Leyden), Dr. H. van den Berghe (Louvain), Dr. T.W.J. Hustinx (Nijmegen), Dr. V.H.G.J.

KIRKELS (Nijmegen) and Dr. C. VAN KEMPEN for the cytogenetic part of this paper; to
B.A. LELIVELD for processing material from the files of the CBS at The Hague to arrive
at our anencephaly data; to Prof. T.D. STAHLIE for reading and commenting on the
manuscript; to Dr. E.J. BIJNEN for commenting on the statistics; to J.G.M. MARTENS
for preparing the tables; to M.H.F. DERKSEN for preparing the text; to J. KONINGS for
the drawings; and to F. LAMPE for the translation.

References

ARRATA, W.S.M. and IFFY, L.: Normal and delayed ovulation in the human. Obstet.
gynec. Surv. 26: 676 (1971).

BARRY, H. and BARRY, H., jr.: Season of birth: an epidemiological study in psychiatry.
Arch. gen. Psychiat. 5: 292 (1961).

BARRY, H. and BARRY, H., jr.: Season of birth in schizophrenics: its relation to social class.
Arch. gen. Psychiat. 11: 385 (1964).

BLUMBERG, B.S.; SUTNICK, A.I.; LONDON, W.T., and MILLMAN, I.: Australia antigen
and hepatitis (Butterworths, London, 1971).

BOAZ, D.; MACE, J.W., and GOTLIN, R.W.: Poland's syndrome and leukaemia. Lancet
i: 349 (1971).

BOLK, L.: Naar aanleiding der erfelijkheid van tuberculose. Ned. T. Geneesk. 38: 1023
(1902).

BORDAHL, P.F.: Anencephalus, forekomst i tre svangerskap has samme kvinne. T. norske
Laegeforen. 91 (1940). Anencephalus in three pregnancies in the same women.
Excerpta med. hum. Genet. 11 (1971).

CBS: Anencephalie in Nederland 1951–1968 (Staatsuitgeverij, The Hague 1971).

COHEN, B.: Is there a relationship between birth month and maternal ABO blood type?
Amer. J. hum. Genet. 20: 197 (1968).

COLLMAN, R.D. and STOLLER, A.: A survey of mongoloid births in Victoria, Australia,
1942–1957. Amer. J. pbl. Hlth 52: 813 (1962).

COURT-BROWN, W.M.; HARNDEN, D.G.; JACOBS, P.A., et al.: Abnormalities of the sex
chromosome complement in man. Spec. Rep. Ser. Med. Res. Coun., No. 305 (1964).

DALÉN, P.: Month of birth and schizophrenia. Acta psychiat. scand. Suppl. 203: 55 (1968).

DOORNBOS, K.: Geboortemaand en schoolsucces. (Wolters-Noordhoff NV, (Groningen
1971).

DUDLEY, F.J.; FOX, R.A., and SHERLOCK, S.: Cellular immunity and hepatitis-associated,
Australia antigen liver disease. Lancet i: 723 (1972).

Editorial: Brit. med. J. i: 695 (1958).

Editorial: Brit. med. J. ii: 1041 (1962).

EDWARDS, J.H.: Seasonal incidence of congenital disease in Birmingham. Ann. hum.
Genet. 25: 89 (1961).

EMME, A.M.: Photoperiodic response in reproduction. Russ. Rev. Biol. 49: 223 (1960).

EYK, H.H. van: De tweekoppigheid der geboortecurve. Ned. T. Geneesk. 40: 1304 (1904).

ENGLE, E.T. and SHELESNYAK, M.C.: First menstruation and subsequent menstrual cycles
of pubertal girls. Human Biol. 6: 431 (1934).

FITT, A.B.: Seasonal influence on growth function and inheritance. New Zealand Council for Educ. Res. Ser., No.17 (Oxford University Press, London 1941).

FRØLAND, A.: Seasonal dependence in birth of patients with Klinefelter's syndrome. Lancet *ii:* 771 (1967).

GIUSTINO, V.; DUDLEY, F.J., and SHERLOCK, S.: Thymus-dependent lymphocyte function in patients with hepatitis-associated antigen. Lancet *ii:* 850 (1972).

GREENBERG, R.C.: Two factors influencing the birth of mongols to younger mothers. Med. Offr. *109:* 62 (1963).

GROOT, M.J.W. DE: Epidemiologische aspecten van de aangeboren misvormingen. Huisarts en wetenschap *8:* 121, 176, 211 (1965).

HAMERSMA, K.: Anencephalie en spina bifida (Romijn, Apeldoorn 1966).

HARE, E.H. and PRICE, J.S.: Mental disorder and season of birth; comparison of psychoses with neurosis. Brit. J. Psychiat. *115:* 533 (1968).

HARE, E.H.; PRICE, J.S., and SLATER, E.: Schizophrenia and season of birth. Brit. J. Psychiat. *120:* 124 (1972).

HARTMAN, C.G.: Studies in the reproduction of the monkey *Macacus rhesus* with special reference to menstruation and pregnancy. Contrib. Embryol. Carneg. Inst. *23:* 38 (1932).

HOLLAND, W.W.; DOLL, R., and CARTER, C.O.: The mortality from leukaemia and other cancers among patients with Down's syndrome and among their parents. Brit. J. Cancer *16:* 177 (1962).

HUNTINGTON, E.: Season of birth (J. Wiley & Sons, Chichester 1938).

INGALLS, T.: Maternal health and mongolism. Lancet *ii:* 213 (1972).

JANERICH, D.T.; PORTER, J.H., and LOGRILLO, V.: Season of birth and neonatal mortality. Amer. J. publ. Hlth *61:* 1119 (1971).

JONGBLOET, P.H.: Overripeness of the egg. Maandschr. Kindergeneesk. *36:* 352 (1968). cf. IDEM. Chapter 1 in Mental and physical handicaps in connection with overripeness ovopathy (H.E. Stenfert Kroese N.V., Leiden 1971).

JONGBLOET, P.H.: The intriguing phenomenon of gametopathy and its disastrous effects on the human progeny. Maandschr. Kindergeneesk. *37:* 261 (1969).

JONGBLOET, P.H.: An investigation into the occurrence of overripeness ovopathy in the normal population. Maandschr. Kindergeneesk. *38:* 228 (1970).

JONGBLOET, P.H.: Month of birth and gametopathy. Clin. Genet. *2:* 315 (1971a).

JONGBLOET, P.H.: Status Bonnevie-Ullrich and Turner's syndrome. Overripeness ovopathy as a unifying concept. Parts 1 and 2 Mental and physical handicaps in connection with overripeness ovopathy (H.E. Stenfert Kroese, Leiden 1971b).

JONGBLOET, P.H.: Diagnostic criteria for overripeness ovopathy. Maandschr. Kindergeneesk. *39:* 251 (1971c).

KAPLAN, A.R. and ZSAKO, S.: Biological variables associated with mothers of children affected with G_1-trisomy syndrome. Amer. J. ment. Defic. *4:* 745 (1970).

KIRCHOFF, H.: Jahreszeiten und Belichtungen in ihrem Einfluss auf weibliche Genitalfunktionen. Arch. Gynäk. *163:* 141 (1937).

KNOBLOCH, H. and PASAMANICK, B.: Seasonal variation in the birth of the mentally deficient. Amer. J. publ. Hlth *48:* 201 (1958).

KOBAYASHI, N.; FURUKAWA, T., and TAKATSU, T.: Congenital anomalies in children with malignancy. Paediat. jap. *16:* 31 (1968).

KÖNIG, K.: Der Mongolismus (Hippokrates-Verlag, Stuttgart 1959).

LANDER, E.; FORSSMAN, H., and AKESSON, H.O.: Season of birth and mental deficiency. Acta genet., Basel *14:* 265 (1964).

LECK, I.: Incidence and epidemicity of Down's syndrome. Lancet *ii:* 457 (1966).

LILIENFELD, A.M.: Epidemiology of mongolism (Hopkins Press, Baltimore 1969).

LINDSTEN, J.: The nature and origin of X chromosome aberrations in Turner's syndrome. A cytogenetical and clinical study of 57 patients. (Almqvist & Wiksell, Stockholm 1963).

LISCHNER, H.W.: DiGeorge syndrome(s). J. Pediat. *81:* 1042 (1972).

McDONALD, A.D.: Seasonal distribution of abortions. Brit. J. prev. soc. Med. *25:* 222 (1971).

McDONALD, A.D.: Yearly and seasonal incidence of mongolism in Quebec. Teratology *6:* 1 (1972).

MENSER, M.A. and PURVIS-SMITH, S.G.: Dermatoglyphic defects in children with leukaemia. Lancet *i:* 1076 (1969).

MIKAMO, K.: Mechanism of non-disjunction of meiotic chromosomes and of degeneration of maturation spindles in eggs affected by intrafollicular overripeness. Experientia *24:* 75 (1968).

MILIC, A.B. and ADAMSONS, K.: The relationship between anencephaly and prolonged pregnancy. J. Obstet. Gynaec. Brit. Cwlth *76:* 102 (1969).

MILLER, R.W.: Childhood cancer and congenital defects. Pediat. Res. *3:* 389 (1969).

MILLER, R.W.: Neoplasia and Down's syndrome. Ann. N.Y. Acad. Sci. *171:* 637 (1971).

MILLER, D.R.; NEWSTEAD, G.J., and YOUNG, L.W.: Perinatal leukemia with a possible variant of the Ellis-van Creveld syndrome. J. Pediat. *74:* 300 (1969).

MUTTON, D.E.: Origin of the trisomic 21 chromosome. Lancet *i:* 375 (1973).

NIELSEN, J. and FRIEDRICH, U.: Seasonal variation in non-disjunction of sex chromosomes. Human Genet. *8:* 258 (1969).

NOMURA, T.; OHSAWA, N.; TAJIMA, Y.; TANAKA, T.; KOTERA, S.; ANDO, A., and NIGI, H.: Reproduction of Japanese monkeys; in DICZFALUSY and STANDLEY The use of non-human primates in research on human reproduction. Proc. Symp. WHO in collaboration with the Ministry of Health of the USSR, Sukhumi 1971. Acta endocrin., Kbh. Suppl. *166:* 473 (1972).

NORRIS, A.S. and CHOWNING, J.R.: Season of birth and mental illness. Arch. gen. Psychiat. *7:* 206 (1962).

ORME, J.E.: Intelligence, season of birth. Brit. J. med. Psychol. *25:* 233 (1962).

ORME, J.E.: Intelligence, season of birth, and climatic temperature. Brit. J. Psychol. *54:* 273 (1963).

ORME, J.E.: Ability and season of birth. Brit. J. Psychol. *56:* 471 (1965).

OVERBEKE, J.: Anencephalie in Nederland, 1951–1968 (Staatsuitgeverij, The Hague 1971).

PFEIFFER, R.A.: Die kriminologische Bedeutung der Chromosomenanomalien. Kriminol. Gegenwartsfragen *9:* 119 (1971).

PRIEST, J.H.: Parental dermatoglyphs in age-independent mongolism. J. med. Genet. *6:* 304 (1969).

ROBINSON, J.: Origin of the trisomic 21 chromosome. Lancet *i:* 131 (1973).

SAUVAGE-NOLTING, W.J.J. DE: Considerations regarding the possible relation between the vitamin C content of the blood of pregnant women and schizophrenia, debilitas mentis, and psychopathia. Folia psychiat. neerl. *57:* 347 (1954).

SAUVAGE-NOLTING, W. J. J. DE: Seasonal variations in birth-rates of cancer patients. Int. J. Biometeor. *12:* 293 (1968).

SCHULZ, F. W. und HIENZ, H. A.: Zur Häufigkeit gonosomaler Chromosomenaberrationen beim Menschen. Med. Welt., Stg. *39:* 2105 (1969).

SLATIS, H. M. and DE CLOUX, R. J.: Seasonal variation in stillbirth frequencies. Human Biol. *39:* 284 (1967).

STARK, C. R. and MANTEL, N.: Lack of seasonal- or temporal-spatial clustering of Down's syndrome births in Michigan. Amer. J. Epidem. *86:* 199 (1967).

STARK, C. R. and MANTEL, N.: Maternal-age and birth-order effects in childhood leukemia. J. nat. Cancer Inst. *42:* 857 (1969).

STEINBACH, J. and BALOGUN, A. A.: Seasonal variations in the conception rate of beef cattle in the seasonal-equatorial climate of Southern Nigeria. Int. J. Biometeor. *15:* 71 (1971).

STEWART, A. M. and DRAPER, G. J.: X-rays and childhood cancer. Lancet *ii:* 828 (1968).

STEWART, A. M.; WEBB, J., and HEWITT, D.: A survey of childhood malignancies. Brit. med. J. *i:* 495 (1958).

TIMONEN, S.; FRANZAS, B., and WICHMANN, K.: Photosensibility of the human pituitary. Ann. Chir. Gynaec. Fenn. *53:* 165 (1964).

TÜNTE, W. and NIERMANN, H.: Incidence of Klinefelter's syndrome and seasonal variation. Lancet *i:* 641 (1968).

UOHASHI, T.: The EEG in cases of Down's syndrome. Bull. Osaka med. Sch. *16:* 1 (1970).

VAN DEN BERGHE, H.; FRIJNS, J. P., and VERRESEN, H.: Congenital leukaemia with 46, XX,t (Bq+, Cq–) cells. J. med. Genet. *9:*468 (1972).

Vital and Health Statistics: Seasonal variation of births, United States, 1933–1963, ser. 21, No. 9 (National Center for Health Statistics, Washington 1966).

WAHRMAN, J. and FRIED, K.: The Jerusalem prospective newborn survey of mongolism. Ann. N. Y. Acad. Sci. *171:* 341 (1971).

WERTELECKI, W.; FRAUMENI, J. F., and MULVIHILL, J. J.: Nongonadal neoplasia in Turner's syndrome. Cancer, Philad. *26:* 286 (1970).

WILLIAMS, P.: Date of birth, backwardness and educational organization. Brit. J. educ. Psychol. *34:* 247 (1964).

WITSCHI, E.; NELSON, W. C., and SEGAL, S. J.: Genetic developmental and hormonal aspects of gonadal dysgenesis and sexinversion in man. J. clin. Endocrin. *17:* 737 (1957).

WOLDA, G.: Akklimatisierung und Deklimatisierung. Genetica, s'Gravenh. *9:* 157 (1927).

WOLDA, G.: Interperiodizität. Genetica, s'Gravenh. *11:*453 (1929).

ZÜBLIN, W.: Chromosomale Aberrationen und Psyche (Karger, Basel 1969).

Author's address: Dr. P. H. JONGBLOET, Huize 'Maria Roepaan', Institute for Observation and Treatment of the Mentally Retarded, Siebengewaldseweg 15, *Ottersum* (The Netherlands)

Aging Gametes. Int. Symp., Seattle 1973, pp. 330–348 (Karger, Basel 1975)

The Epidemiology of Human Spontaneous Abortions with Chromosomal Anomalies

J. Boué, A. Boué and P. Lazar

Centre International de l'Enfance, Laboratoire de la SESEP, Paris, et Unité de Recherches Statistiques, Institut Gustave Roussy, Villejuif

The various aspects of aging of gametes have been recognized in mammals as possible predisposing factors to reproductive failures, especially those involving chromosome anomalies. To study these phenomena in the human is extremely difficult. Malformations of some kind are present in 2–3% of newborn infants; their causes, for the most part, are obscure, and only 0.5% of newborn infants have chromosome anomalies. Epidemiologic studies on events that may predispose toward the birth of infants with chromosome anomalies must pool case reports from different sources in order to accumulate a sufficient number of observations. Consequently, the evaluation of the data becomes very difficult. Certain types of aging of gametes are very difficult to specify in humans on account of the nature of their sexual physiology. Furthermore, the information gathered requires recall of events long past in a domain in which precise data are always difficult to obtain.

It seemed to us that epidemiological studies on early spontaneous abortions might constitute a more rewarding approach to the problem for the following reasons: (a) there is a high frequency of chromosome anomalies in abortions; (b) these anomalies may result from a variety of mechanisms, and (c) information obtained at the time of the abortion concerning the conceptional period is more reliable because it is more recent.

The majority of the chromosomal studies on human spontaneous abortions have been based on too few observations to permit an epidemiologic study on a single series. The cytogenetic survey of 1,500 abortuses that was carried out in our laboratory from 1966 to 1972, however, provides the material for both retrospective and prospective epidemiological studies.

I. Population Studied

We studied abortions in which the development of the embryo was less than 12 weeks (14 weeks gestational age). This limit was chosen for two reasons: (1) such abortions represent at least 80% of all spontaneous abortions, and (2) pathologic studies have clearly demonstrated that it is in these abortions that abnormalities in the development of the embryo are the most frequent [Mikamo, 1970; Miller and Poland, 1970]; thus these are the abortions that are most likely to be due to zygotic causes. In our experience gestational age is a poor criterion by which to date the conceptus. This figure may be inexact because the interval between the last menstrual period and conception is not known, and the length of time the conceptus is retained in the uterus may be very long, as much as an average of 7 weeks after the arrest of development.

Table I shows the number of specimens per year that have been karyotyped and the proportion of chromosomal anomalies. A certain number of provoked abortions were undoubtedly included in our study during the first 2 years since the majority of abortions analyzed came from public hospitals. Consequently, the proportion of chromosomal anomalies rose. In the following years the proportion remained stable. Efforts have been made to (a) obtain specimens from abortions that occurred at home (a special flask is given to the patient when she consults her obstetrician for a threatened abortion), and (b) have the specimens brought to the laboratory by a member of the patient's family.

Table I. Number of specimens from spontaneous abortions studied from 1965 to 1972

Year	Number of abortuses karyotyped	Abnormal karyotype	
		number	%
1965	4	1	
1966	57	27	47.3
1967	84	42	50.0
1968	170	100	64.7
1969	264	165	62.5
1970	343	212	61.8
1971	362	226	62.5
1972	214	138	64.4
Total	1,498	921	61.48

This change in collection technique accounts for the increase in frequency of anomalies since very few provoked abortions were collected and a great number of early specimens were obtained.

II. Methods of Inquiry

Retrospective study: At the time of the abortion (before the karyotype of the abortus is known) a questionnaire is completed by the parents. This questionnaire contains numerous questions concerning the medical histories of the 2 parents, the gynecological and obstetrical history of the mother, and, if feasible, the circumstances surrounding conception (temperature curves, date of ovulation, dates of sexual intercourse . . .).

Prospective studies: Two prospective studies have been carried out: one in May, 1971 [BOUÉ *et al.*, 1973] and a second in October, 1972 in which a questionnaire was sent to women who had previously had abortions karyotyped in our laboratory.

III. Frequency of Chromosomal Anomalies in Abortuses and Estimation of their Frequency at the Time of Conception

Table II shows the results of chromosomal analysis of the 1,498 abortuses studied; 921 of them had chromosome anomalies. Several observations emerge from a study of table II. Structural anomalies were observed in 3.8% of abortuses with anomalies. In only one third of these observations was the anomaly transmitted by one of the parents. So nearly all these chromosomal aberrations are the results of errors either at the time of gametogenesis or at the time of fertilization.

The chromosomal anomalies observed at birth are much less frequent than those revealed in early spontaneous abortions, and those in early spontaneous abortions represent only a portion of the total number of anomalies conceived. An estimation of this total will be attempted based on data from the karyotypic analysis of our survey study, in particular that concerning chromosomal nondisjunctions.

Monosomies, almost exclusively monosomy X, are 15% of the anomalies encountered. Only one autosomal monosomy has been observed. Autosomal trisomies are very frequent and account for more than half of the anomalies observed. The relative frequency of the different trisomies varies al-

Table II. Karyotypes of 1,498 abortuses studied from 1965 to 1972

	Number		%
Normal	577		38.52
Abnormal	921		61.48

Details of abnormal karyotypes

Monosomy			
45,X	140	} 141	15.30
45,G–	1		
Trisomy			
A+	12		
B+	6		
C+	86		
D+	109	} 479	52.00
E+	172		
F+	7		
G+	87		
Double trisomy	16		1.73
Triploidy			
XXY	92		
XYY	7	} 183	19.86
XXX	57		
Unkaryotyped	27		
Tetraploidy	57		6.18
Translocations	35		3.80
Mosaicism	10		1.08

though trisomies A, B, and F are consistently rare and trisomies D, E, and G are common.

Formerly cytogenetic techniques could not in general distinguish individual chromosomes within the same group except for trisomy 16 (E), which could be identified by the standard staining technique. Trisomy 16 is the most frequently encountered trisomy in abortions. We have observed that trisomy 16 accounts for about 14% of the total of the anomalies found in these abortions.

It can thus be seen that the only two anomalies resulting from a chromosomal nondisjunction for which a precise identification has been possible, monosomies X and trisomies 16, are present in similar numbers, each one representing about 15% of the anomalies observed. The observations on the relative frequencies of the various anomalies that result from chromosomal nondisjunction at meiosis and on the high frequency of monosomy X and trisomy 16 have been confirmed in all the surveys. The identification of chromosomes by banding techniques has confirmed the exactitude of these observations.

To account for the absence of autosomal monosomies and the low frequency of certain trisomies it has been suggested that these anomalies must lead to a very early developmental arrest, most of the zygotes being eliminated before the pregnancy is recognized. This postulation is supported by morphological examination of zygotes with rare chromosome anomalies; they show very precocious developmental arrests, either a complete absence of embryonic formation (blighted ovum) or a malformed embryonic formation only a few millimeters long [BOUÉ and BOUÉ, 1970]. This hypothesis of precocious elimination of zygotes with autosomal monosomies and certain autosomal trisomies has recently been experimentally confirmed in translocated mice (Mus poschiavinus) by GROPP [1973] and FORD and EVANS [1973].

If one accepts the hypothesis that meiotic nondisjunction (in male or in female) occurs with equal probability for each chromosome pair, an identical number of zygotes should be conceived with monosomy and trisomy for each chromosome pair and, in accordance with the observations of FORD and GROPP, most of these would be eliminated before pregnancy becomes evident. Thus, the total number of monosomies and trisomies conceived can be estimated from the data for monosomy X and trisomy 16, assuming an equal frequency of nondisjunction for the other chromosome pairs.

In general, 15% of clinically recognized pregnancies terminate in abortion. (This figure is higher in prospective studies.) Thus for every 1,000 clinically recognized pregnancies there are 850 births and 150 abortions. Of these 150 abortions, we know that 60% (about 100) have a chromosome anomaly. Among these 100 anomalies there are 15 monosomies X and 15 trisomies 16 on the average. This leads to an estimate of $15 \times 23 = 345$ monosomies and $15 \times 23 = 345$ trisomies or a total of 690 anomalies resulting from meiotic nondisjunction. To this figure can be added the other chromosome anomalies observed in abortions (table II), in particular the triploidies, which accounts for about 20% of the anomalies found in abortions. A number of factors lead one to believe that there are many more 69,XYY karyotypes than have actually been observed. Statistical studies on the frequency of the different types of triploidy vary according to the responsible mechanism (diandry or digyny [BOUÉ *et al.*, 1967; SCHINDLER and MIKAMO, 1970]. Laboratory studies encounter great difficulties in culturing 69,XYY cells and consequently are not a fruitful source of information. When the other anomalies are added to the 690 trisomies and monosomies, the resulting figure for total chromosome anomalies conceived is quite close to that of the 850 births at term, an estimate in agreement with those deduced from other observations on humans. The fundamental work of HERTIG [1967], who was the first to measure the extent of these errors of reproduction at a time when chromosomal anomalies were still unknown, consisted of an anatomical study of zygotes of 1–17 days development. In examining these zygotes, which he collected from hysterectomies performed on women of normal fertility, he was able to demonstrate a high frequency of abnormal zygotes. He estimated that in couples of proven fertility in cases in which the ovum had definitely been in contact with spermatozoa, only 30–50% of the zygotes are of 'good quality' and will go to term.

More recently, new staining techniques have made possible the recognition of certain chromosomes in human spermatozoa; first the Y chromosome by fluorescence techniques, then chromosome 9 by Giemsa staining at pH 11.6. PAWLOWITZSKI and PEARSON [1972] have demonstrated the presence of either 2 Y chromosomes or 2 chromosomes 9 in spermatozoa in which DNA estimation showed a haploid constitution. In extrapolating these results to the rest of the chromosomes, they compute the frequency of such abnormal spermatozoa to be as high as 38%.

The results of all these different approaches to an estimation of the frequency of errors of reproduction are in agreement. The figures are perforce imprecise considering the data on which they are based, but they give an idea of the order of magnitude of these chromosomal accidents that lead to reproductive failure; about one conception out of every two. Although this estimate may be valid for the population as a whole, for each couple the risk of conceiving zygotes with chromosomal anomalies is extremely variable. These variations have been revealed by a study of the obstetric events preceding or following the abortions that have been analyzed in our laboratory.

In this study 43 cases in which two consecutive karyotyped abortions occurred were analyzed [BOUÉ and BOUÉ, 1973 b]. Retrospective analysis of the obstetrical history of these women showed one or more deliveries at term in 17/43 (39.5%) and one or more spontaneous abortions in 27/43 (62.7%). In a control group composed of 590 women with only one karyotyped abortion (this being already a high-risk group), 46% had had one or more deliveries at term and 41% one or more abortions.

Table III. Frequency of recurring spontaneous abortions in relation to obstetrical history

Obstetrical events before the karyotyped abortion	Frequency of abortion in the following pregnancy	
	number of pregnancies	abortions, %
No obstetrical event	146	13.9
Delivery, one or more without previous spontaneous abortion	97	11.4
Spontaneous abortion, one or more with or without delivery	184	24.3

Prospective studies on the outcome of pregnancies following a spontaneous abortion have clearly shown a difference between women with no previous history of abortion (excepting the karyotyped abortion studied) and those with previous abortions. Whether or not there had been previous pregnancies to term the frequency of subsequent abortion in the former group is less than 15%, whereas in the group of women with a history of previous abortion (with or without pregnancy to term) the subsequent abortion frequency is about 25% (table III). One might therefore suppose that in a given couple there exists predisposing factors for these accidents that lead to repeated abortions.

IV. Epidemiologic Study of Predisposing Factors

The epidemiologic study that we have undertaken is an attempt to reveal possible predisposing factors; some of these factors may have only a transitory influence whereas others, because of their constant presence, may be primary causes of repeated abortions.

One of the most troublesome problems in such an epidemiologic study is the absence of a control group of normal pregnancies. To obviate the lack of this control group, we have compared two groups: abortions with normal karyotype and those with abnormal karyotype. As for the group with normal karyotype we do not really know what is included in the classification 'apparently normal'. Abortions with a conceptus of normal karyotype, due to nonzygotic factors, certainly exist, yet often the pathologic examination reveals morphologic anomalies comparable to those found in a conceptus with chromosomal aberrations, implicating a zygotic cause. Certain structural anomalies of chromosomes (such as small deletions or pericentric inversions) were not revealed by cytogenetic techniques until recently, and lesions at the level of the gene itself must also be responsible for development arrests. For these reasons the 'normal karyotype' group cannot be considered a well-defined entity.

V. Maternal Age

The increased incidence of mongolism with advancing maternal age is based on well-substantiated observations. The analysis of the maternal age distribution of mongoloid children has shown a bimodality in the curve of maternal age distribution, an early peak for the younger mothers and a later large peak for the older ones. PENROSE and SMITH [1966] have shown that this bimodal curve can be broken down into 2 curves corresponding to 2 different classes of risk of having a mongoloid child: class A, in which the risk is independent of maternal age, and class B, which is age-dependent.

Similarly, there appears to be a maternal age effect in Patau's syndrome (trisomy 13) and in Edwards' syndrome (trisomy 18) [HAMERTON, 1971]. As for the sex chromosome aberrations, maternal age influence has been demonstrated for XXY males and XXX females [COURT-BROWN et al., 1969] but not for Turner's syndrome (monosomy X).

Studies of chromosomal anomalies in abortions should shed more light on the influence of maternal age on the incidence of these anomalies. The first series of karyotyped abortions showed that the average maternal age is higher in abortions with chromosomal anomalies than in those with normal karyotype, in which the average maternal age is about the same as that for normal infants (table IV) [ARAKAKI and WAXMAN, 1970; CARR, 1967; LAZAR et al., 1971].

Analysis of maternal age in relation to the different types of anomaly,

Table IV. Comparison of the mean maternal age in abortions with normal and abnormal karyotypes

Study		Abortuses with normal karyotype	Abortuses with abnormal karyotype
CARR [1967]	n = 195	27.1	28.9
ARAKAKI [1970]	n = 127	27.2	28.3
BOUÉ [1970]	n = 1374	27.51	29.48

Table V. Maternal and paternal ages in relation to the different types of chromosomal anomalies

Karyotype	Number	Mean maternal age, years	Number	Mean paternal age, years
Monosomy X	134	27.57 ± 0.88	104	29.48 ± 1.10
Autosomal trisomy	448	31.25 ± 0.60	345	33.54 ± 0.72
Triploidy	167	27.38 ± 0.79	131	30.44 ± 1.04
Tetraploidy	53	26.79 ± 1.40	40	29.38 ± 1.71
Translocation	26	26.96 ± 2.32	23	28.04 ± 1.77
Normal	509	27.48 ± 0.45	343	30.57 ± 0.64

Table VI. Maternal age in abortuses with autosomal trisomies

Karyotype	Number	Mean maternal age, years
47,A+	13	29.62 ± 2.18
47,B+	7	33.43 ± 7.13
47,C+	72	30.93 ± 1.67
47,D+	92	32.49 ± 1.33
47,E+	157	29.58 ± 0.88
47,F+	8	30.13 ± 5.32
47,G+	78	33.17 ± 1.40
48	14	35.00 ± 6.09

however, indicates clear differences. No maternal age influence can be demonstrated for monosomy X, triploidies, tetraploidies, or translocations. An age influence is found only for the autosomal trisomy group, for which the mean maternal age is 31.25 as compared to 27–27.5 for the other categories (table V). The large number of trisomies permits a more detailed analysis of maternal age (table VI). It can be seen that it is primarily the trisomies involving acrocentric chromosomes in which the influence of maternal age is marked. For the other trisomies this influence is less significant, especially in trisomy E (most of which are trisomies 16). Average maternal age is most markedly increased (35 years) for the double trisomies; among these are 5 in which both supplementary chromosomes are acrocentric and 8 in which one of them is an acrocentric chromosome.

The maternal age distribution can best be illustrated graphically. In each group of abortuses, the observations were separated into two classes: class A, in which the risk is independent of maternal age, and class B, which includes

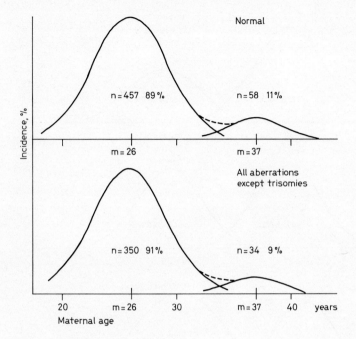

Fig. 1. Maternal age percentage distributions of abortuses with normal karyotype and abortuses with monosomy X, triploidy, tetraploidy and translocations.

the age-dependent cases. The mean maternal age for the class A curve is about 26.5 years, and for class B 37.5 years (fig. 1, 2).

Figure 1 shows the curves of maternal age distribution in abortuses with normal karyotype and in the group of abortuses with monosomy X, triploidy, tetraploidy, and translocations. The distribution is very similar in the 2 populations. Class B observations represent around 10% and seem mostly linked to the incidence of all the conceptions that normally give an asymmetric distribution that shows an excess in the older maternal age group.

The curves of maternal age distribution of abortuses with trisomy (fig. 2) show that class B includes 37% of the cases. When the curves of maternal age distribution are established for trisomy D and trisomy G the differences are more striking. The maternal age distribution of 79 cases of trisomy G shows a pattern that is very similar to the observations of PENROSE and SMITH [1966], who found that 60.2% of 9,441 cases of Down's syndrome belong to the age-dependent group (class B). In our series this percentage is 62%.

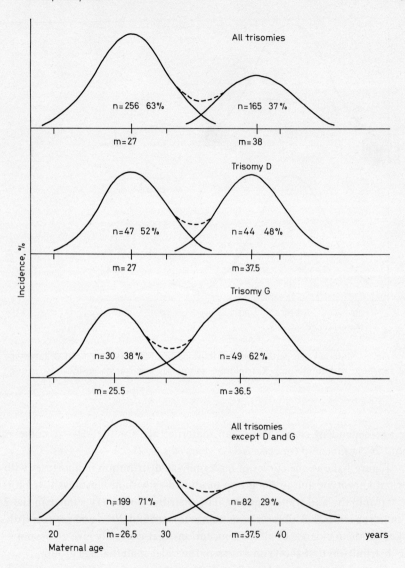

Fig. 2. Maternal age percentage distributions of abortuses with trisomies. Hypothetic distribution in two classes: A, independent of age; B, age-dependent. For further details see text.

When such curves are established for the total number of trisomies minus D and G trisomies, the age-dependent group includes only 29% of the cases. It should be noted that this group includes most of the double trisomies, many of which involve an acrocentric chromosome.

Studies on the maternal age distribution in spontaneous abortions permit the clarification of several important points. The magnitude of maternal age influence can be adequately assessed. There is no influence of maternal age in many anomalies: monosomy X, triploidy, and tetraploidy. The mean maternal age in tetraploidy seems to be even lower than that of control groups; however, the number of observations is not large enough for the difference to be significant.

Some trisomies are clearly influenced by maternal age, but the proportion that is age-dependent varies for each kind of trisomy: less than 30% for trisomies A, B, C, E, and F, 48% for trisomy D, and 62% for trisomy G (for some groups of trisomies the number of observations is so small that it is impossible to draw definitive conclusions). Thus, the age influence is preponderant only in trisomies of the acrocentric chromosomes.

The striking agreement between the class A and class B curves for Down's syndrome and in abortuses with trisomy G demonstrates that whether a zygote with trisomy G evolved towards a spontaneous abortion or a delivery at term does not depend on the age of the mother.

Paternal age: Table V shows the mean paternal age in relation to the karyotype of the abortus. So far no influence of paternal age has been demonstrated in relation to chromosomal aberrations.

VI. Delays at the Time of Conceptions

In the human species it is extremely difficult to assemble a large number of observations in which a delay in fertilization involving aging of the gametes can be demonstrated. We have attempted this analysis, however, utilizing the questionnaires that are filled out by the parents at the time of the abortion when the karyotype of the abortus is still unknown.

In an early study of 530 observations we had analyzed the characteristics of the menstrual cycles in the months before the conception of the karyotyped abortus (regularity and length). No influence of regularity or irregularity of the cycles was found, but a group of 72 women was selected on the basis of a minimum length of 32 days of the menstrual cycle and in this group the percentage of abortuses with chromosomal anomalies was 78%, com-

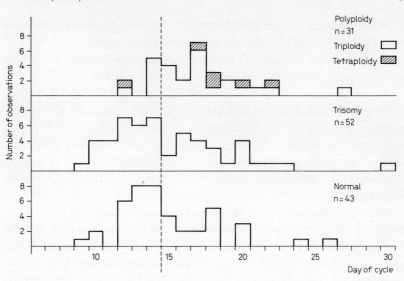

Fig. 3. Distribution of presumed day of ovulation in relation to the karyotype of the abortus.

pared with 62% in the 458 controls. In these 72 women, 20 were more than 30 years old, the chromosomal anomalies were age-dependent, and 14 trisomies were observed. In the 52 younger women (less than 30 years old) an increase in the frequency of polyploidy was noted: 9 triploidies and 4 tetraploidies, 25% in contrast to 16% polyploidies in the controls.

To try to clarify this point we then analyzed all the questionnaires of the study to select the cases in which it was plausible to suppose that fertilization occurred at the time of ovulation. In these cases the date of ovulation was usually estimated from temperature curves, and the couples had daily intercourse during this period or kept a record of the dates of intercourse. We compared the interval between the first day of the last menstrual period and the probable date of ovulation for the various different classes of chromosomal anomalies (fig. 3). The average interval found in this first part of the cycle was 14.95 days for normal karyotypes and 15.0 days for trisomies. For polyploidies (triploidies and tetraploidies), however, this interval was markedly longer: 17.06 days. A detailed analysis of these results has been attempted, even though the number of cases is not large enough to yield significant differences. When we compared warm season conceptions (April to September) with those occurring during the colder months (October to March),

Table VII. Seasonal influence on the presumed day of ovulation in relation to the karyotype of the abortus

Karyotype of the abortus	Mean day of ovulation			
	conceptions from April to September		conceptions from October to March	
Normal	14.3	(20)	15.6	(23)
Trisomy	14.0	(25)	15.4	(28)
Triploidy, tetraploidy	15.5	(14)	18.3	(18)

Number of observations in parentheses.

we found that the presumed date of ovulation is generally later in winter. This difference is small for normal and trisomic karyotypes but especially marked in the cases of polyploidy (table VII). These observations suggest that a delay in the presumed date of ovulation may play a role in the determination of polyploidies. This delay may reflect an anomaly of ovulation leading to intrafollicular overripeness.

Through an analysis of the questionnaires we have also looked for delays between ovulation and fertilization. Only cases in which a temperature curve was available and in which the dates of intercourse of the couples seemed sufficiently reliable were studied. There were only 24 observations in which there were intervals of 2 days or more before or after the probable date of ovulation and the possible day of fertilization. Karyotypes of the abortuses were: 5 normal, 1 monosomy X, 11 autosomal trisomies, 6 triploidies, and one tetraploidy. The frequency of anomalies increased to 79% and there was an increased incidence of polyploidy.

These analyses suggest that when delay in fertilization can be demonstrated there seems to be an influence primarily on those mechanisms that lead to the formation of polyploidies.

VII. Conceptions after Oral Contraceptives

It has been supposed that abnormalities in the maturation of the oocytes during the first cycles following contraceptive steroid treatment might reproduce conditions that are favorable to the occurrence of accidents that may lead to chromosome anomalies. This effect was first suggested by CARR [1970] who collected 54 karyotyped abortions from women who conceived

Table VIII. Chromosomal anomalies in abortuses from women who conceived after an inhibition of ovulation (physiologic or therapeutic)

Karyotype of abortuses	Normal delivery		Spontaneous abortion		Oral contraception		Controls	
	0–6 months	7–12 months	0–6 months	7–12 months	0–6 months	7–12 months	inhibition of ovulation > 12 mos	no previous inhibition of ovulation
Normal	9 (36)	10 (31)	22 (33)	24 (35)	20 (32)	11 (38)	82 (35)	75 (41)
Monosomy	2	4	6	5	5	4	26	16
Trisomy	11	12	29	25	23	11	79	55
Triploidy	1 ⎱ (12)	6 ⎱ (19)	9 ⎱ (16)	10 ⎱ (21)	11 ⎱ (20)	2 ⎱ (10)	37 ⎱ (19)	22 ⎱ (18)
Tetraploidy	2 ⎰	0 ⎰	2 ⎰	5 ⎰	2 ⎰	1 ⎰	8 ⎰	11 ⎰
Translocation	0	0	1	0	2	0	1	1
Total	25	32	68	70	63	29	233	180

Percentages in parentheses.

within 6 months of the discontinuation of oral contraceptive treatment. He concluded: 'Chromosome analysis of the abortuses showed an increase in triploidy which was highly significant statistically when compared with a control series.'

Among our observations there were 520 in which conception followed a period of inhibition of ovulation, either physiologic or therapeutic (180 after pregnancy with birth at term, 220 after pregnancy terminating in spontaneous abortion, and 120 after steroid contraceptives).

Table VIII gives the frequency of abortuses with normal karyotype according to the cause of inhibition of ovulation and according to the time elapsed between cessation of treatment and conception. No significant difference has been shown. Abortions following a conception occurring 0–6 months after discontinuation of treatment are more numerous (63 abortuses) than those occurring 6–12 months afterwards (29 abortuses), which is in correlation with the frequency of conception in the year following the cessation of treatment.

There is a slight difference in the frequencies of chromosomal anomalies among the 3 groups of women who had an inhibition of ovulation (either physiologic or therapeutic) and those who never had an ovulatory inhibition. This difference, which is very small, can be explained simply by the difference in average age of the groups of women (normal delivery, 30.46 years; spontaneous abortion, 30.13 years; oral contraceptives, 28.18 years; no ovulatory inhibition, 26.41 years).

The relative frequencies of each type of chromosomal anomaly are not different; in particular there is no significant increase in the frequency of polyploidy.

VIII. Discussion

In spite of the difficulties inherent in these studies, epidemiologic analysis of the observations of karyotyped spontaneous abortions reveals a certain amount of information on the influence of factors related to aging of gametes.

It must be emphasized that a comparison has been made between 2 categories of spontaneous abortions: those with normal karyotype and those with chromosome anomalies. In such studies it is impossible to establish a comparison with conceptions resulting in the birth of a normal infant at term; and the frequency of abortions in relation to conceptions is unknown. If such a comparative study were possible, the influence of some factors would probably become more evident.

In relation to the different types of chromosomal aberrations observed in spontaneous abortions some remarks can be made. In the case of monosomy X, no influence of a process of aging of gametes could be demonstrated, neither aging related to maternal age nor aging resulting from delays at the time of conception. This agrees well with observations in Turner's syndrome in which a study of the Xg^a antigen, which is an X-linked dominant character, has shown that about 74% of the patients have a maternal X chromosome [FRASER, 1963]. Along the same lines, the studies of PAWLOWITZKI and PEARSON [1972] have shown that about 1% of spermatozoa with a normal haploid DNA complement have 2 Y chromosomes; logically it might be postulated that there must exist an at least equivalent number of spermatozoa with no sex chromosome.

In the case of autosomal trisomies, the important role of aging of the oocyte has clearly been demonstrated for trisomies D and G. This selective activity on acrocentric chromosomes may be in favor of mechanisms involving an effect of aging on the nucleolus. The marked influence of maternal age on trisomies of acrocentric chromosomes in contrast to its minor influence on trisomies involving metacentric or telocentric chromosomes leads to possible speculation regarding the causes of these nondisjunctions. The mechanism that seems to fit in best with this selective action of aging has been proposed by FORD [1960], who implicates the nucleolus :'The acrocentric chromosomes remain attached to the nucleolus throughout interphase, and it is likely that its presence may interfere mechanically with their pairing in early meiotic prophase. So if an aging factor interferes with the rapid breakdown of the nucleolus in meiotic prophase of ovogenesis, nondisjunction of the associated chromosome pair would be increased.' Other processes of aging of gametes have not been demonstrated for trisomies, but theoretically this remains a possible mechanism for nondisjunction in the second meiotic division of the oocyte.

One must always remember that these trisomies may also result from nondisjunctions in the male gametes. The recent work of PAWLOWITZSKI and PEARSON [1972] demonstrated existence of spermatozoa with 2 chromosomes. It seems that chromosomal accidents of male gametogenesis are more sensitive to environmental influences, irradiations for instance [BOUÉ and LAZAR, personal observations].

In polyploidies (triploidy and tetraploidy) the studies fail to show any marked maternal age effect, but it seems that all events that may lead to delays at the time of fertilization increase the frequency of polyploidies. This has been observed (1) in young women with abnormally long menstrual cycles, or when the day of ovulation is later than normal, and (2) in observations in which a delay of 2 days or more between ovulation and fertilization has been suspected.

In CARR's observations a high frequency of polyploidy after steroid contraceptive treatment was noted in abortuses.

Recently, we have reported [BOUÉ and BOUÉ, 1973 a] an increased frequency of chromosomal anomalies after induced ovulation. In these observations it is mainly the frequency of polyploidy that is increased (17 polyploidies, 28%, in 61 cases in which drugs were given during either the cycle in which conception occurred or the cycle just previous to it).

These different observations have to be compared with laboratory studies in different animals in which experimental triploidy can be produced by various means.

IX. Conclusion

The high percentage of chromosomal disorders in human spontaneous abortions and the fact that some of these aberrations (such as polyploidy) are never seen in living newborns has permitted epidemiological studies that shed some light on predisposing factors linked to different processes of aging of gametes.

The role of maternal age, which had been previously clearly demonstrated in Down's syndrome, is significant only in trisomies and mainly in trisomies involving an acrocentric chromosome.

In spite of the difficulties inherent in epidemiological studies of human reproduction limiting the number of well-documented observations, different approaches show that disturbances in the timing of fertilization are conducive to the occurrence of polyploidy.

Acknowledgments

These studies have been supported by research grants from INSERM (Institut National de la Santé et de la Recherche Médicale) from DGRST (Délégation Générale à la Recherche Scientifique et Technique) and from private funds.

We are greatly indebted to NICOLE PERRAUDIN and CHRISTIANE DELUCHAT who provided fine technical assistance, to Mrs. S. GUEGUEN for her statistical work and to SUSAN CURE for her helpful assistance in writing the English text.

References

ARAKAKI, D.T. and WAXMAN, S.: Effect of gestational and maternal age in early abortion. Obstet. Gynec. *35*: 264 (1970).

BOUÉ, A. and BOUÉ, J.: Actions of steroid contraceptives on gametic material. Geburtsh. Frauenheilk. *33:* 77 (1973).

BOUÉ, J.G. et BOUÉ, A.: Les aberrations chromosomiques dans les avortements spontanés humains. Presse méd. *78:* 635 (1970).

BOUÉ, J.G. and BOUÉ, A.: Increased frequency of chromosomal anomalies in abortions after induced ovulation. Lancet *i:* 679 (1973a).

BOUÉ, J.G. and BOUÉ, A.: Chromosomal analysis of two consecutive abortuses in 43 women. Humangenetik *19:* 275 (1973b).

BOUÉ, J.G.; BOUÉ, A. et LAZAR, P.: Les aberrations chromosomiques dans les avortements. Ann. Génét. *10:* 179 (1967).

BOUÉ, J.G.; BOUÉ, A.; LAZAR, P., and GUEGUEN, S.: Outcome of pregnancies following a spontaneous abortion with chromosomal anomalies. Amer. J. Obstet. Gynec. *116:* 806 (1973).

CARR, D.H.: Chromosome anomalies as a cause of spontaneous abortion. Amer. J. Obstet. Gynec. *97:* 283 (1967).

CARR, D.H.: Chromosomal studies in selected spontaneous abortions. I. Conception after oral contraceptives. Canad. med. Ass. J. *103:* 343 (1970).

COURT-BROWN, W.M.; LAW, P., and SMITH, P.G.: Sex chromosome aneuploidy and parental age. Ann. hum. Genet. *33:* 1 (1969).

FORD, C.E.: Chromosomal abnormality and congenital malformation. Ciba Found. Symp. Congenital Malformations, p. 32 (J. & A. Churchill, London 1960).

FORD, C.E. and EVANS, E.P.: Non expression of genome imbalance in haplophase and early diplophase of the mouse and incidence of karyotypic abnormality in post-implantation embryos; in Chromosomal errors in relation to reproductive failure (INSERM, Paris 1973).

FRASER, G.R.: Parental origin of the sex chromosomes in the XO and XXY karyotypes in man. Ann. hum. Genet. *26:* 297 (1963).

GROPP, A.: Fetal mortality due to aneuploidy and irregular meiotic segregation in the mouse; in Chromosomal errors in relation to reproductive failure (INSERM, Paris 1973).

HAMERTON, J.L.: Human cytogenetics. II. Clinical cytogenetics (Academic Press, New York 1971).

HERTIG, A.T.: The overall problem in man; in Comparative aspects of reproductive failure, p.11 (Springer, Berlin 1967).

LAZAR, P.; GUEGUEN, S.; BOUÉ, G. et BOUÉ, A.: Sur la distribution des âges de 715 mères ayant eu un avortement spontané précoce. C.R. Acad. Sci. *272:* 2852 (1971).

MIKAMO, K.: Anatomic and chromosomal anomalies in spontaneous abortion. Amer. J. Obstet. Gynec. *106:* 243 (1970).

MILLER, J.R. and POLAND, B.J.: The value of human abortuses in the surveillance of development anomalies. I. General overview. Canad. med. Ass. J. *103:* 501 (1970).

PAWLOWITZKI, I.H. and PEARSON, P.L.: Chromosomal aneuploidy in human spermatozoa. Humangenetik *16:* 119 (1972).

PENROSE, L.S. and SMITH, G.F.: Down's anomaly (J. & A. Churchill, London 1966).

SCHINDLER, A.M. and MIKAMO, K.: Triploidy in man, report of a case and a discussion on etiology. Cytogenetics *9:* 116 (1970).

Authors' addresses: Dr. J. BOUÉ and Dr. A. BOUÉ, Centre International de l'Enfance, Laboratoire de la SESEP, Château de Longchamp, Bois de Boulogne, *75016 Paris;* Dr. P. LAZAR, Unité de Recherches Statistiques, Institut Gustave Roussy, *94800 Villejuif* (France)

Aging Gametes. Int. Symp., Seattle 1973, pp. 349–368 (Karger, Basel 1975)

Prenatal versus Postnatal Malformations Based on the Japanese Experience on Induced Abortions in the Human Being

Hideo Nishimura

Department of Anatomy, Faculty of Medicine, Kyoto University, Kyoto

I will first briefly cover the procedures used in our 10-year epidemiological teratological study on early human conceptuses mainly garnered from induced abortion, and some of its results; then, my further studies with the same materials relevant to the general topic of the aging of gametes. I chose such a scheme of presentation because I believe that the development of knowledge on overripeness of the gametes in man could benefit by specific techniques and that our approach might provide a clue as to how to attack an admittedly difficult problem.

I. Exploration into Early Overall Human Prenatal Populations

Most of the knowledge on normal and abnormal human development has been obtained through examination of the abortuses and stillborns of mothers with pathological conditions. Needless to say, more reliable standards of normal development should be established by observation of embryonic specimens from healthy pregnancies. It should be noted that malformations occur in most cases in the stage of organogenesis. It can be assumed that spontaneous termination of pregnancy occurs more frequently when fetuses with anomalies are present because aborted conceptuses show a very high frequency of structural abnormalities [reviewed by Stratford, 1970]. Therefore, the malformations found during the perinatal stage or in newborns are only one part of the whole range of maldevelopments. The real incidence of malformations can be found only by examining all embryos from all abortions. Certainly, a systematic survey of the occurrence of maldevelopments among specimens at the organogenic stage in relation to various parental factors would be an approach that has never been attempted.

Legal abortion in postwar Japan has provided an exceptional opportunity for human embryonic studies (Japanese Eugenic Protection Law in 1952). A large number of induced abortions have been performed mainly for socio-economic reasons. Interruption of the pregnancies in most abortion cases (more than 90%) has been accomplished by dilatation and curettage in the second to the fourth month of pregnancy, and a small number have been done by means of induced delivery at a later stage. Generally, the number of such operations has been far larger at private clinics than at municipal, national, or university hospitals. It occurred to me to conduct a systematic study on normal and abnormal development by using these embryonic specimens from almost unselected mothers. The aims of the project were: to establish more reliable normal standards as diagnostic criteria of embryonic materials; to find the real incidence of all anomalies and loss during the early gestational stage by thorough external and internal observations with the aid of histological studies; to monitor a potential role of some new teratogens by continued surveillance; to clarify the initiating processes of various anomalies and, in cases of specimens with multiple defects, to determine the successive chains of teratogenesis; to find the probable relationship between the occurrence of the specific type of anomalies and some genetic or extrinsic factors affecting gametes or embryos.

At the beginning of our study we encountered three obstacles to obtaining conceptuses for experimental purposes: the traditional Buddhist prohibition against the destruction of life, the belief that the body and its soul will resurrect if the dead body has not been impaired, and the parental emotional attachment to the intrauterine child. We solicited the cooperation of the obstetricians who explained to their clients the significance of medical research and the contributions the parents could make by leaving the embryos with them. In most cases the mothers acceded to the requests of the obstetricians in whom they had trust. We regarded ourselves as an extension of the obstetrician's clinic and could accept the specimens in good faith.

A technical problem existed as well. It was almost inevitable that the embryos were crushed by the operation of curettage and were not suitable for anatomical survey. Rarely was an undamaged embryo a chance product. We found that some obstetricians exercise more skill in obtaining undamaged embryos than others and stored such embryos as specimens for teaching nurses or patients. By seeking out these skilled doctors we were able to collect embryonic specimens of about 5–20 weeks of menstrual age. Our materials thus obtained could be regarded as approximately a nonselected sample of the total embryonic population.

As mentioned in my previous report [NISHIMURA, 1970], the socioeconomic rank of the patients was generally the so-called middle class; the frequency of declared consanguinous marriage was lower than the reported figure of overall Japanese; the average maternal age was only 2.5 years older than the average for Japan; and the average parity was higher by one than the figures for total deliveries in Japan. The obstetricians did not examine the embryos for external defects or signs of intrauterine death before providing us with them. It was in our favor that the operation of curettage was usually finished within 30 min of its initiation and, therefore, those specimens could be considered free of artificial changes, such as slowing of the growth rate, prior to their recovery. They were fixed in Bouin's fluid or 10% formalin immediately after their recovery. Obstetricians provided us a record covering general information and the obstetric history.

We have now set up the largest collection of normal and abnormal human embryonic and early fetal specimens, described as follows:

A. Number of Specimens Obtained

Fixed embryos: 30,200 (about one fifth of those are undamaged specimens); fixed early fetuses: 2,900 (the majority undamaged).

B. Anomalies Found in the Fixed Specimens:

1. Malformed and Deviated Embryos

a) Externally malformed embryos (ca. 500 cases) with some of the following types: exencephaly, microcephaly, myeloschisis, hydromyelia, nuchal blebs, holoprosencephaly, microtia, low set ear, anomalies of pharyngeal arches, cleft lip, micrognathia, hypoplasia of the pelvic region, anomalies of the anus and external genitalia, overgrowth of the tail, amelia of the upper limb, hypoplasia of the upper limb, split hand, oligodactyly of the hand, syndactyly of the hand, polydactyly of the hand, macrodactyly of the hand, hypoplasia of the lower limb, split foot, polydactyly of the foot.

b) Embryos with suspected external anomalies (ca. 230 cases),

c) Malformations found by microdissection: heart anomalies (ca. 40 cases), kidney anomalies (ca. 15 cases),

d) Anomalies found by cartilage and skeletal staining: anatomical variants of ribs (ca. 30 cases).

2. Malformed Early Fetuses

Approximately 60 cases fell into this category with external malformations of some of the following types: chondrodystrophy, oxycephaly, anencephaly, exencephaly, meningocele, holoprosencephaly, spina bifida, anotia, other anomalies of the ear auricle, cleft lip, cleft palate, micrognathia, omphalocele, single umbilical artery, hypoplasia of the external genitalia, atresia ani, reduction deformities of the upper limb, polydactyly of the hand, syndactyly of the hand, oligodactyly of the hand, hip joint dislocation (?),polydactyly of the foot.

C. Histological Embryonic and Fetal Specimens

a) Normal embryos: serial sections, from Streeter's horizon VIII–XXIII including some dead embryos (ca. 500 cases).

b) Abnormal embryos (ca. 340 cases): externally malformed – whole embryos or malformed parts only (ca. 190 cases), specimens with suspected external anomaly or anomalies (ca. 150 cases).

c) Miscellaneous: gonads of embryos (ca. 2,550 cases), anal region of embryos (ca. 62 cases), some histochemically stained embryos (ca. 65 cases), fetal hip joints (ca. 45 cases), various fetal organs (ca. 20 cases), chorion (ca. 600 cases).

II. Prevalence of Malformations among Embryonic and Early Fetal Population as Compared with that in Newborns

Unlike spontaneously aborted specimens, our specimens from induced abortion provide almost unbiased sampling and allow thorough examination of maldevelopments owing to their small size and no postmortem changes in most cases. Detection of various malformations was made by the criteria set by our studies on normal standards for various stages of development.

Since we are dealing with early malformations, prevalence of stage differences should be considered. Table I shows prevalences of malformed specimens among total undamaged cases that are judged alive *in utero*. Our figures are more than two times higher than the corresponding prevalences in Japanese newborns shown in table II, notwithstanding the several types, such as cleft palate, hip joint dislocation, club foot, etc., not included in our series.

Next, the prevalence of each of several malformations obtained by our group (fig. 1–11) will be compared with that in newborns.

Table I. Prevalence of externally malformed embryos by developmental stage (summation of specimens from 1961 to 1971)

Streeter's horizon	Total number	Number of malformed	Prevalence, %
VIII–XV	1,794	23	1.28
XVI–XVIII	1,870	44	2.35
XVIII–XXIII	2,169	46	2.12
Unknown	2	1	–

Table II. Some reported prevalences of malformed Japanese newborns

Authors	Period	Source of statistics	Number of births	Newborns affected	
				number	%
MITANI and KITAMURA [1968]	1922–67	hospital records	155,222	1,295	0.83
SAITO and KANDACHI [1954]	1930–52	hospital records	15,996	72	0.45
SHIRAKAWA *et al.* [1963]	1946–63	hospital records	11,716	108	0.92
NEEL [1958]	1948–54	physical examination soon after birth	64,569	659	1.02
TSUKAMOTO [1956]	1953–55	hospital records	105,730	823	0.78
BABA *et al.* [1967]	1955–65	hospital records	37,723	344	0.91
MORIYAMA [1964]	1957–61	hospital records	334,529	2,209	0.66
OSHIMA [1966]	1959–66	hospital records	11,982	117	0.98

A. Holoprosencephaly

TANIMURA and UWABE [1971] in our laboratory found 81 cases of holoprosencephaly among 11,068 embryos at Streeter's horizons XIV–XXIII. This prevalence (0.73%) is about 70 times higher than 14 cases among 144,670 newborns (0.01%) reported by MITANI and KITAMURA [1968]. The prevalence is especially high in the group of threatened abortion (3.7%). 45 cases (56%) showed signs of intrauterine death. Histological examination of cyclopic embryos revealed univentricular hypoplastic telencephalon in all cases, frequently hypoplastic hypophysis in primordium, occasional fusion of the oculomotor nerves of both sides, and dilatation of the fourth ventricle. 29 cases (36%) had malformations such as polydactyly (17 cases) and myeloschisis (7 cases), combined with face malformations. Several cases of cardiac and meta-nephrotic anomalies were found.

B. Exencephaly and Myeloschisis

These anomalies were first detected by external observation and con-firmed histologically. Further study after our preliminary report [NISHIMURA *et al.*, 1969] revealed that prevalences of exencephaly and myeloschisis among 5,835 undamaged embryos were 16 cases (0.27%) and 20 cases (0.34%), respectively. These figures are far higher than the reported figures of 0.06 and 0.02% among 144,670 newborns [MITANI and KITAMURA, 1968]. Histological studies revealed that both anomalies can be classified into at least 2 types, nonclosed and closed neural tubes.

C. Cleft Lip and Cleft Palate

Among 5,117 undamaged embryos at horizons from XVIII to XXIII, 22 specimens with cleft lip (0.43%) (8 bilateral, 13 unilateral, and 1 median type) were observed [IIZUKA, 1973]. Again, this prevalence is 2 times or more higher than the figure in newborns, 0.17% [MITANI and KITAMURA, 1968] or 0.21% [NEEL, 1958]. The tendency we noted that unilateral cleft is more frequent than the bilateral type coincides with the finding in Japanese infants [KOBAYASHI, 1958].

616 early fetuses (46–160 mm in crown-rump length) were examined for detection of cleft palate. Two cases of this defect with cleft lip (0.32%) and 2 with isolated cleft palate (0.32%) were found [IIZUKA, 1973]. Since the reported frequency of isolated cleft palate in Japanese infants was 0.02% [MITANI and KITAMURA, 1968] and 0.06% [NEEL, 1958], it is clear that the incidence in our series is several times higher than that in infants.

Fig. 1. Embryo with holoprosencephaly (No. 4540; horizon XVIII).

Fig. 2. Embryo with exencephaly (No. 7176; horizon XX).

Fig. 3. Embryo with cervical and lumbosacral myeloschisis accompanied with holo-prosencephaly (No. 21973; horizon XVII).

Fig. 4. Embryo with left unilateral cleft lip (No. 28090; horizon XX).

Fig. 5. Fetus with cleft palate with cleft lip (No. 468; 57 mm in crown-rump length).

Fig. 6. Embryo with preaxial polydactyly of right hand (arrow) and normal left hand (No. 27053; horizon XVIII).

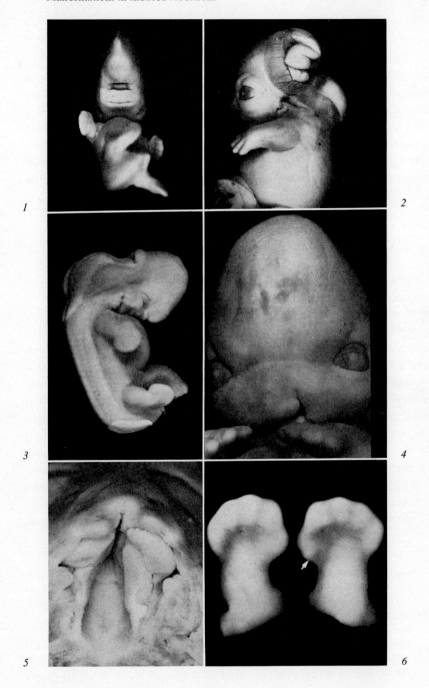

D. Polydactyly

Among 2,631 undamaged embryos at horizons XVII–XXIII, 37 cases with polydactyly of the hand (1.41%) were found, and among 2,169 undamaged embryos at horizons XVIII–XXIII, 8 cases with polydactyly of the foot (0.37%). Comparing these figures with the prevalences in newborns, 0.093% for the hand and 0.043% for the foot [MITANI and KITAMURA, 1968], frequencies of polydactyly of the hand in the embryos are about 15 times higher than those in newborns and polydactyly of the foot 9 times higher. Similar to the recognized tendency in newborns, preaxial polydactyly of the right thumb was most frequent among overall polydactylous cases.

E. Cardiac Malformations

The heart, the pulmonary trunk, ductus arteriosus, and aortic arch were examined in 1,289 externally normal embryos at horizons XVIII–XXIII by means of microdissection by SEMBA and co-workers [unpublished]. Ventricular septal defect was identified on specimens at and over horizon XXI. The occurrence of malformed hearts was 8 (1.16%) among 687 embryos at horizons XVIII–XX and 21 (3.5%) among 602 cases at horizons XXI–XXIII, whereas the corresponding prevalence in live infants was reported as 0.14% by NEEL [1958]. Such types as patent foramen ovale and patent ductus arteriosus that appear in the perinatal stage could not be included in our series. The type of defects and its frequency in our series were: persistent ostium I (2), persistent A–V canal (5), tricuspid valve defect (1), mitral valve defect (1), ventricular septal defect (10), Fallot's tetralogy (1), transposition of great vessels + ventricular septal defect (2), overriding aorta (2), pulmonary stenosis (1), aortic valve defect (2), aortic valve defect + pulmonary valve defect (1), coarctation of aorta (1). The ventricular septal defect was most common,

---

Fig. 7. Heart with ventricular septal defect (No. 4145; horizon XXI).

Fig. 8. Embryo with prominent nuchal bleb (No. 21698; horizon XXI).

Fig. 9. Embryo with tubercle (arrow) on the tail accompanied with postaxial polydactyly of the left foot (No. 31962; horizon XXI).

Fig. 10. Embryo with perforated pharyngeal cleft II (No. 21136; horizon XIII).

Fig. 11. Embryo with deformed pharyngeal arch I and hypoplastic pharyngeal arch II (No. 27230; horizon XIV).

Fig. 12. Embryo with normal pharyngeal arches (No. 28786; horizon XIII).

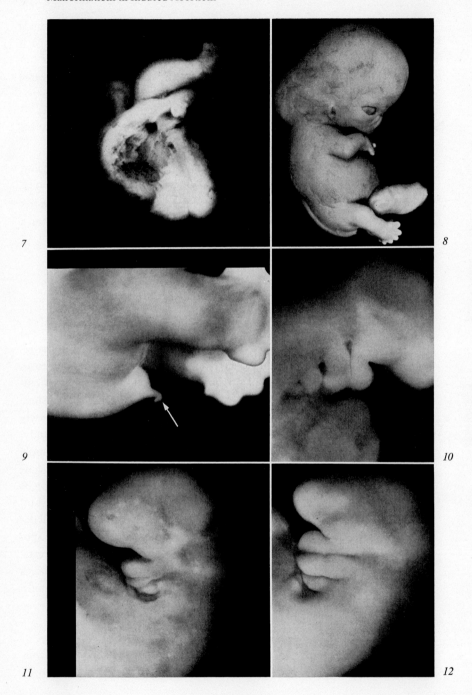

7   8

9   10

11   12

which is in accord with the reported finding among the perinatal and clinical cases. The persistent atrioventricular canal was also common in our specimens; this anomaly has been very rare in infants. It is interesting that our specimens included several other severe types that are reported as very scarce in infants.

F. True Hermaphroditism

A large scale histological study on gonads of 1,525 embryos at horizons XVIII–XXIII by LEE [1971] revealed 16 true hermaphrodites (1.08%): 9 lateral, 4 unilateral and 3 bilateral types. This figure is far higher than the frequency 0.2–0.3% in the total postnatal population projected by OVERZIER [1963].

G. Some Other Anomalies without Unequivocal Counterparts in Newborns

1. Nuchal Blebs

An unusually high incidence of external vesicular projections in the region of cervical flexure was found at a particular embryonic stage. If the cases with slight projection are included, 85 embryos were affected among 564 embryos at horizons XIX–XXIII (ca. 15%). Horizon XXI seems to be a stage of the highest predisposition to this anomaly. Our findings are approximately in accord with those of TÖNDURY et al. [1959]. After histological study, SHIOTA et al. [1973] classified these anomalies as five types: (a) simple subcutaneous blebs; (b) submeningeal blebs; (c) subcutaneous blebs associated with defects of the skull and primitive meninx; (d) subcutaneous blebs with perforation of the roof of the rhombencephalon but without skull defects, and (e) subcutaneous blebs with brain defects and additional skull defects. Judging from the unusually high incidence of these anomalies at the specific embryonic stage, the nuchal region seems to be the locus minoris resistentiae of causation of damage at this stage. The exact fate of these anomalies are not known, but it may be that some of these cases develop later into meningoencephalocele, exencephaly, or anencephaly.

2. Anomalies of the Pharyngeal Arches

Observation of the pharyngeal arches on 1,680 specimens at horizons XIII–XVII before the appearance of recognizable ear auricle revealed 21 cases with anomalous unilateral or bilateral pharyngeal arch or cleft (1.25%), of which 14 were cases with perforated pharyngeal cleft I or II, 5 were cases with hypoplastic arch I, II or III, and 2 were cases with retarded regression of arch III. Twelve cases with these anomalies were accompanied by some other external malformations. Such anomalies of the early primordia of the branchial organs have never been reported, and it is difficult to estimate their development.

3. Some Minor Anomalous Formations

The following anomalous formations, which have never been described in the literature, were occasionally found in embryos at a certain stage.

a) Small Tubercles on the Body Surface

One or 2 small tubercles were found on the postaxial side of the foot plate of human embryos at only horizons XVIII–XIX. Their frequency was about 20% (32 among 175 cases) and most of them appeared to be bilateral. Similar formations existed on the basal part of the hyoid arch of embryos at only horizons XIV–XVI with the frequency of 14.2% (54 among 379 cases), and on the caudal end of the tail in embryos at only horizons XX–XXIII with the frequency of 15.6% (32 among 205 cases). Histologically, most of those formations were characterized by localized epithelial proliferation; those of the tail were occasionally accompanied by duplication of the caudal neural tube.

b) Endocardiac Protrusion at the Conal Region

Usually 1, sometimes 2–3 endocardiac protrusions in the conal region were found (about 30%) among the embryos at only the horizon XIX [SEMBA and NISHIMURA, 1972]. Those are located around the portion where the 2 conal ridges fuse. Presumably, the protrusions are only transitional in most cases, but there is a possibility that they could later lead to a malformation, such as conal stenosis.

H. High Frequency of Combined Internal Defects in Externally Malformed Cases

23 externally malformed embryos at horizons XIV–XXIII showing no operative damage or signs of death *in utero* were serially sectioned and examined histologically for internal defects [TANIMURA, 1972]. Nine cases (39%)

showed one or more internal anomalies. Organs affected were the digestive system (3 cases), the urogenital system (3), the heart (2), the endocrine organs (2), the skeletal system (1) and the central nervous system (1). The other 4 cases showed blood stasis in various organs, which may indicate threatened death *in utero*. Such a high rate of combined internal anomalies with external malformations suggests that clinically there exists a number of undiscovered cases of malformation syndromes.

Now, looking over the above-mentioned findings, the following two facts are noteworthy: the especially high incidence of most types of malformation over that in newborns and the presence of some characteristic anomalies that have never been found in newborns. Such discrepancies between the findings on embryos and on newborns could be explained in 2 ways. First, a large proportion of certain malformations may be incompatible with live births. The fact that a high rate of combined internal anomalies accompanies the high incidence of externally malformed embryos in spontaneously aborted and stillborn fetuses may support this thesis. Second, the anomalous structure may recover (e.g., the delayed closure of ventricular septal defect), or the abnormal development may not progress further (e.g., the lack of noticeable growth of polydactyly).

It is to be emphasized that the embryonic population is the earliest human material that affords epidemiological study. Such a study can reveal aspects of maldevelopments thus far hidden. Therefore, it may be concluded that continued study along these lines may uncover more accurate information on the role of early human prenatal factors.

III. Analysis of Defective Early Embryos for Possible Role of Aged Gametes

Since the earliest work by BLANDAU and YOUNG [1939] there has been considerable evidence that when aged gametes take part in fertilization in animals, developmental defects and chromosomal aberrations increase [CARR, 1971]. IFFY [1963, 1965] and DE MORAES-RUEHSEN *et al.* [1969] advocated that delayed ovulation could occur in the woman and lead to pathological pregnancies, such as ectopic gestation, placenta previa, hydatidiform mole, early abortion, stillbirth, and congenital anomalies. JONGBLOET [1970] mentioned that in view of his human studies the chance of pathological progeny seems increased in certain situations where overripeness ovopathy may be expected. Based on a reanalysis of the unique series of Carnegie speci-

mens, HERTIG [1967] reported that a high incidence of abnormal human ova
is related to ovulations that had occurred after the 14th day of the cycle. An
appreciable proportion of these ova may undergo degeneration and be eliminated at a very early stage of gestation; others may manifest congenital defects compatible with at least an early intrauterine life. Since some of the defects can be commonly found in embryos, but very rarely in the perinatal
stage, an embryonic population appears to be one of the reliable sources to
verify the overripeness theory in man. Among our embryonic collections, 8
cases whose pregnancy was judged to occur by a single coitus were singled
out. Their dates were the 7th, 7th, 10th, 11th, 15th, 16th, 25th, and 30th day
of the menstrual cycle. This seems to suggest at least an existence of fertilization of the aged gametes in the human embryonic population.

In view of these considerations, we attempted to examine indirectly the
possible role of delayed ovulation on malformations at the embryonic stage
by detecting discrepancies between the morphological stage and the 'ovulation age' of defective embryos in our collection. 'Ovulation age' refers to the

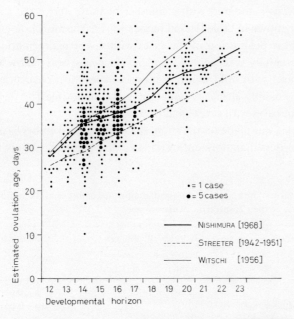

Fig. 13. Curves illustrating ovulation age of normal embryos by developmental
horizons (Streeter). 694 embryos from mothers with regular menstrual cycles. From
NISHIMURA *et al.* [1968]. Reprinted courtesy of Teratology.

period between the date 14 days prior to the expected onset of the next menstrual period and the date of recovery of an embryo. We adopted this method of assessing the embryonic age, because in the case of induced abortion, unlike the complaint of infertility, the basal body temperature was usually not measured.

We reasoned that if the general development of certain pathological embryos was less advanced than the calculated 'ovulation age' would indicate, the 'actual embryonic age' was shorter than the calculated 'ovulation age'; i.e., fertilization may have occurred later than the expected date. Such an inference is based on the premise that the rate of development of pathological embryos at an early stage differs little from that of normal embryos. An appreciable number of embryos with a certain type of malformation but no sign of intrauterine death were morphologically staged according to Streeter, and the relationship between the morphological stage and the ovulation age was compared with the standard for normal Japanese embryos shown in figure 13. Embryos with 4 types of malformations, holoprosencephaly, exencephaly and myeloschisis, preaxial polydactyly of the hand and cleft lip, were examined. The number of embryos below the standard morphological stage for their ovulation age was compared with a number of those above the standard. The results are shown in table III and figures 14–17. The morphological development of a large proportion of the cases with severe malformations, such as holoprosencephaly, exencephaly and myeloschisis, was below the standard; that of cases with mild malformations was less so [YASUDA and NISHIMURA, 1973]. Possibly delayed ovulation was responsible for developmental delay in the cases with severe malformation.

A similar analysis was made on the spontaneously aborted embryos and on the early embryos (less than horizon XVII) of ectopic pregnancy. Only the

Table III. Comparison of morphological stage of malformed embryos to the standard of normal embryos at their respective 'ovulation age'

Type of malformation	Number of embryos		Significance
	below standard	above standard	
Holoprosencephaly	22	10	p < 0.05
(with polydactyly)	(7)	(1)	(p < 0.05)
Exencephaly and myeloschisis	19	11	p > 0.1
Preaxial polydactyly	16	10	p > 0.1
Cleft lip	6	8	p > 0.5

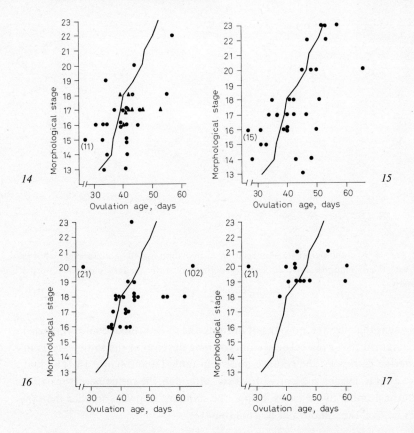

Fig. 14–17. Morphological stage in relation to ovulation age of malformed embryos as compared with standard curve for normal embryos. *14* Holoprosencephaly (▲ with polydactyly); *15* exencephaly and myeloschisis; *16* preaxial polydactyly; *17* cleft lip.

Table IV. Comparison of morphological stage of embryos from spontaneous abortion or ectopic pregnancy to the standard of normal embryos at their respective 'ovulation age'

Category of embryos	Number of embryos		Significance
	below standard	above standard	
Spontaneous abortion	14	6	0.05 < p < 0.1
Ectopic pregnancy	11	7	0.3 < p < 0.5

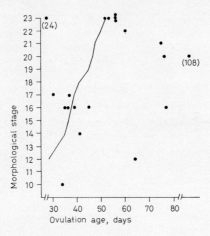

Fig. 18. Morphological stage in relation to ovulation age of spontaneously aborted (nonmacerated) embryos alive *in utero* as compared with standard curve for normal embryos.

specimens that showed no signs of intrauterine or intratubal death were used. We assumed that even ectopic embryos may develop at the same rate as intrauterine embryos. The result is shown in table IV and figure 18. The findings in table IV are suggestive because, although the difference is insignificant, the number of the cases 'below' the standard is always smaller than the cases 'above' the standard as it is in table III.

IV. Maternal Age Effect on Incidence of Defective and Dead Embryos

Clinically, it has been noted that the initiation and the end of ovarian functional life are not abrupt. In fact, anovulatory cycles are common in the beginning of the menstrual period and just before its end. The 2 extremes of the menstrual period can be separated from the intermediate period. There seems to be a possibility that delayed ovulation occurs more frequently in very young and very old women when changes in the hypothalamic-pituitary-ovarian relationship may be taking place.

In order to examine the effects of extreme maternal age on early conceptuses, we studied the overall occurrence of malformed and dead embryos retained *in utero* among both the very young and very old mothers and compared it with the corresponding occurrence among the median-aged mothers.

Table V. Maternal age and prevalence of pathological embryos

Groupe	Maternal age, years	Embryos number of normal	number of malformed[1] (%)	number of dead[2] (%)
I	17	8 ⎫	0 ⎫	1 ⎫
	18	40 ⎬ 125	0 ⎬ 1 (0.79)	6 ⎬ 27 (17.7)
	19	77 ⎭	1 ⎭	20 ⎭
II	27–29	1,705	33 (1.90)	344 (16.5)
III	41	108 ⎫	1 ⎫	22 ⎫
	42	99	0	17
	43	51	2	20
	44	30	1	15
	45	15	0	3
	46	8 ⎬ 316	0 ⎬ 5 (1.56)	3 ⎬ 84 (20.7[3])
	47	3	1	2
	48	–	–	–
	49	1	0	0
	50	1	0	1
	53	0 ⎭	0 ⎭	1 ⎭

1 Among total embryos alive *in utero*.
2 Among total normal, malformed and dead embryos.
3 p < 0.05 (compared with group II).

The results are shown in table V. The obstetric records showed no notable differences in menstrual cycles among the 3 groups; however, some differences were noted in the number of pregnancies. Almost all of the youngest group had no previous experience of pregnancy; the median age group were ca. 7% primigravid and ca. 93% multigravid; the old group were all multigravid. Table V shows that there is little difference in prevalence of malformed or dead embryos between the youngest and the median-aged group, a finding that may be influenced by the absence of mothers under 17 years of age in the study. The oldest group suffered a significant increase of early embryonic death compared to the median-aged group. Contrary to several observations in newborns, including the statistics by Japanese Ministry of Health and Welfare in 1971, we did not find a correlation between age and early malformations, probably because we could not examine such anomalies as Down's syndrome and congenital heart defects in this study. According to a recent large scale study on maternal age effect by HAY and BARBANO [1972] positive age effects were shown most dramatically in Down's syndrome and to a less degree congenital heart defects, and a positive association in other congenital malformations was observed among first births only. Our old group did not include a primigravid case. However, further analysis revealed these interesting figures: 99 old mothers whose interval between previous and present pregnancy was 10 years or more showed an occurrence of 3 malformed embryos (3.9%) and 22 dead (22.2%). Such results encourage us to collect more cases in this category to determine whether such old mothers with an unusual pregnancy history indeed show the highest prevalence of malformed embryos.

Summary

1. The embryonic population showed an unusually high incidence of most types of malformation and the presence of some anomalies without exact counterpart in newborns. Such findings suggest that an epidemiological teratological study with an overall embryonic population provides information not available elsewhere, and therefore continuation of such studies as ours is useful in analyzing the roles of various human prenatal factors, including the aging of gametes.

2. We sought for indirect evidence of possible effects of overripeness of human eggs in 2 ways. First we examined malformed embryos and embryos from spontaneous abortion and ectopic pregnancy to determine whether the morphological development, assessed from various developmental characteristics was less than the 'ovulation age', calculated from menstrual history, would lead us to expect. The results caused us to speculate that delay of ovulation may be responsible for the occurrence of some severe malformations. Second, we tried to determine whether the embryonic population from mothers of extreme child bearing age showed a higher occurrence of malformed or dead embryos than those from median-aged mothers, probably with regular ovulatory function. In spite of a limited number of specimens from the extreme-aged group, a significantly increased tendency was recognized with respect to early embryonic death in older mothers. Moreover, there seemed to be a tendency for malformation to occur more in the older mothers with a long interval between the last 2 pregnancies.

3. To continue the study of overripeness of human gametes, we expect to accumulate and examine thoroughly embryonic specimens with a history of a single and fruitful coitus. Such specimens will be obtained as chance products from induced abortuses. Specimens from mothers of extreme reproductive ages and from those whose pregnancy was an unsuccessful outcome of the use of an oral contraceptive or was preceded by the use of some central depressant drug with antiovulatory effects will also be collected for this purpose.

Acknowledgments

This study was supported by grants from the National Institute of Child Health and Human Development (HD 01401-01-06), the Association for the Aid of Crippled

Children, New York, the Population Council, New York, World Health Organization (Human Reproduction Unit) and Japanese Ministry of Health and Welfare (Section of Child and Maternal Welfare). I gratefully acknowledge the continued help of the collaborating obstetricians and the participation of my associates, Drs. T. TANIMURA, M. YASUDA, O. TANAKA and other co-workers in the Department.

References

BABA, K.; TAKEYA, H.; OKADA, T.; NAKAMURA, J., and OTSUKA, S.: Twenty-year review of congenital abnormalities born in a hospital in Tokyo (in Japanese). Nichidai Igaku Zasshi (Med. J. Nippon University) 26: 420 (1967).

BLANDAU, R.J. and YOUNG, W.C.: The effects of delayed fertilization on the development of the rat ovum. Amer. J. Anat. 64: 303 (1939).

CARR, D.H.: Chromosome abnormalities in the preimplanting ovum; in BLANDAU The Biology of the Blastocyst, vol. 20, p. 349 (University of Chicago Press, Chicago 1971).

HAY, S. and BARBANO, H.: Independent effects of maternal age and birth order on the incidence of selected congenital malformations. Teratology 6: 271 (1972).

HERTIG, A.T.: The overall problem in man; in BENIRSCHKE Comparative aspects of reproductive failure, vol. 11 (Springer, Berlin 1967).

IFFY, L.: Time of conception in pathological gestation. Proc. roy. Soc. Med. 56: 1098 (1963).

IFFY, L.: Embryologic studies of time of conception in ectopic pregnancy and first-trimester abortion. J. Obstet. Gynec. 26: 490 (1965).

IIZUKA, T.: High incidence of cleft lip and cleft palate in the human embryos and early fetuses. Folia anat. jap. 50: 259 (1973).

Japanese Ministry of Health and Welfare: White paper on Japanese welfare in 1971 (in Japanese) (Japanese Finance Ministry Press, Tokyo 1971).

JONGBLOET, P.H.: An investigation into the occurrence of overripeness ovopathy in the normal population. Maandschr. Kindergeneesk. 38: 228 (1970).

KOBAYASHI, Y.: A genetic study on harelip and cleft palate (in Japanese). Jap. J. hum. Genet. 3: 73 (1958).

LEE, S.: High incidence of true hermaphroditism in the early human embryos. Biol. Neonat. 18: 418 (1971).

MITANI, S. and KITAMURA, Y.: Malformations and their classification (in Japanese). Sanfujinka-Chiryo (Obstet. gynec. Ther.) 17: 265 (1968).

MORAES-RUEHSEN, M.D. DE; JONESE, G.S.; BURNETT, L.S., and BARAMKI, T.A.: The aluteal cycle. Amer. J. Obstet. Gynec. 103: 1059 (1969).

MORIYAMA, Y.: Statistical study on congenital malformations (in Japanese). Sanfu no Sekai (The World of Obstetrics and Gynecology) 16: 139 (1964).

NEEL, J.V.: A study of major congenital defects in Japanese infants. Amer. J. Obstet. Gynec. 10: 398 (1958).

NISHIMURA, H.: Incidence of malformations in abortions; in FRASER and McKUSICK Congenital malformations, vol. 4, p. 275 (Excerpta Medica, Amsterdam 1970).

NISHIMURA, H.; TAKANO, K.; TANIMURA, T., and YASUDA, M.: Normal and abnormal development of human embryos. First report of the analysis of 1,213 intact embryos. Teratology 1: 281 (1968).

NISHIMURA, H.; TANIMURA, T., and SWINYARD, C.A.: A study of 26 human embryos (horizon 11–22, Streeter) with central nervous system defects. Teratology 2: 267 (1969).

OSHIMA, K.: On congenital malformations surveyed from viewpoints of the public health (in Japanese). Senten-Ijo (Congenital Anomalies) 6: 5 (1966).

OVERZIER, C.: Intersexuality (Academic Press, London 1963).

SAITO, S. and KANDACHI, Y.: Incidence of the deformities of the newborns in our clinic (in Japanese). Nippon Sanka-Fujinka Gakkai Zasshi (Organ jap. Soc. Obstet. Gynec.) 6: 573 (1954).

SEMBA, R. and NISHIMURA, H.: Endocardiac protrusions in the conal region occasionally found in five week human embryos. Teratology 6: 118 (1972).

SHIOTA, K.; UWABE, C.; TANIMURA, T., and NISHIMURA, H.: Nuchal blebs occasionally found in human seven week-embryos. Teratology 8: 105 (1973).

SHIRAKAWA, K.; ISHIZAKA, K.; GONJO, N., and AMAGASE, Y.: Congenital malformations observed in our clinic during past 17 years (in Japanese). Senten-Ijo (Congenital Anomalies) 3: 71 (1963).

STRATFORD, B.F.: Abnormalities of early human development. Amer. J. Obstet. Gynec. 107: 1223 (1970).

TANIMURA, T.: Internal anomalies combined with external malformations in human embryos. Teratology 6: 121 (1972).

TANIMURA, T. and UWABE, C.: Eighty one cases of holoprosencephaly in Japanese embryos (in Japanese). Senten-Ijo (Congenital Anomalies) 11: 130 (1971).

TÖNDURY, G.; SCHENK, R. und MORGER, R.: Menschliche Keimlinge mit Nackenblasen. Biol. Neonat. 1: 68 (1959).

TSUKAMOTO, S.: Round table discussion on congenital malformations (in Japanese). Sanfu no Sekai (The World of Obstetrics and Gynecology) 8: 843 (1956).

YASUDA, M. and NISHIMURA, H.: Substandard intrauterine development shown in some of the malformed human embryos. Teratology 7: A-30 (1973).

Author's address: Dr. HIDEO NISHIMURA, Department of Anatomy, Faculty of Medicine, Kyoto University, Kyoto 606 (Japan)

Aging Gametes. Int. Symp., Seattle 1973, pp. 369–392 (Karger, Basel 1975)

Perspective on the Etiology of Anomalous Development[1]

KURT BENIRSCHKE and DETLEV H. BUSCH

Department of Reproductive Medicine, University of California, San Diego, La Jolla, Calif., and Department of Obstetrics and Gynecology, University of Bonn, Bonn

A primary reason for gathering information on the 'Biology and Pathology of Aging Gametes' is the recognized relationship of some human congenital anomalies, particularly trisomies, such as mongolism, with advancing maternal age. No clearcut correlation exists in this respect to advancing paternal age, and it is this discrepancy that has led to the notion that aging of oocytes *per se* may be deleterious. In preceding chapters we have examined our current understanding of some of the possible causes of abnormal development of ill-timed fertilization, the possible nature of aging of gametes, and of other cellular events. The relationship of some of these considerations to reproductive failure is not immediately known, but this knowledge is thought to provide fundamental insight into the problem of the maternal age effect upon reproduction.

In these concluding remarks it is our obligation to draw attention to some other aspects of defective development that bear on this question and to put the issues examined into proper perspective.

I. Incidence of Anomalies in Man

It is difficult to assess the frequency of malformations accurately. The reasons for this difficulty are many and they have been carefully analyzed by LAMY and FRÉZAL [1961]. Assessments made from birth records showing autopsy results differ from those made from records lacking such information. The incidence in neonates and stillborns is estimated to be close to 1.5 %

1   Work reported in this contribution was supported by grant RF 70029 from the Rockefeller Foundation.

but by age 1 year it is much higher, 4–5%. Investigators who count minor anomalies, not usually detailed in birth records, give even higher figures. It is recognized that most statistics do not include a careful assessment of anomalies in stillborns, particularly those macerated. The frequency of single umbilical artery alone is 1% in the newborn population [BENIRSCHKE and DRISCOLL, 1967], and its occurrence is never counted in these statistics. It is thus probably a conservative statement by LAMY and FRÉZAL [1961] that: 'The overall incidence of major malformations is higher than 5%.'

This statement was made at a time when one of the pathogenetic mechanisms of mongolism, trisomy 21, had just been discovered. In subsequent years the contribution of chromosomal errors to congenital anomalies has been more fully explored, and we now recognize the numerical enormity of this etiology, particularly among spontaneous abortions. Probably it is best to consider the concentration of these errors in the population of abortuses as reflecting a selective mechanism. Nevertheless, the frequency with which chromosomal errors are still encountered in the newborn population, 0.5%, is a remarkable and recent finding to which we need to return. Here it is relevant only to stress the known relationship to advanced maternal age of some of these chromosomal errors and to consider next whether such an association exists for anomalies other than those caused by aneuploidy.

The incidence of human congenital anomalies differs with seasons, with locations, with sex, with birth order, and with maternal age. MCKEOWN [1961] has analyzed sources of these variations and separated the effect of age from that of birth order for several common congenital anomalies. He concludes that, in general, a correlation exists between anomalies and primogeniture and between anomalies and increasing maternal age. The age effect is slight in anencephaly, marked in hydrocephaly, marked in harelip (with or without cleft palate), and absent in isolated cleft palate, spina bifida, and patent ductus arteriosus. Of course, the well known age effect associated with mongolism, first described by PENROSE [1934], was substantiated and, despite the recent recognition of its chromosomal basis, MCKEOWN [1961] suggested that the described 'U-shaped pattern' may be the sequel of significant environmental influences. These, he deduced, operated at different stages of fetal or neonatal development.

JANERICH [1972] has reexamined the situation for anencephaly from birth records in New York State and finds an overall U-shaped curve with maternal age. When the data were broken into sequential time intervals, however, there was no consistently increased risk with advancing maternal age, particularly in the years between 1945 and 1949. The risk was more directly relatable to the year of maternal birth, and he suggests the possibility that an environmental etiologic factor may act early in the mother's life, perhaps as early as her intrauterine life.

The principal interest in these relationships of course is our desire to dissect possible environmental agents as causes of congenital anomalies in order that they can ultimately be controlled. And the belief that some of these effects accumulate in the gametes with advancing age is provocation for making this book. Some of the prevalent hypotheses will now be examined in greater detail.

II. Chromosomal Errors

It is estimated that at least 7% of known pregnancies yield chromosomally abnormal offspring [JACOBS, 1972]. The majority is aborted, presumably as a result of aneuploidy, and of the 0.5% of newborns harboring a chromosomal anomaly, well over 50% are clinically silent at birth; some of the 'translocation carriers' remain asymptomatic through life. The only known positive relationship to these anomalies is that of increasing maternal age. The effect is apparent only in newborn autosomal trisomics and those individuals with additional X chromosomes. It is absent with structural rearrangements, X monosomy, and the common trisomy 16 of abortions [ARAKAKI and WAXMAN, 1970], although this population (29 specimens) may be bimodal and too small for analysis. Considering the possibility that in X monosomy the missing sex chromosome may often be the paternal one (and evidence for this has been advanced), the deleterious relationship of most common errors to increased maternal age is even more striking. Why the 'aging ovary' should give rise to aneuploid gametes, however, is unknown. The absence of maternal age effect upon triploid conceptuses, so frequently aborted, suggests that a gross disturbance of the meiotic events (which would lead to polyploidy) is an unlikely progenitor of the common chromosomal errors (trisomies) in man. Is it possible that mutagenic events or chemical substances accumulate in the oocyte whose prolonged prophase arrest differs so much from that of males, and that thereby the maternal age effect upon trisomies and perhaps other congenital anomalies can be explained?

Chromosomal damage can readily be induced by *irradiation* in a variety of species. These include mutations, breaks, rearrangements, nondisjunction, etc. A direct or indirect effect upon the spindle apparatus can be envisaged. Of prime relevance at a time when increased radiation usage by society can be anticipated is the question: What is the potentially mutagenic effect of exposure to a variety of radiation? This concern has led to the thoughtful BEIR Report [1972]. The issues are exceedingly complex, and it is apparent that not enough data are available from the study of man to answer the rhetorical question unequivocally and that those answers derived from experimental animals, largely Drosophila and Mus, cannot be used with certainty to extrapolate the situation for man. In reviewing this evidence carefully it appears that neither the increased risk of aging mothers to have a trisomic child nor that of producing other anomalous children (e.g., with cleft lip) can be related to an accumulation of mutagenic radiation effects in oocytes. BAKER [1971] and NEWCOMBE [1972] have summarized the state of knowledge in 2 well documented reviews. Although dose-related linear increase of radiation-induced germ cell mutation occurs, the effect of low dose irradiation on the gamete of the human is unknown. In specific inbred lines of mice 200 rad administered to each of 35 successive generations yielded no measurable changes in fertility, mortality, or body characteristics. In fruitflies, monosomies are induced above a threshold of 1,000 rad but not trisomies, to which our attention is directed by the maternal age effect. Similarly, the XO anomaly in the mouse has been induced by oocyte irradiation, the mouse oocytes being apparently considerably more radiosensitive than those of primates. Following the atomic explosions in Japan no significant deleterious effect upon the offspring of irradiated mothers has been detected. (A slight increase in sex ratio was noted.) Nevertheless, a higher abortion and still birth rate occurred. Most remarkable perhaps is the finding that following intense (therapeutic) irradiation of female and male gonads apparently normal offspring are produced. It has been hypothesized that 'germinal selection' may be the basis for these findings or that damage to chromosomes is quickly repaired by the dictyate-stage oocyte.

The radiation exposure of mothers of children with trisomy 21 has been specifically reviewed in one retrospective and one prospective study. In 216 cases SIGLER et al. [1965] found a 9.7-percent exposure rate to all types of irradiation and a 4.6-percent rate in controls, that of X-ray therapy being most markedly different (14.5 versus 7.0%). In a prospective study of 972 radiated mothers and age-matched controls UCHIDA et al. [1968] also demonstrated a higher frequency of mongols in the experimental group. There were 10 aneuploids (8 mongols) as against only 1 aneuploid in the controls, a statistically valid difference. No differences were observed with respect to other congenital anomalies or perinatal deaths. It has been pointed out that the total exposure in this latter group was remarkably low, and also that other series have not shown such an association. Moreover, it is totally unclear why primarily an effect on chromosome 21 should be apparent, the two other newborns having trisomy 18. More explicable perhaps might be the finding of chromosomal damage in one infant suffering from anomalies probably secondary to translocations and ring chromosomes. Clearly, this subject needs more direct inquiry than it has received to date. However one may look upon this, the cumulative evidence suggests that: (a) radiation-induced mutations possibly accumulating in aging gametes cannot explain satisfactorily the age-effect upon anomalies or most chromosomal aneuploidy; and (b) some contribution to the mutational load probably is incurred by exposure to irradiation, and translocations may be one such event.

The fact is that we are largely ignorant as to how important irradiation is in the balance of genetic disease and wellbeing although we suspect that 'too much' irradiation will tip the balance unfavorably. Similar questions arise on chemicals, pollutants, etc. On the other hand, no doubt exists that irradiation, by even small doses, is teratogenic to the embryo, a consideration that need not be pursued further at this point.

It may be mentioned here parenthetically that the increased usage of ultrasonic equipment during pregnancy-diagnostic procedures has raised the question of its potential harm. The effect has been analyzed by lymphocyte cultures of mother and the therapeutic abortus in 35 patients [ABDULLA et al., 1971]. No increase in chromosomal abnormalities was found over 11 controls, but it must be remembered that the finding of such abnormalities as induced chromatid breaks bears an unknown relationship to somatic or gametic effects upon the fetus. It is only inferred to have some significance from detection of similar aberrations following mutagenic irradiation and from general comparisons of plant and animal experiments with drugs to be discussed below.

Alterations of chromosomes are also a frequent sequel to *virus infections* and, of the three main types observed, so-called pulverization, chromosome breakage, and spindle effects, NICHOLS [1970] considers the chromosome breakage as the most significant. Although some fetal virus infections, particularly fetal rubella, are teratogenic and although chromosome damage has been identified in some appropriate circumstances, it is not at all clear as yet that this chromosomal effect leads to the organogenetic deficits. NAEYE and BLANC [1965] have identified a reduced number of somatic cells in these infants, many of whom are significantly runted. SAXÉN [1970] considers this effect not so much secondary to a loss of cells during infection as to mitotic inhibition. Others have argued that embolic occlusion, secondary to placental and other endothelial damage, may be the immediate cause of the anomalous development [Töndury, 1962]. The difference in fetal effects between early infection and infection after fetal immunologic competence makes it even more difficult to support this interpretation of the primacy of chromosomal damage as the cause of anomalous development. One must further consider that fetal damage is caused by other agents, such as the cytomegalovirus, toxoplasma, etc., for which chromosomal sequelae have not been found. In any event, no solid support has been provided to prove that the virus infection of mammalian germinal cells is causative in the nondisjunction or the U-shaped effect of spontaneous anomalies. The case has been advanced that such a relationship may hold for maternal infection with hepatitis virus. This putative relationship of antecedent maternal hepatitis to trisomy 21 [Stoller and Collmann, 1965] has found no support in several subsequent inquiries [Burch, 1969].

Much more difficult still is an answer to the questions: Do *chemical agents* that are known to cause chromosome breakage *in vitro* have a teratogenetic effect in embryos? Do similar agents accumulate their chromosomal effect in oocytes to result in the observed age effect?

A very large number of chemicals, drugs, and environmental substances can be shown to cause types of chromosomal damage *in vitro* as well as *in vivo*. They have been compiled in an exhaustive review by Barthelmess [1970], and new effects are continually being described. Proof of a transmissible mutagenic effect has only very rarely been provided for any of these chemicals, even in experimental mammals. This is not to say that such chemicals do not exist, only that this lack of recognition probably reflects the inadequacy of registration methods for man and the paucity of information on agents in general. Most is known about the most powerful chemicals which, on the whole, are rarely employed. Moreover, whereas point mutations doubtless can be so induced, their effect is even more difficult to ascertain by current methods than that of gross chromosomal damage. For, unlike such singular teratogenic effects as the thalidomide embryopathy, point mutations are similar to those mutations already present in the gene pool and their (slight) increase is extremely difficult to ascertain.

The review of 'chemical mutagenesis' [Vogel and Röhrborn, 1970] is an exceedingly complete assessment of most questions under consideration here, and it should be consulted for details, particularly for the practicality of the assessment of chemical mutagenesis by chromosomal analysis. It emerges from this review that adult female mammals are less likely to have induced germ cell mutations than adult males, at least so far as chromosomal aberrations are concerned. Some specific and powerful mutagens (Cytoxan and trenimon) produce their damage after meiosis during spermiogenesis, whereas in female mice the trenimon damage can be induced only in embryonic oogonia and in very young oocytes. It is clear from these and other studies that only very specific stages of the meiotic cycle seem to be affected by various agents, a parameter that is virtually unknown for most suspected mutagens. New approaches in this area are probably most needed.

In this connection the recent work by LAVAPPA and YERGANIAN [1971] is pertinent. They treated male Armenian hamsters *(Cricetulus migratorius)* with a single intraperitoneal dose (100 mg/kg body weight) of ethyl methanesulfonate (EMS) and bred them to normal females. Two of 15 F_1 males had chromosomal errors upon meiotic study undertaken on testes obtained by unilateral castration, and they were excluded. The remainder was bred to cytologically normal females, and cytologic analysis of the males F_2 (No. 56) showed that they possessed the normal number of 11 bivalents at diakinesis. These animals and other controls were then given a single intraperitoneal dose of urethan (100 mg/kg), an otherwise poor mutagen. Diakinesis was studied daily for 2 weeks. Control animals were not affected; however, in those whose grandsires had received EMS two types of meiotic anomalies were observed with 2 sharp temporal peaks. On the sixth day X-chromosome breakage was found, and on the eighth day various bivalent associations occurred in diakinesis. The precise reasons for these events are not understood at present but the authors suggest that EMS treatment had led to a cytologically undefinable premutation that was retained over two generations and that the latent damage was expressed only after an additional impetus, supplied in this case by the otherwise harmless urethan.

This newly described latency of a mutagenic effect, presumably accumulating in germ cells, is alarming in the face of the enormous number of potential mutagens to which man is exposed [BARTHELMESS, 1970]. At present we are ignorant as to whether such events occur in man; nor do we know that, if they did occur, they would lead to anomalous offspring. However, the experiment has opened the door for a new look at chemical mutagenesis.

As has been indicated, the powerful mutagens, such as cytoxan, are rarely employed in procreative individuals, and therefore general concern is more relevant perhaps for the more widely administered drugs whose mutagenicity is poorly understood at present. We will refer here only briefly to 3 agents to which wide attention has been paid: contraceptives, antiepileptics, and LSD. Much of what has been learned of these agents may hold for others whose mechanisms have not been explored so extensively.

Concern over possible mutagenic effects of *oral contraceptives* stems from CARR's [1967] observation of an increased frequency of polyploid abortuses following cessation of therapy. Some subsequent studies have tended to confirm these findings, others have failed to support the results and have pointed out that this population studied was not comparable to controls. These aspects have been discussed earlier in this book. Results of studies seeking a direct chromosomal effect of contraceptives *in vitro* have been variable. SINGH and CARR [1970] tested in lymphocyte cultures a wide variety of hormone additives, finding no effect whatever, other than a mitotic inhibition through FSH. BISHUN *et al.* [1972], although not confirming the putative breaking effect of contraceptives in lymphocyte mitoses described by others, observed a significantly increased satellite association among D chromosomes in former pill users. This effect was not transmitted to the offspring and no translocations have apparently been engendered by this association. Long-term oral contraceptive users had a significantly depressed PHA response in lymphocyte cultures [FITZGERALD *et al.*, 1973]. The mechanism is not fully understood, although a direct effect upon DNA replication has been suggested. Other effects upon mitosis (depression) and meiosis (clumping, stickiness, giant cells) of estrogen and progesterone have been described in experimental animals [WIDMEYER and SHAVER, 1972], including the increased incidence of aneuploid rabbit blastocysts when these agents were applied shortly after mating. A systematic study of cell kinetics under defined conditions is yet to come, however. This would seem to be all the more urgent since some such agents now given intentionally are known to be teratogenic as shown by the recent association between vaginal adenocarcinoma in young women and maternal stilbestrol treatment [HERBST *et al.*, 1972]. Moreover, it is currently suspected that the (inadvertent) administration of contraceptives and other hormones in early pregnancy may have deleterious consequences. Thus LEVY *et al.* [1973] find in a retrospective analysis of 76 mothers of children with transposition of great vessels that 7 were treated in early pregnancy with sex hormone preparations and 3 had other hormonal medication; none of the matched controls had been so treated. A retrospective study by NORA and NORA [1973] shows similar results. Fortunately, in those cases in which therapy was discontinued prior to conception, no adverse effects of former contraceptive therapy on the neonatal outcome has yet been found [ROBINSON, 1971]. In light of the knowledge of fractional mutation cited above, however, this should not be viewed with complacency as, clearly, subtle effects cannot be assessed at this time.

Anticonvulsive agents might be mentioned briefly because of the frequently very long-term administration of these drugs. Therefore, if they prove mutagenic, the possibility of the accumulation of adverse effects in germ cells must be considered. Studies *in vitro* and in treated patients suggest that some of these agents can affect chromosomal behavior. NEUHÄUSER *et al.* [1970] confirmed the finding of earlier investigators that mothers and the children of mothers treated with hydantoin and the commonly used oxazoli-dinediones have increased chromatid breakage frequencies in leukocyte cul-tures. More disturbing perhaps is the finding of occasional translocations and deletions. A suspected relationship also exists between maternal treat-ment with the latter types of anticonvulsive agent (trimethadione) and a vari-ety of birth defects [GERMAN *et al.*, 1970]. Of 14 pregnancies during which this drug was taken, 8 yielded defective children, only 3 of whom survived. In ad-dition there were 3 abortions. It is important to point out that in later preg-nancies, when the drug therapy was discontinued, the initial family with 4 successive malformations produced 2 normal children. It appears from these initial and very sporadic data that, whatever the mutagenic effect of these drugs may be, it applies to the developing embryonic cells and does not accu-mulate in the maternal oocytes. Of course no information exists as yet about the possibility of premutations as discussed above.

Similar difficulties exist in attempts to ascertain whether *LSD* has a mu-tagenic effect in man. The question is relevant because of the long-term expo-sure to this agent in some parents and the need for proper counseling to prospective foster parents of children conceived to such parents. A portion of the conflicting LSD studies has been reviewed by JACOBSON and BERLIN [1972]. That chromosome breakage as a result of pure LSD administra-tion has occurred in man and in experimental species has been suggested by some and denied by others. A direct effect upon DNA has been demonstrat-ed, and its teratogenetic effect has been studied in man and experimental spe-cies with conflicting results. One problem is the very frequent simultaneous use of other drugs by the parents whose progeny is under investigation; some of these drugs may have the effects commonly attributed to LSD. The study by JACOBSON and BERLIN [1972] suggests that (a) chromosomal breakage that quickly disappears is observed more often in the leukocyte cultures of one half of the newborns of LSD users; (b) more congenital anomalies occur, both among newborns and abortuses; (c) reproductive performance of the users may be decreased, and (d) no 'runting' of newborns results. Since the purity of the drug used by the probands of this study is unknown, since var-ious infectious diseases were increased, and because poor nutrition was an additive variable, the implications of these (and other) findings are difficult to substantiate. Others have reported that mothers of children with a variety of congenital anomalies have significantly higher intakes of a variety of drugs such as aspirin, amphetamines, barbiturates [NELSON and FORFAR, 1971]. Thus, a true mutagenic effect (aside from the teratogenic sequel) can at present not be accepted, let alone cumulative effects in germ cells.

These examples suffice to demonstrate the complexity of the problem. Its universality becomes apparent when one considers the exposure to *pollutants* of air, water, and foods, the exposure to metals and chemicals from numerous sources, and the exposure to naturally occurring substances, such as mycotoxins and plant-contained agents. For instance, the cause of Itai-Itai disease, a sequel to industrial pollution, is ingestion of water containing cadmium sulfide. In leukocyte cultures from patients with the disease CdS induced high frequencies of chromosome breaks and translocations [SHIRAISHI and YOSIDA, 1972]. These authors point out that very short term exposure (4 h) of cultures caused the effect, whereas *in vivo* the material is accumulated over long periods. Potentially this may have an effect upon the germ cells. Another element, mercury, is accumulating in food sources and is the cause of Minamata disease, which has deleterious effects upon the human embryo [PIERCE *et al.*, 1972] without as yet known chromosomal or mutagenic sequelae. Continuous exposure to such heavy metals should come under as strict surveillance as the drugs referred to above. Best explored perhaps of the heavy metals is lead [NEEDLEMAN and SCANLON, 1973]. Although lead content in certain segments of the population is markedly increased (for example, in traffic police), and a stunning increase in lead consumption and pollution are documented, the levels of lead have not changed in man over the past 3 decades. Moreover, no evidence exists that current lead levels adversely affect health [HANLON, 1972]. This is surprising since various diseases of fetuses, children, and adults, can be attributed to lead intoxication [NEEDLEMAN and SCANLON, 1973]. No chromosomal effect was found in traffic policemen with elevated lead levels [BAUCHINGER *et al.*, 1972]. Gonadal effects (testicular atrophy, cystic ovaries) can be produced in rats by lead administration and lead to reduced reproductive activity [HILDEBRAND *et al.*, 1973].

In fact, the fetal and mutagenic effects of various metals are very difficult to anticipate, and much more investigation is needed, particularly of possible mutagenicity. Deficiency and excess of various metals can induce congenital abnormalities in experimental animals, and various metals interact to potentiate or to counteract individual effects [FERM, 1972]. Indeed, it has been postulated that because of their chelating capabilities and binding to DNA some metals may protect against chemical mutagenesis [SCANLON, 1972].

Other pollutants may be even more ubiquitous, such as nitrates in the air and food (fear of conversion of nitrosamines), and insecticides (considerable accumulation for instance in zoo animals [MILLER-BEN-SHAUL, 1971]. The polychlorinated biphenyls (PCB) are extremely stable compounds that have become very widely dispersed pollutants from various industries (plastic, electric, lubricant, etc.). They are known to cause disease in man and in experimental animals and to traverse the placenta [KOLLER and ZINKL, 1973]. These are diverse chemicals with differing chlorine content and variable cellular toxicity. Some interfere with reproduction and cause uterine atrophy. A mutagenic effect has not been discovered.

Thus, the potential number of substances with teratogenic or mutagenic effect is enormous and steadily increasing. Investigation of these effects is commonly begun only after some serious sequelae have been recognized accidentally, such as the thalidomide tragedy, the Minamata disease occurrences, but the mutagenic potential has not really been approached because of the overwhelming nature of such study. The needs, the known facts, and the suggestions for such studies are carefully considered in a recent Conference Report [SUTTON and HARRIS, 1972]. It is suggested there that germ cell mutations might be ascertained in man as follows:

1. Point Mutations

a) Comparison of groups of children, exposed and unexposed. This is difficult because of the ubiquity of chemicals and pollutants, and useful only in drastic situations, such as massive doses of radiation.

b) Monitoring of frequency of known specific diseases, e.g., retinoblastoma, chondrodystrophy. It was estimated that in order to ascertain a 50-percent increase in mutation rate of some diseases with an incidence of 0.5/1,000 births a population of 6 million persons would have to be monitored.

c) Utilization of biochemical techniques (electrophoresis) to ascertain variants. Large populations, many laboratories, and enormous support are needed.

2. Chromosomal Errors

a) Surveillance of newborn populations by blood culture. For the ascertainment of insults leading to a doubling rate (from 0.5 to 1 %) at least 7,500 consecutive newborns are needed in different geographical areas, a feasible, albeit costly, undertaking.

b) Surveillance of only sex chromosomal errors by buccal smears, a cheaper process but one requiring a vastly larger number of newborns.

Abortuses might also be studied by more sophisticated techniques, and numerous experimental studies, such as meiosis in oocytes, are suggested as means of future inquiries [COHEN, 1970; VOGEL and RÖHRBORN, 1970]. Most importantly, as HANLON [1972] has stated, 'there is great need for reliable methods of extrapolating from animal experiments to man' and for future exploration of the possible synergistic toxicity of various compounds.

These aspects are all of very great concern, in part, of course because of the natural guilt feelings we possess as consumers or producers, because of economic pressures, and because they may constitute 'attackable' problems. It must be remembered though that, with the possible exception of germ cell radiation, no proof exists yet that the U-shaped curve referred to at the outset can be explained by accumulating mutagens or accumulation of their effect upon the gamete. Are there other possible interactions whose contribution is overlooked because of our concern for environmental (pollutant) mutagenesis?

A variety of data suggests that only a minor portion of so-called congenital anomalies can be explained by single events, such as mutations. Most congenital defects must be considered as the result of complex interactions between environmental and genetic factors. They fall into the realm of multifactorial processes with threshold. The deciphering of individual components is very complex in man; it is more readily accomplished in inbred strains of mice where considerable progress has been made toward the understanding of these complex phenomena. Nevertheless, some studies in man suggest avenues for future approaches toward which we now direct attention. Relationship to age, though not necessarily of gametes, is germane to these approaches and thus relates to the general theme of this book.

III. Twins and Disturbed Placentation

There is reliable indication that the twinning phenomenon increases with maternal age, and it is apparent upon analysis of this phenomenon that only dizygotic twinning (littering, polyovulation) is so affected [BENIRSCHKE and KIM, 1973]. Although multiple pregnancies are related to increased gonadotropin stimulation of the ovary, their relationship to increasing age has never been studied directly. Present techniques allow precise quantitation of gonadotropins. The single older study of an age-related increase of urinary gonadotropic substances needs to be reinvestigated with these techniques. Twinning is also positively related to congenital anomalies. Discordant anomalies of

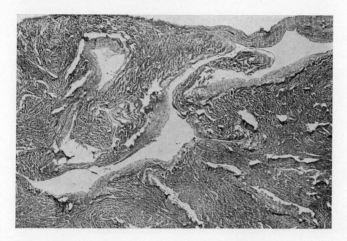

Fig. 1. Ventricle of human 'acardiac' twin [BENIRSCHKE, 1972] showing normal general histologic organization of this heart that lacked auricles. Focal thickening of endocardium is evident. HE, × 16.

monozygous twins can be understood rationally only by considering them the result of subtle deleterious influences presumably of disturbed placentation. In particular the development of the acardiac twin is so construed to be the end-effect of prenatal vascular reversal. Discordances are often observed in anomalies for which a familial or hereditary basis is established, such as cleft lip, anencephaly, and congenital heart disease. It is suggested that discordant development of twins serves as a model from which insight may be gained into the causes of abnormal development of singletons.

Bearing this point of view in mind, further correlations can be suggested. Thus, BOUÉ and BOUÉ [1973] found a significant increase in chromosomal errors in abortuses of women whose pregnancy had been achieved by very recent stimulation of ovulation (gonadotropins or clomiphene), but not in the abortuses of those whose treatment with these drugs was in the past. This suggests that these agents have no mutagenic effect upon the oocytes but that perhaps they induce unfavorable timing of ovulation and conception.

Amplification of our view of the genesis of the acardiac fetus is warranted because of the recent publication of an alternate concept [SEVERN and HOLYOKE, 1973]. The etiology and pathogenesis of this severest form of anomalous development are unknown. The acardiac is always one of twins whose circulation, indeed development, depends upon that of the co-twin who has always been normal. In man the anomaly occurs only in monozy-

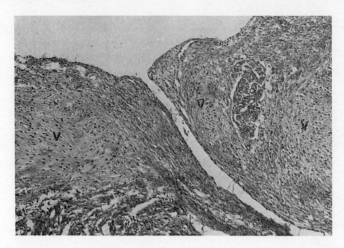

Fig. 2. Same as figure 1 showing rudimentary deformed valves (V) that have a hyaline, cartilage-like appearance. HE, × 100.

gous twins, but in ruminants it is found in dizygous twins, presumably because in these species placental anastomoses form frequently among fraternal twins [BENIRSCHKE and KIM, 1973]. Why it has not been seen in marmosets with a similar placental vasculature is an intriguing question.

It has been suggested that 'unequal splitting' in a zygote may lead to this anomaly; however, its discovery in dizygous ruminants speaks against this. For various reasons, because of the anastomoses, the very variable developmental perfection that favors proper development of the lower extremity, and the analogy to discordant development of other monozygous twins, we have assumed with most older authors that the circulatory reversal is the original cause of the monstrosity [BENIRSCHKE, 1972]. The term 'acardiac', like most related denominations (acephalus, acormis, etc.), must not be taken too literally. Thus, the absence of a heart cannot be taken as evidence of primacy of a failure of the paired structures to meet, as SEVERN and HOLYOKE [1973] view the pathogenesis. Indeed, remnants of hearts and of most other organs have been reported; the anomaly is then referred to as a 'hemicardiac'. Figures 1 and 2 show the microscopic features of the heart in a typical 'acardiac' monster; many others are on record. This fetus also possessed a lung (fig. 3), an unusual finding. Commencement of fetal circulation (about day 22 in the human embryo) occurs when paired primordia fuse. Thus, if

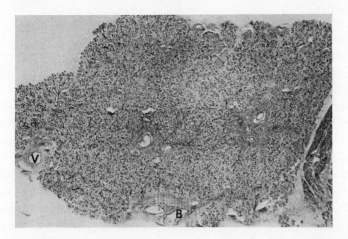

Fig. 3. Lung of same acardiac fetus. The rudimentary nature of the lung with poor alveolar expansion is evident. There was no amniotic fluid; larger spaces are bronchi and bronchioles (B) and vessels (V). Tissues were slightly macerated. Unlike many other acardiacs, this one possessed, among other organs, an atrophying second umbilical artery, pancreas, and remnant of trachea. HE, × 16.

reversal of circulation were to occur at this time, it would be optimal for disturbed cardiac development.

Others have suggested that cytogenetic error in only that monozygous twin destined to become the acardiac may be the etiologic mechanism. Indeed chromosome mosaicism has been described in some but not in all of these anomalies [BENIRSCHKE and KIM, 1973; DUNN and ROBERTS, 1972]. It is interesting that the anomalies were always mosaic in constitution and that the anomalous cell line was a small one. An alternative possibility then exists that these abnormal cell lines may have formed *in vivo* as a result of unfavorable conditions (which exist), and are analogous to some changes occurring in cell cultures *in vitro*. This is surely an important area for further investigation. ARMENDARES *et al.* [1971] have made the only study of the possible relationship of malnutrition to chromosome errors, a most difficult area of investigation. They found in lymphocyte cultures and marrows of children with kwashiorkor and marasmus a much higher incidence of chromatid breaks and other anomalies, notably dicentrics, than in those of the controls. They were unable to control such aspects as virus infections, therapeutic medication, etc., in the study; however, antecedent radiation was excluded. Finally, the surprising number of heterokaryotic monozygous twins discovered suggests that early embryonic experiences may result in chromosomal sequelae.

Although our knowledge in this area is grossly imperfect, some sporadic evidence has been gathered to indicate that abnormal development occurs because of faulty implantation and development. KRONE [1961] has been a principal proponent of this thesis in largely ignored contributions that suggest expansion in prospective and experimental studies. He finds a much increased frequency of malformed embryos in ectopic gestations and a relationship of anomalies with maternal age and with abnormally constructed placentas. In particular the association with aberrant cord insertion, which in itself correlates with single umbilical artery, is taken as evidence that very early implantational disturbances lead to defective embryonic development.

Only one type of experimental study bearing directly on this hypothesis is known to us [TALBERT and KROHN, 1965], the results of which tend to confirm the notion that aging uteri may present a more unfavorable environment for embryonic development. TALBERT and KROHN [1965] transplanted fertilized ova from old mice to young, from young mice to young mice, and from young to old mice. The viability varied greatly. In the first 2 groups it was around 50%; in the last group only 14%. For our purposes it is important to recognize that the zygotes of older mice were not seemingly deleteriously affected, a notion that warrants considerable further inquiry with cytogenetic techniques in different species and perhaps with other controlled variables. Of course, it is easy to visualize the possible nature of such aging; decreased blood flow and altered hormonal support come to mind, but these have not been proved.

The purpose of these statements in this context is to emphasize that a variety of teratogenetic pathways may correlate with maternal age. These are more subtle and also more difficult to analyze within our current conceptualization of the problem. This is not to say that they are invalid; indeed, our inability to have explained satisfactorily the maternal age effect upon trisomies may lie in the mutagenic approach. For these and other reasons a study of cytogenetic findings in ectopic pregnancies was undertaken [BUSCH and BENIRSCHKE, 1973].

IV. Ectopic Gestation

71 cases of tubal ectopic pregnancies were collected as fresh as possible from various hospitals. In 5 cases no fetal or placental tissue was found. Of the remaining 66 cases, 44 established some growth in tissue culture; the other 22 were infected or apparently too long in transport for success. Only 25

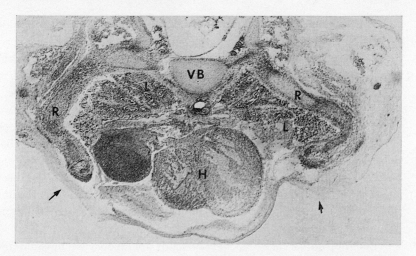

Fig. 4. Cross section through chest of slightly macerated 2-cm embryo of tubal ectopic pregnancy. Macroscopically the anterior chest wall was translucent, lacking sternum and ribs, and heart was bulging anteriorly beneath very thin skin covering. Maternal age 31; karyotype of embryo 46, XX. Cleft palate was also present. VB = Vertebral body; R = rib; H = heart; L = lung. Arrows denote ends of ribs. HE, × 16.

cultures, however, succeeded to final karyotyping of sufficient numbers of cells to satisfy our criteria. It appeared early that more mosaic conceptuses were present than in the usual abortion material, for which reason a very large number of cells was karyotyped. There were 7 chromosomal anomalies: One a trisomy G, the other 6 mosaics (G+; D+; 2 C+E+; 2 X/XX). There may have been one XO/XY but we were uncertain about it. The maternal ages varied from 18 to 31 years (average 27). Histologic examination of tubal tissue apart from the implantation showed chronic inflammation in 80% (35 of 44). In 9 of 66 specimens an embryo was found. Three showed congenital anomalies but had normal chromosomes. One had only one umbilical artery; one had rachischisis and cervical myelocele (incipient craniorachischis); one had cleft palate and an absent anterior bony chest wall (incipient ectopia cordis; fig. 4). Maternal age of the latter two was 28 and 31 years, respectively.

Only few ectopic pregnancies have been included in previous cytogenetic studies of spontaneous abortions, and the efforts involved to collect our cases yielded only a relatively small return. The findings, different from those of spontaneous abortion material, was both expected and surprising. We interpret them as indicating the following:

1. Ectopic pregnancies are caused primarily by pathological conditions of the fallopian tube, usually of chronic inflammatory nature.

2. The poor culture results are the sequel of infection and often long-standing degenerative and hemorrhagic changes.

3. The finding of three congenital anomalies, one a most unusual type, in only 9 embryos confirms previous observations [KRONE, 1961] and may well be the sequel of the subtle influences of a disturbed nidation of the blastocyst.

4. Chromosomal errors are very different from those in intrauterine abortions, only 1 trisomy having been found. In particular, no polyploidies were observed, and there was an unusual number of apparent mosaics. We speculate that the large numbers of mosaics may have resulted also from the unusual (poor) nutritional environment, but in the absence of experimental support this must remain hypothetical.

Poor nutritional environment is currently not favored as a possible etiology of chromosomal errors but is certainly subject to experimental verification or exclusion. Its study would be useful in explaining further the relationship of maternal age effect to fetal development. The problem has been approached surgically by WIGGLESWORTH [1964] who ligated the uterine artery of rats and found that the adjacent embryos developed in a remarkably stunted fashion. GRAUWEILER and LEIST [1973] found significant fetal wastage on the 14 th day of pregnancy in rats that had been given ergotamine, an effect that could be partially counteracted by phenoxybenzamine. Doubtless, other approaches to this complex problem are possible and cytogenetic study of such embryos is desirable.

V. Plant Toxins

The teratogenic activity of some plant-contained substances must also be mentioned briefly as the effects are remarkably age dependent. Perhaps best known is *Veratrum californicum* whose ingestion by cows and ewes, among other species, leads to multiple and complex fetal anomalies [BINNS *et al.*, 1972]. Work stemming from this poisoning has led to the recognition that fetal endocrine activity may trigger the onset of labor since fetuses whose CNS and pituitary were malformed frequently had atrophic adrenals and were carried much beyond term. Plants in different countries contain other poisonous substances whose destructive action in fetuses has become well known. Perhaps one of the most interesting plant groups are the Cycadaceae, the widely distributed cycads. Their reproductive units contain starch with variable quantities of poisonous substances, a prominent one being cycasin [MICKELSEN, 1972]. The plants were first investigated because of the unexplained high frequency of amyotrophic lateral sclerosis (ALS) on Guam. Extensive work with the poisons of several species shows a variety of toxic effects in different animals: micrencephaly in embryonic life; neonatal cerebellar damage and, in adult animals fed cycad flour, neurotoxicity, tumors of liver, lung, kidneys, a variety of brain tumors, and widespread necrotic lesions. It appears fairly certain that ALS and perhaps a few other chronic brain diseases in Guam are at times the result of ingestion of cycad flour. Probably only the natives' practice of leaching the cycad flour with water and testing the supernatant in chickens has prevented more widespread damage. No clearcut evidence exists as yet that some congenital anomalies as well as tumors in man have resulted from these poisons. Their very wide distribution in nature, however, suggests that plant toxins should be considered when the etiology of geographically inexplicable frequencies of anomalies, etc., are studied.

The recent attempt to unravel the mystery of anencephaly serves as a good example. RENWICK's [1972] hypothesis that some toxin, developing upon insults (e.g. the potato blight in stored potato tubers), is responsible for the difference in incidence of anencephaly in the various parts of the British Isles is widely debated now. From many corners of the world come reports that failed to find a correlation between potato blight and anencephaly, possibly in part because potatoes were not consumed in all areas. POSWILLO *et al.* [1972] induce similar skeletal defects in marmoset monkey fetuses with food containing blighted potato concentrate. Rats were not susceptible. What is interesting is their finding that the most significant effects were achieved in those animals that were conceived after the longest preconception exposure to the putative teratogen. These are results that, conventionally, might be attributed to a mutagen acting upon the germ cells, although this is presumably incorrect, and the next few years should bring clarification of the agent(s) responsible for this phenomenon. Here it is only important to recognize the difficulties that exist in separating mutagenic from teratogenic effects, particularly when toxins are involved that are very widespread in nature.

VI. Hybrid Germ Cells

Although the primary aim of this book is the understanding of the effect of aging upon the gamete, it may be useful to direct attention briefly to the model of 'aging' germ cells that exists in some hybrids. It is known that mules and hinnies, the reciprocal crosses of horse and donkey, are completely sterile. No truly substantiated fertile hybrid of this type has been described, the occasional claim notwithstanding [SHORT, 1972]. Sterility is, doubtless, the result of asynapsis at meiosis because of the grossly different structural characteristics of the parental chromosomes. In males the mitotic activity of germ cells is normal, and meiosis is attempted but fails to complete. The cells degenerate long before meiosis I. In adult female mules the ovaries are usually devoid of ova, at best a very isolated oocyte can be detected. In the embryonic stages, however, the germinal cell complement appears to be entirely normal, degeneration occurring in the latter stages of gestation and in neonatal life [TAYLOR and SHORT, 1973].

This situation is not unlike that observed in human XO conceptuses. In early embryos, ovaries of fetuses with the karyotype 45,X contain a normal complement of oocytes, subsequent degeneration of which with advancing fetal age leads to the usually depleted streak at birth [SINGH and CARR, 1966]. An occasional ovum is found, an occasional patient even with Turner's syndrome has produced offspring, but usually the gonads are devoid of oocytes. The temporal similarity of the degenerative event in these 2 situations is striking, and one may inquire into the reasons. By analogy one may assume that germ cell death in the female mule is the result of asynapsis as it appears to be in the male after puberty. Is then embryonic or neonatal oocyte survival dependent upon the attainment of a specific stage of meiosis? And is degeneration the sequel if, by a certain age, the programmed synapsis has not been achieved? If this were clarified then a better understanding of the death of germ cells in the ovaries of gonadal dysgenesis might be at hand. This phenomenon is currently not comprehended, and the nature of oocytes' dictyate stage with its possible control not understood at all. It appears that the fetal mule, and perhaps other hybrids of chromosomally divergent species, may be useful models in the study of this aspect of the effect of aging upon reproductive phenomena.

In reviewing the evidence presented here and in the literature, it is fair to conclude that some progress has been made in our understanding of age effects upon reproductive processes. Nevertheless, in the individual case of a clinical malformation the contribution made by aging can almost never be assessed directly. We have seen the deleterious effect upon the zygote when aging of gametes is induced experimentally but have failed to be able to measure it. Most disappointingly, the precise means by which the age effect upon trisomies is translated still escapes our grasp. The suggestion, perhaps only to

be called the hint, of an accumulation of mutations in oocytes through antecedent irradiation [UCHIDA *et al.*, 1968], has not yet been confirmed. In fact,
the experience of the reproductive performance of A-bomb survivors shows
no measurable deleterious effects of this irradiation [BLOT and SAWADA,
1972]. Although mutagens affect chromosomal behavior adversely in experimental animals, it has never been possible to shown a similar reaction in
man. These aspects may be frustrating to the scientist who is working in this
field, but it is comforting to know that, by and large, reproductive functions
are seemingly so well protected from environmental agents and that the
prenatal selection by spontaneous abortion is so efficient.

References

ABDULLA, U.; CAMPBELL, S.; DEWHURST, C. J., and TALBERT, D.: Effect of diagnostic
  ultrasound on maternal and fetal chromosomes. Lancet *ii:* 829 (1971).
ARAKAKI, D. T. and WAXMAN, S. H.: Effect of gestational and maternal age in early
  abortion. Obstet. Gynec. *35:* 264 (1970).
ARMENDARES, S.; SALAMANCA, F., and FRENK, S.: Chromosome abnormalities in severe
  protein caloric malnutrition. Nature, Lond. *232:* 271 (1971).
BAKER, T. G.: Radiosensitivity of mammalian oocytes with particular reference to the
  human female. Amer. J. Obstet. Gynec. *110:* 746 (1971).
BARTHELMESS, A.: Mutagenic substances in the human environment; in VOGEL and RÖHR-
  BORN Chemical mutagenesis in mammals and man, p. 69 (Springer, Berlin 1970).
BAUCHINGER, M.; SCHMID, E. und SCHMIDT, D.: Chromosomenanalyse bei Verkehrspoli-
  zisten mit erhöhter Bleilast. Mutation Res. *16:* 407 (1972).
BEIR Report: The effect on populations of exposure to low levels of ionizing radiation
  (US Government Printing Office, Washington 1972).
BENIRSCHKE, K.: Prenatal cardiovascular adaptation; in BLOOR Comparative patho-
  physiology of circulatory disturbances, p. 3 (Plenum Publishing, New York 1972).
BENIRSCHKE, K. and DRISCOLL, S. G.: The pathology of the human placenta (Springer,
  Berlin 1967).
BENIRSCHKE, K. and KIM, C. K.: Multiple pregnancy. New Engl. J. Med. *288:* 1276 (1973).
BINNS, W.; KEELER, R. F., and BALLS, L. D.: Congenital deformities in lambs, calves, and
  goats resulting from maternal ingestion of *Veratrum californicum:* hare lip, cleft
  palate, ataxia, and hypoplasia of metacarpal and metatarsal bones. Clin. Toxicol. *5:*
  245 (1972).
BISHUN, N.; MILLS, J.; LLOYD, N.; WILLIAMS, D. C., and GRISTWOOD, E.: Chromosomal
  satellite association in women using oral contraceptives and their progeny. Cytologia,
  Tokyo *37:* 639 (1972).
BLOT, W. J. and SAWADA, H.: Fertility among female survivors of the atomic bombs of
  Hiroshima and Nagasaki. Amer. J. hum. Genet. *24:* 613 (1972).
BOUÉ, J. G. and BOUÉ, A.: Increased frequency of chromosomal anomalies in abortions
  after induced ovulation. Lancet *i:* 679 (1973).

BURCH, P.R.J.: Down's syndrome and maternal age. Nature, Lond. *221:* 173 (1969).

BUSCH, D.H. and BENIRSCHKE, K.: Cytogenetic study of tubal ectopic conceptuses. Virchows Archives (submitted, 1974).

CARR, D.H.: Chromosomes after oral contraceptives. Lancet *ii:* 830 (1967).

COHEN, M.M.: Drugs and chromosomes. Ann. N.Y. Acad. Sci. *171:* 467 (1970).

DUNN, H.O. and ROBERTS, S.J.: Chromosome studies of an ovine acephalic-acardiac monster. Cornell Vet. *62:* 425 (1972).

FERM, V.H.: The teratogenic effects of metals on mammalian embryos. Adv. Teratol. *5:* 51 (1972).

FITZGERALD, P.H.; PICKERING, A.F., and FERGUSON, D.N.: Depressed lymphocyte response to P.H.A. in long-term users of oral contraceptives. Lancet *i:* 615 (1973).

GERMAN, J.; KOWAL, A., and EHLERS, K.H.: Trimethadione and human teratogenesis. Teratology *3:* 349 (1970).

GRAUWEILER, J. and LEIST, K.H.: Impairment of uteroplacental blood supply by ergotamine as a cause of embryotoxicity in rats (abstr.). Teratology *7:* 16 (1973).

HANLON, J.J.: Environmental hazards. Fed. Proc. *31:* 101 (1972).

HERBST, A.L.; KURMAN, R.J.; SCULLY, R.E., and POSKANZER, D.C.: Clear-cell adenocarcinoma of the genital tract in young females. Registry Report. New Engl. J. Med. *287:* 1259 (1972).

HILDEBRAND, D.C.; DER, R.; GRIFFIN, W.T., and FAHIM, M.S.: Effect of lead acetate on reproduction. Amer. J. Obstet. Gynec. *115:* 1058 (1973).

JACOBS, P.A.: Human population cytogenetics; in DE GROUCHY, EBLING and HENDERSON Human genetics, p. 232 (Exerpta Medica, Amsterdam 1972).

JACOBSON, C.B. and BERLIN, C.M.: Possible reproductive detriment in LSD users. J. amer. med. Ass. *222:* 1367 (1972).

JANERICH, D.T.: Anencephaly and maternal age. Amer. J. Epidem. *95:* 319 (1972).

KOLLER, L.D. and ZINKL, J.G.: Pathology of polychlorinated biphenyls in rabbits. Amer. J. Path. *70:* 363 (1973).

KRONE, H.A.: Die Bedeutung der Eibettstörungen für die Entstehung menschlicher Missbildungen (G. Fischer, Stuttgart 1961).

LAMY, M. and FRÉZAL, J.: The frequency of congenital malformations. Proc. 1st Int. Conf. Congenital Malformations, p. 34 (Lippincott, Philadelphia 1961).

LAVAPPA, K.S. and YERGANIAN, G.: Latent meiotic anomalies related to an ancestral exposure to a mutagenic agent. Science *172:* 171 (1971).

LEVY, E.P.; COHEN, A., and FRASER, F.C.: Hormone treatment during pregnancy and congenital heart defects. Lancet *i:* 611 (1973).

MCKEOWN, T.: Sources of variation in the incidence of malformation. Proc. 1st Int. Conf. Congenital Malformations, p. 45. (Lippincott, Philadelphia 1961).

MICKELSEN, O.: Introductory remarks. 6th Int. Cycad Conf. Fed. Proc. *31:* 1465 (1972).

MILLER-BEN-SHAUL, D.: Residual organochlorine insecticides in the body fat of zoo animals and in foods fed to zoo animals. Int. Zoo Yb. *11:* 236 (1971).

NAEYE, R.L. and BLANC, W.: Pathogenesis of congenital rubella. J. amer. med. Ass. *194:* 1277 (1965).

NEEDLEMAN, H.L. and SCANLON, J.: Getting the lead out. New Engl. J. Med. *288:* 466 (1973).

NELSON, M.M. and FORFAR, J.O.: Associations between drugs administered during pregnancy and congenital abnormalities of fetus. Brit. med. J. *i:* 523 (1971).

NEUHÄUSER, G.; SCHWANITZ, G., und ROTT, H.D.: Zur Frage mutagener und teratogener Wirkung von Antikonvulsiva. Fortschr. Med. *88:* 819 (1970).

NEWCOMBE, H.B.: Effects of radiation on human populations; in DE GROUCHY, EBLING and HENDERSON Human genetics, p. 45 (Exerpta Medica, Amsterdam 1972).

NICHOLS, W.W.: Virus-induced chromosome abnormalities. Annu. Rev. Microbiol. *24:* 479 (1970).

NORA, J.J. and NORA, A.H.: Preliminary evidence for a possible association between oral contraceptives and birth defects (abstr.). Teratology *7:* 24 (1973).

PENROSE, L.S.: A method of separating the relative aetiological effects of birth order and maternal age with special reference to mongolian imbecility. Ann. Eugen. *6:* 108 (1934).

PIERCE, P.E.; THOMPSON, J.F.; LIKOSKY, W.H.; NICKEY, L.N.; BARTHEL, W.F., and HINMAN, A.R.: Alkyl mercury poisoning in humans. Report of an outbreak. J. amer. med. Ass. *220:* 1439 (1972).

POSWILLO, D.E.; SOPHER, D., and MITCHELL, S.: Experimental induction of fetal malformation with 'blighted' potato: preliminary report. Nature, Lond. *239:* 462 (1972).

RENWICK, J.H.: Hypothesis. Anencephaly and spina bifida are usually preventable by avoidance of a specific but unidentified substance present in certain potato tubers. Brit. J. prev. soc. Med. *26:* 67 (1972).

ROBINSON, S.C.: Pregnancy outcome following oral contraceptives. Amer. J. Obstet. Gynec. *109:* 354 (1971).

SAXÉN, L.: Defective regulatory mechanisms in teratogenesis. Int. J. Gynaec. Obstet. *8:* 798 (1970).

SCANLON, J.: Human fetal hazards from environmental pollution with certain nonessential trace elements. Clin. Ped. *11:* 135 (1972).

SEVERN, C.H. and HOLYOKE, E.A.: Human acardiac anomalies. Amer. J. Obstet. Gynec. *116:* 358 (1973).

SHIRAISHI, Y. and YOSIDA, T.H.: Chromosomal abnormalities in cultured leucocyte cells from Itai Itai disease patients. Proc. jap. Acad. *48:* 248 (1972).

SHORT, R.V.: Germ cell sex; in BEATTY and GLUECKSOHN-WAELSCH Proc. Int. Symp. Genetics of the Spermatozoon, Copenhagen 1972, p. 325, Bogtrykkeriet Forum.

SIGLER, A.T.; LILIENFIELD, A.M.; COHEN, B.H., and WESTLAKE, J.E.: Radiation exposure in parents with mongolism (Down's syndrome). Bull. Johns Hopk. Hosp. *117:* 374 (1965).

SINGH, R.P. and CARR, D.H.: The anatomy and histology of XO human embryos and fetuses. Anat. Rec. *155:* 369 (1966).

SINGH, O.S. and CARR, D.H.: A study of the effects of certain hormones on human cells in culture. Canad. med. Ass. J. *103:* 349 (1970).

STOLLER, A. and COLLMANN, R.D.: Virus aetiology for Down's syndrome (mongolism). Nature, Lond. *208:* 903 (1965).

SUTTON, H.E. and HARRIS, M.I. (eds): Mutagenic effects of environmental contaminants (Academic Press, New York 1972).

TALBERT, G.B. and KROHN, P.L.: Effect of maternal age on viability of ova and on ability of uterus to support pregnancy. Anat. Rec. *151:* 424 (1965).

TAYLOR, M. J. and SHORT, R. V.: Development of the germ cells in the ovary of the mule and hinny. J. Reprod. Fertil. *32:* 441 (1973).

TÖNDURY, G.: Embryopathien (Springer, Berlin 1962).

UCHIDA, I. A.; HOLUNGA, R., and LAWLER, C.: Maternal radiation and chromosomal aberrations. Lancet *ii:* 1045 (1968).

VOGEL, F. and RÖHRBORN, G.: Chemical mutagenesis in mammals and man (Springer, Berlin 1970).

WIDMEYER, M. A. and SHAVER, E. L.: Estrogen, progesterone, and chromosome abnormalities in rabbit blastocysts. Teratology *6:* 207 (1972).

WIGGLESWORTH, J. S.: Experimental growth retardation in the foetal rat. J. Path. Bact. *88:* 1 (1964).

Authors' addresses: Dr. KURT BENIRSCHKE, Department of Reproductive Medicine, University of California at San Diego, *La Jolla, CA 92037* (USA); Dr. DETLEY H. BUSCH, Department of Obstetrics and Gynecology, University of Bonn, *Bonn* (FRG)

List of Contributors

ADAMS, C.E., A.R.C. Unit of Reproductive Physiology and Biochemistry, 307 Hunting-don Road, Cambridge CB3 0JQ (England)

BENIRSCHKE, K., Department of Reproductive Medicine, University of California at San Diego, La Jolla, CA 92037 (USA)

BLAHA, G.C., Department of Anatomy, College of Medicine, University of Cincinnati, Cincinnati, OH 45219 (USA)

BOUÉ, A., Centre International de l'Enfance, Laboratoire de la SESEP, Château de Long-champ, Bois de Boulogne, F-75016 Paris 16 (France)

BOUÉ, J., Centre International de l'Enfance, Laboratoire de la SESEP, Château de Long-champ, Bois de Boulogne, F-75016 Paris 16 (France)

BUSCH, D.H., Department of Obstetrics and Gynecology, University of Bonn, D-5300 Bonn (Germany)

BUTCHER, R.L., Departments of Obstetrics-Gynecology and Anatomy, School of Medi-cine, West Virginia University, Morgantown, WV 26506 (USA)

CHANG, M.C., Worcester Foundation for Experimental Biology, Shrewsbury, MA 01545 (USA)

DONAHUE, R.P., Departments of Obstetrics-Gynecology and Medicine, School of Medi-cine, University of Washington, Seattle, WA 98195 (USA)

FOOTE, R.H., Department of Animal Science, Cornell University, Ithaca, NY 14850 (USA)

HAMAGUCHI, H., Department of Biological Sciences, Asahikawa Medical College, Asahi-kawa (Japan)

HUNT, D.M., Worcester Foundation for Experimental Biology, Shrewsbury, MA 01545 (USA)

JONGBLOET, P.H., Huize 'Maria Roepaan', Institute for Observation and Treatment of the Mentally Retarded, Siefengewaldseweg 15, Ottersum (The Netherlands)

KOHN, R.R., Department of Pathology, School of Medicine, Case Western Reserve University, Cleveland, OH 44106 (USA)

LAZAR, P., Unité de Recherches Statistiques, Institut Gustave Roussy, F-94800 Villejuif (France)

LORENZ, F.W., Department of Animal Physiology, University of California at Davis, Davis, CA 95616 (USA)

LUTWAK-MANN, C., Agricultural Research Council's Unit of Reproductive Physiology and Biochemistry, University of Cambridge, Cambridge CB2 3EZ (England)

MANN, T., Agricultural Research Council's Unit of Reproductive Physiology and Biochemistry, University of Cambridge, Cambridge CB2 3EZ (England)

MARTIN-DeLEON, P. A., Department of Anatomy, University of Western Ontario, London, Ontario (Canada)

MIKAMO, K., Department of Biological Sciences, Asahikawa Medical College, Asahikawa (Japan)

NISHIMURA, H., Department of Anatomy, Faculty of Medicine, Kyoto University, Kyoto 606 (Japan)

NIWA, K., Worcester Foundation for Experimental Biology, Shrewsbury, MA 01545 (USA)

ROWSON, L. E. A., Agricultural Research Council's Unit of Reproductive Physiology and Biochemistry, University of Cambridge, Cambridge CB2 3EZ (England)

SATO, H., Program in Biophysical Cytology, Department of Biology, University of Pennsylvania, Philadelphia, PA 19104 (USA)

SHAVER, E. L., Department of Anatomy, University of Western Ontario, London, Ontario (Canada)

SMITH, K. D., Program in Reproductive Biology and Reproductive Endocrinology, The University of Texas Medical School at Houston, 6400 West Cullen Street, Texas Medical Center, Houston, TX 77025 (USA)

STEINBERGER, E., Program in Reproductive Biology and Reproductive Endocrinology, The University of Texas Medical School at Houston, 6400 West Cullen Street, Texas Medical Center, Houston, TX 77025 (USA)

STULTZ, D. R., Program in Reproductive Biology and Reproductive Endocrinology, The University of Texas Medical School at Houston, 6400 West Cullen Street, Texas Medical Center, Houston, TX 77025 (USA)

SZOLLOSI, D., Institut National de la Recherche Agronomique, Station de Recherches de Physiologie Animale, F-78350 Jouy-en-Josas (France)

Author Index

Subject Index